# Uncertain Suffering

D0940792

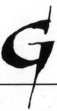

THE GEORGE GUND FOUNDATION
IMPRINT IN AFRICAN AMERICAN STUDIES

The George Gund Foundation has endowed
this imprint to advance understanding of
the history, culture, and current issues
of African Americans.

# Uncertain Suffering

*Racial Health Care Disparities and Sickle Cell Disease*

Carolyn Moxley Rouse

UNIVERSITY OF CALIFORNIA PRESS
*Berkeley · Los Angeles · London*

University of California Press, one of the most
distinguished university presses in the United States,
enriches lives around the world by advancing
scholarship in the humanities, social sciences, and
natural sciences. Its activities are supported by the
UC Press Foundation and by philanthropic
contributions from individuals and institutions.
For more information, visit www.ucpress.edu.

University of California Press
Berkeley and Los Angeles, California

University of California Press, Ltd.
London, England

© 2009 by The Regents of the University of California

Library of Congress Cataloging-in-Publication Data

Rouse, Carolyn Moxley, 1965–.
 Uncertain suffering : racial healthcare disparities
and sickle cell disease / Carolyn Moxley Rouse.
  p.  cm.
 Includes bibliographical references and index.
 ISBN 978-0-520-25911-9 (cloth : alk. paper)
 ISBN 978-0-520-25912-6 (pbk. : alk. paper)
  1. Sickle cell anemia—Patients—United States.
2. Discrimination in medical care—United States.
3. Health services accessibility—United States.
4. Minorities—Medical care—United States.  5. Race
discrimination—United States.  6. Social medicine—
United States.  I. Title.
RC641.7.S5R68  2009
362.196'15270089—dc22          2008054125

Manufactured in the United States of America

18  17  16  15  14  13  12  11  10  09
10  9  8  7  6  5  4  3  2  1

This book is printed on Cascades Enviro 100, a 100%
post consumer waste, recycled, de-inked fiber. FSC
recycled certified and processed chlorine free. It is
acid free, Ecologo certified, and manufactured by
BioGas energy.

*For Skylar and Marieke*

# Contents

# Preface

What does it mean that the life expectancy of blacks in the United States is on average five to six years shorter than that of whites? I once joked in my course entitled "Race and Medicine" that the black students could leave class ten minutes early in order to make up for what would eventually be a shortened life. Two weeks later a student from the Bahamas called my bluff, saying that she wanted to take advantage of the early dismissal.

We lament the gaps in longevity between whites and blacks, but my student from the Bahamas had the same life expectancy as the white men in the class. So, how should we feel about the fact that white men die earlier than white women? Or that Asian women from Bergen County, New Jersey, live on average about twenty years longer than black men from Harlem? Is there a way to quantify suffering and then somehow equalize it to attain some abstract form of social justice by race, class, or gender? *Uncertain Suffering: Racial Health Care Disparities and Sickle Cell Disease* interrogates the cultural assumptions that underlie our quest to equalize health outcomes. Any discourses about why blacks or women or ethnic minorities should have the same health outcomes as white women (for example) are built upon beliefs about what citizens are owed.

It should come as no surprise that the ways clinics organize patient care are built around philosophies about distributive justice or utilitarian notions about individualism and rational action. During my research, when I asked medical professionals to discuss how they standardize equitable treatment given so much medical uncertainty, I elicited conversations invoking everything from the philosophy of Ludwig Wittgenstein to discussions about how placebos produce actual physical responses. Discussions about what constitutes equitable care merged seamlessly into ones about truth versus reality, and perceptions of health and well-being versus actual physical health.

Asking physicians and patients to imagine and describe idealized forms of health care is more than just an intellectual exercise. How medical professionals and patients imagine health care and well-being determines how health care is structured and accessed. *Uncertain Suffering* examines how, in the case of sickle cell disease, the imaginations of medical professionals, patients, families, and disease advocates (the sickle cell disease community) shape the quality and delivery of sickle cell disease care. Based upon three years of ethnographic fieldwork in a pediatric hospital and four years of fieldwork around the country, this book examines the production of discourses about health care justice within the sickle cell community and how these discourses become embedded in evidence-based treatment paradigms that ultimately shape treatment access.

Evidence-based medicine is an approach to medical treatment that relies on legitimated, usually randomized, scientific studies to determine best clinical practices. Given this attempt to standardize best practices, one would assume that scientific rationality would win out over unconscious bias that in part produces health care disparities. *Uncertain Suffering* not only interrogates what we mean by bias (i.e., racial disparities are possible without racists) but also shows that institutionalized evidence-based treatments for sickle cell disease, from treatment for pain to blood transfusion therapy, differ because they are built upon moral understandings about duty and practice. Physicians and hospitals must decide who to treat, how to treat, and the extent of the treatment. Treatment access also involves the social aspects of making patients feel welcome, good communication, patient education, and setting up structures to encourage patients to follow particular treatment regimens. Complicating the issue of evidence and best practices is the question of how to define treatment efficacy.

Scientific discourses are also social discourses, and therefore cultural notions of physician duty are always entangled in the science of sickle cell treatment. With many chronic conditions there is enough medical uncertainty about treatment efficacy that physicians have room to construct different treatment protocols for similar conditions. Uncertainties about treatment efficacy produce enough doubt that it becomes impossible to locate the source of disparate outcomes in one treatment model or another. Uncertainties in medicine allow for variability in treatment access such that certain types of patient neglect and what some might call poor treatment do not actually constitute inappropriate medical care or malpractice. Patient neglect can be couched as teaching patients self-efficacy or teaching patients not to be dependent on health care; and poor treatment can be couched as poor patient education or lack of compliance with medical authority.

Racialized perceptions validate treatment disparities, particularly when it comes to treatments where the outcomes are uncertain and the risks are high. Racial health disparities result from the treatment slippages that arise from medical uncertainty, and from a medical system that rations care by cost. We manage health care for the poor through various forms of charity, but charity is not social justice. Charity requires that those who receive it reward the donors through gratitude and performances of moral character. Charity maintains social hierarchies. In a society where the poor, particularly poor blacks, are perceived as ungrateful and lacking the necessary moral fiber to be self-sufficient, health care charity is a fragile commodity. In this environment, the refusal, for example, to put a black patient on the United Network for Organ Sharing list for a transplant based on the presumption that he or she will be noncompliant with postoperative treatments is not seen as medical neglect. Instead, it is seen as necessary in order to protect scarce resources.

Noncompliance operates in the clinic to reduce patient access to health care services. The term implies, of course, a lack of gratitude on the part of the patient coupled with a bit of hostility and diminished reason or intelligence. Ultimately labeling patients noncompliant orchestrates many of the slippages that produce disparities in care. Simply, the labeling of blacks inside the clinic typically mirrors perceptions of blacks outside the clinic.

By treating health care as a scarce commodity we fuel the production of discourses that legitimate limiting health care access. One can often trace the justification for a particular treatment decision to a resource constraint. Ameliorating racial health care disparities will require unfettering some health care services, which I argue will change how medical professionals understand and treat black patients. In this respect I am a materialist, or a theorist who traces cultural beliefs to the material organization of society. Not a fully committed materialist, however, I believe the imagination also plays a role in producing health care access.

Biomedicine is wonderful, but it is not the primary source of health in the United States. Sewer systems are the largest contributor to health, followed by diet, environment, and vaccines (not necessarily in that order). Once we contain the hype about the miracle of biomedicine, we then need to unfetter medical access through single-payer universal health care. Patients, particularly the growing population of chronically ill patients, need to be educated so that they can use medicine to control what I call lifescapes, or narratives that articulate how actions in the present will contribute to an imagined future. By doing this, we do not control or try to control how someone chooses to ameliorate his or her suffering, and we free ourselves from having to quantify the suffering of various groups in order to attain some abstract form of health care justice. While differences in life expectancy should generate public concern, as they have, *Uncertain Suffering* demonstrates how the data do not reveal much about how race operates in the clinic or how patients experience suffering.

# Acknowledgments

I first want to acknowledge people who have informed this long journey from research to text. Many thanks to Mary-Jo Good, whose theory and analysis of the culture of medicine inspired my research approach. Mary-Jo's body of work creatively engages complexity in the clinic while never losing sight of culture and power. Rayna Rapp, who writes on the narratives women construct in the face of medical uncertainty, has motivated me in ways too numerous to list. In addition, I must thank Rayna's conjoined twin in theory, Faye Ginsburg. Faye not only has been a source of inspiration but also is, I believe, the only one who understands how the study of media, medicine, ethnicity, religion, and gender (MMERG) really constitutes one subdiscipline.

This book would also never have been possible without the input of Lesley Sharp, who always pushes theory by asking questions that others neglect to ask. Lesley's scholarship on exchange in the clinic informs not only this book but also my next project. I want to thank Carol Greenhouse for her intellectual gifts. Carol's work on the varied relationships between states and local culture frames my chapter on medical uncertainty. To have had the opportunity to work with and be mentored by such a brilliant scholar has been both humbling and profoundly enriching.

Julie Livingston, whose work on debility is profoundly attuned to suffering and uncertainty, devoted an extraordinary amount of time to reading my final draft and provided brilliant feedback. I never could have let go of this manuscript without her. Finally, I want to thank Keith Wailoo, who has been a reader and supporter of my work and whose own work on the history of sickle cell disease in the United States makes my intervention possible. Keith's analysis captures the dynamics of the community and the dynamics of race politics in the United States so accurately that *Dying in the City of the Blues* became the unofficial bible for this project.

I also thank my colleagues in my department who challenge the discipline of anthropology in ways that make sense to me: Joao Biehl, Jim Boon, John Borneman, Amy Borovoy, Isabelle Clar-Deces, Abdellah Hammoudi, Alan Mann, Janet Monge, and Larry Rosen. Thanks also to Byron Good, Janet Hoskins, Fred Myers, Arthur Kleinman, Joan Kleinman, and Angela Zito.

Numerous physicians, nurses, psychologists, social workers, hospital administrators, patients, and families made crucial contributions to this book. Although I cannot acknowledge them by name, I must express my gratitude for their participation. I also wish to thank Suzie Lieff, Dr. Kwaku Ohene-Frempong, Dr. Lennette Benjamin, Dr. Thomas Coates, M. Gregg Bloche, Joseph Telfair, the Sickle Cell Disease Association of America, the National Institutes of Health, Cheryl Mattingly, and Mary Lawlor.

Without the financial support of the Woodrow Wilson Foundation, the Mellon Foundation, Wenner-Gren, and Princeton University, this research would not have been possible. In addition, I must include special thanks for Naomi Schneider, Susan Ecklund, and UC Press.

Finally, I am forever grateful to my dear friends/family and family/friends, Betsy Armstrong, Sara Curran, and Mieke Kramer. Also, I need to thank the people who have given their love and support unconditionally throughout: Glenn Schiltz, Cecilia Rouse, Forest Rouse, Lorraine Rouse, Carl Rouse, Eileen Herman, Ford Morrison, Zora, Yahya, and Skylar.

# Introduction

During my first visit to Children's Hospital East (CHE), a pediatric teaching hospital located in an urban center in the Northeast, there were no visual surprises. I had just spent three years conducting fieldwork at Children's Hospital West (CHW) and had become accustomed to everything from the alternating commercial linoleum and broadloom, ultraperformance carpet (in a style named "Traffic") to the young cancer patients hooked up to several intravenous drips, pushed on gurneys or in wheelchairs, who clarify the hospital's moral purpose. Inside CHE, colorful murals and playful structures welcome families in the main entrance while large pictures of smiling multiethnic children line the hallways. The people walking through the hospital mirror the racial diversity of the photos on the wall, and an initial reading of the hospital can make one extremely hopeful that multiculturalism has arrived. At second glance, however, one notices that fairly clear racial and ethnic divisions mark status differentials. Representative of a pattern throughout the United States, the hospital administrators, physicians, nurses, and therapists at CHE are generally *not* representative of the city's ethnic diversity. Instead, the ethnic faces at CHE belong primarily to the black and Latino health care consumers and the low-wage staff.

I was scheduled to visit Eva, a twenty-one-year-old sickle cell patient whom I met through a social worker. Eva, an adolescent with a café au lait complexion, moved her tall, thin body slowly and deliberately, as if her bones were made of lead. Despite the slowness of her gait, she spoke

rapidly. Dressed in a short-sleeved shirt, Eva unself-consciously dis-
played the numerous stretch marks on both her upper arms. Her mot-
tled skin is the result of a steroid that caused her to blow up like a
balloon and signifies her numerous brushes with death. When she was
sick, rather than very sick, Eva was a straight-A student working toward
a degree in psychology and philosophy at a state college close to home
and hospital. When we met, Eva was taking the semester off. She was on
dialysis and as a result had to spend three full days out of every week in
suspended animation waiting for various checkups and treatments. At
each clinic she had to visit within the hospital, Eva would wait patiently
for her name to be called. Sometimes she would meet other adolescent
girls, also black and close to her age, and they would play the "Do you
know. . . ?" game, trying to map each other's social networks, before
falling back into silence. Usually Eva would simply listen to music on
her Discman or read a book. In many ways Eva was like a paper on an
office desk waiting to be a priority. These long waits were necessitated
by the fact that four months prior to our meeting, her kidneys stopped
filtering impurities from her blood.

Kidney failure was perhaps inevitable. Eva had had problems with
her kidneys since the age of twelve. At the time she had been seeing a
doctor from a community hospital who failed to understand the seriousness of her condition. Her parents, who partly out of fear of losing
health care coverage believed in stoicism in the face of illness, were not,
in Eva's words, "the types to go and run to the hospital every five seconds
because you get sick."[1] The opposite of stoicism is understood to be an
inappropriate dependence on health care, and for chronically ill patients
this dependence is often pathologized by medical professionals. Repeated
trips to the hospital for pneumonia would be grounds for the staff to
label Eva a "frequent flyer" or something equally derogatory. Returning
to the emergency department to be treated with an opioid for every one
of her frequent pain crises might have resulted in her being labeled a
"drug seeker" or a "malingerer." The clinic narrative casts patients
as victims, physicians as heroes, and biomedicine as Zeus's thunder-
bolt. When treatments fail to cure disease or relieve suffering, medical professionals often cite patient noncompliance or psychological
dysfunction.

For Eva, staying home was not only stoic but also strategic. Most
sickle cell patients can sense when medical professionals become weary
of their complaints about intractable pain, and some stop seeking help
in order to avoid confrontations. As Eva explained, "My parents just

wanted me to be home. Unless it was really, really severe where I just couldn't handle it anymore, and then I would go to the hospital. I mean, I would have a crisis and it would go away, and I would go on with my life or whatever." Medical professionals label stoic patients like Eva self-sufficient, mature, and rational. But to reward such behavior by calling it courageous, to understand it as a sign of the patient's competence or a family's ability to function, is to turn refusal to access health care into a rational choice.

In the case of Eva's kidneys the problem did not go away, and the lack of follow-up did not help. She continued:

> For years I never really had any trouble. I guess they don't know why I got the kidney infection or whatever. When I was twelve and thirteen then it started going down from there. [Finally] I was like really, really pale. My siblings said I looked white. [That day] I remember parts of it, but I was in and out. I remember my mom holding me. They got me an ambulance and one of the ambulance guys I remember that they kept asking me my name, and of course I didn't understand. When I was twelve, I went to my regular doctor and they're like, "Just take some Tylenol, drink some juice." Because they would usually say drink and they didn't really try to do any tests, or figure out why I was sick. So it was escalating quietly for two years, and that's when it just blew up.

To put Eva's experiences into context, it helps to know that on average blacks develop end-stage kidney failure at 55.8 years of age versus 62.2 years for whites.[2] Blacks, as well as American Indians and Alaska Natives, have four times the rate of end-stage kidney failure as whites, and after three years on the waiting list only 30 percent of blacks have received a kidney transplant, compared with 49 percent of whites, for reasons that may or may not be related to human leukocyte antigen (HLA) matching.[3] Disparities in rates of kidney failure are significant, and at the age of fourteen Eva became one more statistic. But why did it take two years to diagnosis Eva's kidney disease when other patients with the same initial symptoms may have been referred for further testing? A study of preemptive kidney transplantations showed that whites were more than twice as likely as blacks (and patients with private insurance were almost five times more likely than those on Medicare) to receive a kidney transplant before dialysis was required.[4] So, more broadly, why do racial health disparities exist in the United States? Genes? Culture? Poverty? Racism?

The literature on health and health care disparities has grown significantly since President Bill Clinton and Surgeon General David Satcher announced an initiative to end racial and ethnic health care disparities in six disease categories by the year 2010.[5] The literature reveals inequities in pain management, cardiovascular disease care, access to organ transplantation, dialysis, lumbar spine radiographs, and antipsychotic medication, and the list continues to grow.[6] Despite the good intentions, this spillage of ink has amounted to a Rorschach test open to myriad interpretations regarding the source of these inequities. Rather than producing a unified social movement and set of medical practices, publicity surrounding racial health disparities has simply intensified the debate about how race does or does not influence treatment decisions, patient behavior, outcomes, and social responsibility. Racial health disparities, in other words, have become a condensed site for debating the relationship between race and social justice.

The difference in life expectancy between blacks and whites remains undisputed, but policy theorists take extreme positions when it comes to assigning blame. Some hold individuals responsible for their longevity and good health and discount the role of social structures and institutions. The scope and breadth of health care policy are determined by the ways in which analysts assign blame, and the outcomes of these debates are significant for the people at risk for early death. As has been noted in theories of the state, citizens and noncitizens are vulnerable to how states choose to care for their welfare.[7]

Policy analysts argue that finding a solution to health disparities will first require locating an origin. The report *Unequal Treatment: Confronting Racial and Ethnic Disparities in Healthcare* lists probable causes as race and ethnic discrimination (aversive racism); material factors, including insurance, income, and the law (class); the culture of medicine (systems); patient cultural practices and identity (culture); and genetics.[8] Most researchers studying medicine and social justice argue that health care disparities are caused by a confluence of these factors. The solution therefore has been to chip away at each contributing feature. But are we using the right tools? Current attempts to eliminate inequities—cultural competency programs, greater emphasis on family-centered care—have the quality of a sculptor using a chain saw to replicate Michelangelo's *Pietà*. They fail to pay attention to delicate power negotiations that take place in the clinic. Some cultural competency programs, for example, substitute race for culture and end up institutionalizing a strange set of presuppositions that do nothing to change the power dynamics between medical professionals, patients, and families.[9]

The fallback approach has been for institutions to assume particular fiscal and administrative burdens based on the needs of their patient populations, for example, Spanish-language services in communities with large numbers of immigrants from Central and South America. This piecemeal strategy to end disparities has worked in some institutions and has contributed to small gains in access to care at the local level. At the hospitals where I conducted research, the institutional supports created by the sickle cell teams, with the help of the National Institutes of Health (NIH), increased health care access for sickle cell patients.

The local approaches do not, however, tackle the larger issue of health inequities at the national level. The four institutions I observed, for example, are four of only ten comprehensive sickle cell centers across the country. Every five years the NIH awards grants to only ten centers for the development and maintenance of a comprehensive approach to sickle cell care. Given the financial limitations to expand health care services generally, perhaps the public should consider a more radical, nonpiecemeal approach to ending health care disparities, one that focuses on the roots of inequality rather than relying on the novel vision of a handful of physicians. Perhaps this approach might entail stronger public oversight and regulation, or a tax-based universal health care system similar to the one used by the military. In terms of educating the next generation of physicians, the public could also demand that medical schools and hospitals train doctors to become more sensitive to the culture of medicine, with its particular set of presumptions and prejudices about the body and health. Finally, the public could require that cities maintain an optimal ratio of health care facilities to population such that more health care facilities are housed in poor rural and urban neighborhoods.

All these initiatives might help reduce racial disparities in health and health care access, but what if the objects we use to identify unequal treatment—insurance, proximity to a hospital, even life expectancy—obscure a more subtle and important issue? Namely, why do we believe that health care is *the* domain in which issues of social justice and philosophical understandings about a life worth living and a good death must be enacted? Why do we rely on health care to equalize an unequal playing field or to determine what does and does not constitute health and well-being? Perhaps that is asking too much of health care.

Our romance with biomedicine is in part due to a longing that this rational discourse can in Rousseauian fashion locate and unmake our suffering. A moralist and a sentimentalist, Jean-Jacques Rousseau believed that in an enlightened society spectators determine the causes of suffering and deploy means for ameliorating it. Many health care professionals recognize that medicine is far too resource poor to unmake all the social injustice that contributes to racial health care disparities, yet for many it is hard not to believe in the promise of bio-medicine. Unstated is a belief that randomized study trials (medical, psychosocial) that generate statistically significant P values will lead us to a solution to inequities; it is more likely that the data would simply add to the collection of ink blots that people read differently. The uncertainties surrounding how to conduct and apply the science given the complicating factors of cost, treatment side effects, resource distribution, and social value always makes the application of scientific knowledge contingent.

## UNCERTAINTIES

I first tried to address the question of racial health disparities as a research associate studying how African American parents whose children have severe disabilities or illnesses negotiate health care. The health issues of the fourteen children I followed in the late 1990s ranged from cancer to spina bifida, and all but two of the children received care at Children's Hospital West, a renowned teaching facility in California.[10] Observing and interviewing families in the hospital and at home, I was having trouble connecting their experiences to the literature on racial health disparities. In general, the families reported positive encounters with hospital staff and satisfaction with their children's care despite their poverty or lack of private insurance. The physicians also complicated any easy determination that "It's the racism, stupid," as many were aware of racism, and some even initiated institutional correctives.

Because there is so much medical uncertainty in the lives of chronically ill patients, attempting to distill Eva's story down to a parable about racism misses the point that something much more troubling is at work. Racism implies that medical professionals willfully dispense unequal treatment. But most medical professionals are not racists. The problem, I concluded, is not a problem of individuals but one of a collective narrative about race. Americans are still deeply wedded to the notion that blacks are genetically and culturally distinct. The idea that whites and Asians are intellectually and culturally superior to blacks remains such a powerful force in the United States today that psychologist

Linda Gottfredson argues that lower intelligence is to blame for health inequalities.[11] Jonathan Klick and Sally Satel reproduce this same argument in *The Health Disparities Myth*.[12]

To improve health care access, the sickle cell community is faced with the awesome task of trying to rewrite the dominant narratives about their patients whose genetic disease marks them in the United States as quintessentially black.[13] This narrative presumes that sickle cell patients are socially dysfunctional, dependent on narcotics, and poorly educated or, worse, uneducable.[14] Knowing only a patient's race or ethnicity, even a well-meaning doctor may make presumptions that influence how he or she communicates with and medically treats a patient.[15] In the interaction between medical professionals and patients, race emplots individuals in narratives not of their choosing.[16]

In order to demonstrate how imagined cultural narratives produce real outcomes, I turn to prison incarceration for drug offenses. Every year the Substance Abuse and Mental Health Services Administration (SAMHSA), part of the U.S. Department of Health and Human Services, publishes statistics on drug use. In 2005, SAMHSA reported that "among persons aged 12 or older, the rate of substance dependence or abuse was highest among American Indians or Alaska Natives (21.0%) and lowest among Asians (4.5%)." The report goes on to say that the rate was 9.4 percent for whites and 8.5 percent for blacks, representing a fairly consistent yearly finding.[17] Compare these statistics of roughly comparable drug use for blacks and whites to the incarceration statistics cited by Human Rights Watch: "Blacks comprise 62.7 percent and whites 36.7 percent of all drug offenders admitted to state prison, even though federal surveys and other data detailed in this report show clearly that this racial disparity bears scant relation to racial differences in drug offending." The report continues: "Relative to population, black men are admitted to state prison on drug charges at a rate that is 13.4 times greater than that of white men."[18]

Health, education, and incarceration disparities have different sources, but in each case we must ask, What stories do we tell ourselves to justify these inequalities? Genes? Poverty? Culture? Personal responsibility? In *The Health Disparities Myth*, Klick and Satel suggest alternative explanations for racial health disparities to the ones presented in the Institute of Medicine's *Unequal Treatment*.[19] Their critique of the conceptual errors and missing data in the statistical literature is thought-provoking, but it is overshadowed by their mission to release physicians from any blame. Clearly upset that in *Unequal Treatment* physician bias is offered as one of many explanations, Klick and Satel point their fingers at genetic, behavioral, cultural, class, and IQ differences. Defending physicians, they write:

> [W]e question whether negative assumptions about patients are the automatic equivalents of prejudiced attitudes (classically defined as hostility and rigidity and erroneousness). After all, unfavorable impressions can simply reflect realistic group differences in patterns of disease and behavior and imply nothing about the moral disposition of the person who holds such an impression. Indeed, if the doctor's assumptions are unaccompanied by ill will, are paired with efforts to compensate for an unfavorable perception of the patient (such as of poor compliance), and are amenable to change as the doctor sees, for example, a particular patient becoming more conscientious, then is this really prejudice? What harm has been done?[20]

A scary defense indeed, but in many respects "cultural competency" training is predicated on the same assumption that race, culture, and behavior are entangled.[21] Klick and Satel's explanations mirror, in many respects, the multicausal explanation made by liberals: genes, culture, and personal responsibility. Conservatives emphasize IQ and responsibility, and liberals emphasize structures and culture, but the idea that the explanations are reducible to identifiable, isolatable causes is at the heart of most theories. The fact that the first "ethnic" wonder drug for heart disease, BiDil, was embraced by both liberals and conservatives demonstrates that they might disagree on the emphasis but not on the particulars. In the case of BiDil the explanation for the racial disparity in mortality due to heart disease was genes.[22]

My argument is that a multicausal explanation in the sense of isolatable variables is a compromise position. I argue that in order to accept that these disparities are a natural outgrowth of race, culture, behavior, genes, or IQ, one must first accept that the categories are immutable. To accept that genes are responsible for health disparities, one must accept that black people represent a distinct genetic group predisposed to certain health conditions, and that they (perhaps) have on average lower IQs. To accept that culture is responsible for health disparities, one must accept that black people share cultural beliefs and practices that differ significantly from those of the mainstream. If one accepts that the health of black people is determined by their lack of personal responsibility, then perhaps one should also accept that blacks deserve to go to prison at 13.4 times the rate of whites even though their substance abuse rates are slightly lower than those of whites. Incarceration statistics demonstrate how disconnected public perceptions of black "personal responsibility" are from fact.

Far from being immutable, as explanatory categories personal responsibility, race, and culture are themselves ambiguous. If blacks are 13.4 times more likely than whites to go to prison for the same offense, personal responsibility means something different for blacks and whites, rich and poor. If first-generation black immigrants from South Africa are lumped together with first-generation blacks from Haiti, then race is a poor proxy for genes or culture. The categories used to identify the source of health disparities must themselves be questioned.[23]

The explanations we offer for racial health disparities—genes, poverty, culture, personal responsibility—continue to blind us to the suffering we as a society create by simply believing what we want to believe about race. This discourse of otherness does not simply exist in the imaginations of nonblacks. Many black scholars blame black culture or the discourse of victimization for racial disparities.[24]

Despite our tremendous disparities in education, incarceration, and medicine, we remain wedded to the categories that we think explain the differences. But each of these explanations has historically been used as a tool for reproducing patterns of racial exclusion. Genetic explanations or culture of poverty theories have been used in the past to justify black disfranchisement. Therefore, any researcher interested in reducing racial health disparities should look askance at genetic, cultural, and behavioral explanations for higher rates of morbidity and mortality. Instead we must ask ourselves, What discourses and practices are operative in the clinic to turn a cultural story about race and difference into health and health care inequities?

SICKLE CELL DISEASE

To get a sense of how sickle cell disease and sickle cell patients are understood in the clinic, one first needs to appreciate the history of sickle cell anemia in the United States. Sickle cell disease occupies an important place in the history of medicine in this country. Characteristics of the disease were first identified in 1910 by Chicago physician James B. Herrick. A twenty-year-old patient of Herrick's had ulcerative lesions and scabs that went undiagnosed for a year. Observing the patient's blood under a microscope, Herrick noted that the red blood cells were crescent-shaped or sickle-shaped. In 1917, Dr. Victor E. Emmel was able to confirm that the cells were neither parasites nor other physiological artifacts and named the oddly shaped hemoglobin *sickle cells*.[25] In the 1920s, Dr. Verne Mason officially linked the symptom of anemia to the abnormal hemoglobin by coining the clinical term *sickle cell anemia.*

The attention given sickle cell anemia in the 1920s and 1930s by the scientific community seems to belie a common perception that the health of blacks did not matter to the white community. At the time, de jure segregation, or legally sanctioned institutionalized racism, was still the accepted norm throughout the United States. In the realm of medicine this meant that the available health care for blacks was generally provided in inadequately resourced colored hospitals, by medical professionals trained at poorly funded black colleges and universities.[26] Paradoxically, despite a lack of concern for the overall health of the black community, sickle cell anemia captured the imagination of research scientists. One could argue that sickle cell anemia was exciting because it was one of the first identified diseases that could be studied scientifically. New tools for blood analysis coupled with the discoveries about inheritance made by Gregor Mendel (1822–84) made sickle cell anemia an interesting, potentially solvable, medical mystery. The excitement over new technologies does not, however, fully explain why sickle cell disease became the most studied genetic disease in the first half of the twentieth century. Anthropologist Melbourne Tapper and medical historian Keith Wailoo argue that the passion to understand the disease was fueled in large part by a desire to know how it is transmitted; the fear was that bad Negro blood, absent proper social controls, would contaminate the health of the white community.[27] To prevent future contagion, the scientific community would have to quickly assess the origin of the disease.

Consistent with the race politics of the time, in 1922 and 1923, Mason, Taliaferro, and Huck hypothesized that sickle cell disease is a dominant trait, following Mendelian laws; this meant, of course, that these researchers believed the disease could be inherited if only one parent possessed the trait.[28] What follows from this innocent presumption is that if sickle cell disease is a dominant trait, then intermarriage marks the beginning of a rapid spread of the disease into the white population. For many, sickle cell disease proved that antimiscegenation laws were not simply a quaint custom but necessary for survival.

So tightly were race and disease conceptually bound that physicians literally could not diagnose sickle cell disease in white patients. Instead, the physician would reclassify the patient as black before making the diagnosis. In one case the physician noted in his report on a white six-year-old, "Neither parent knew of the existence of any negro forbears;

the father's maternal grandparents were English and Jewish, and the mother's maternal grandparents were Cuban. . . . However, the facial characteristics of the patient indicated a mixture of colored with white blood."[29]

In 1949, chemist Linus Pauling and geneticist J. V. Neel proved that the disorder is a recessive trait. Scientifically, this simply means that both parents must possess the trait in order to pass sickle cell anemia on to their child, but politically the repercussions were not so simple.[30] Even after the structure of the abnormal hemoglobin was discovered and sickle cell anemia became the first identified "molecular disease," heralding the age of molecular biology, the discourses connecting sickle cell disease to race degeneracy and contagion remained in circulation.[31] For some, it seems, no matter what new discoveries were made, sickle cell disease proved that segregating the races was a matter of urgent public health policy.

In 1950, for example, Dr. John H. Hodges published a paper in the journal *Blood* entitled, "The Effect of Racial Mixtures upon Erythrocytic Sickling." In this rather dry and deceptively innocuous article, Hodges cites a brief history of encounters between Europeans and Africans in order to map out the relative purity of Negro blood. He then describes a correspondence between race mixing and the incidence of sickle cell disease. Using the work of anthropologist Melville Herskovits, already well known for his book *The Myth of the Negro Past,* Dr. Hodges claims that only about 22 percent of American Negroes are "pure" Negroes. Herskovits used these data to disrupt the idea of racial purity and racial superiority. Hodges instead used them to demonstrate that the contagion had already begun, and with terrible repercussions. Hodges concludes that people with six-eighths Negro blood had the greatest incidence of sickle cell anemia. He found zero incidence of the disease in people who were more than six-eighths Negro. In his conclusion Dr. Hodges writes, "The incidence of erythrocytic sickling is less in 'pure' Negroes than in those with small admixtures of white and American Indian ancestry. There is no evidence that the dilution of Negro ancestry, to such an extent that the person is one-half or less Negro, will either increase or decrease the incidence of sickling."[32] One can only conclude that once the Caucasian race is contaminated, there is no chance for a return to purity.

Eugenicists and racists are not the only people to embed race and politics in scientific discourse. The history of the classification of sickle cell trait demonstrates that progressives have also rejected scientific knowledge deemed politically threatening. Beyond the classification of sickle cell trait, other observations about the disease have been rejected for political reasons. As Wailoo writes in *Dying in the City of the Blues: Sickle Cell Anemia and the Politics of Race and Health,* in 1972 Ernestine Flowers, a Memphis schoolteacher, had to essentially sell her observation to the medical community that children with sickle cell disease underperformed in school by saying, "It's not that they have lower intelligence but because they're so tired all the time that they can't listen and learn."[33] Trying to disentangle discourses of racial inferiority from sickle cell disease health care policy, in the early 1970s medical professionals avoided at all costs any discussions of patient IQ. Decades after Ms. Flowers's careful walk through a discursive mine field, new research describing the level of cerebral damage caused by silent strokes is being embraced by the scientific community. At the thirtieth anniversary meetings of the National Heart, Lung, and Blood Institute of the NIH and the Sickle Cell Disease Association of America, the authors of a paper entitled "Neuropsychological Functioning in Infants and Young Children with Sickle Cell Disease" concluded that "age does appear to be related to decrements in specific cognitive functions."[34]

The effect of politics on scientific discourse has been well documented in the literature in medical sociology and the history of medicine.[35] The particular instance of the identification of the trait demonstrates that even nonracist, nonsexist, "do-gooder" scientists and social scientists (labels I claim for myself) have difficulty separating their politics from what they consider to be scientific truth. In research design, data collection, and interpretation, scientific knowledge is framed in political and racial terms.

## LOCATING THE QUESTION

It is against this rich historical background that I began my research on sickle cell disease and racial health care disparities. I had been told by Vanessa Rogers, a black social worker at Children's Hospital West, that adolescent sickle cell patients, particularly the darker-skinned boys, were being discriminated against in the wards. Ms. Rogers described how these patients were more likely to be transferred as teens into adult care, to be denied pain medication, and to be accused of misbehavior. In addition, about five years before I started my research at CHW, a sickle cell patient had died of a morphine overdose, the result of physician neglect. Ms. Rogers was part of CHW's sickle cell clinic run at the time by three physicians (two white men and one Asian woman) and a white female nurse-practitioner. The clinic was housed in a separate outpatient building next to the hospital. Not only was Ms. Rogers concerned, but the entire clinic staff had made it a priority to change the way their admitted patients were treated while on the wards.

The sickle cell community has been frustrated by patient reports of medical practitioner hostility, neglect, and reduced treatment access. Many adult hospitals even refuse to open sickle cell clinics because they consider the patients to be difficult, and physician tolerance is made worse by the fact that reimbursements from insurance companies for treatment are extremely low. One of the sources of frustration for the sickle cell community has to do with not knowing what or who to blame. At CHW many nonclinic nurses and residents blamed the patients.[36] They felt that sickle cell patients exaggerated their pain in order to receive higher dosages of pain medicine. The perception was that patients were drug seeking. As drug seekers, they were manipulative and often hostile to the nurses and residents. When I asked a white nurse at a mixed-disease teen support group what one could learn by comparing the hospital experiences of adolescent cystic fibrosis patients, who are typically European American, with sickle cell patients, who in the United States are typically African American, she said that the comparison was impossible, explaining, "Their experiences are different because their illnesses are different."[37] This professional, like many, argued that any prejudices she may harbor had less to do with race than with pain and patient demands for pain treatment.

Many of the black families I spoke to also held patients and their guardians responsible for mistakes, neglect, or poor communication. This self-blame was consistent with my fieldwork experiences in the black community generally. Something rarely noted by social scientists or journalists is how much the black community blames itself for its problems. So in many ways this sense of responsibility is not surprising, but it needs to be problematized. One must ask how the patients know whom to blame given that they have no basis for comparison when it comes to determining the quality of their experiences. They are not privy to decisions that determine how care is distributed across the institution. In contrast, many of the professionals I spoke to who are aware of how resources and care are distributed blamed unequal health treatment and outcomes on institutional racism. But does the fact that patients and their families have less institutional knowledge make their generally positive perceptions any less valid?[38] For researchers interested in closing the racial health care gap, the dissimilarity in the perceptions of families and professionals complicates the question of who or what to blame and how to find a solution. Whose reality should matter to a social scientist? The parents who only occasionally noted racism as a factor in their own experiences? Or the hospital staff who are knowledgeable about institutional dynamics and who blamed the institution?

In addition to the question of whose perception should be privileged, the distribution of material resources at my primary field sites also produced competing truth claims and more research questions. On the one hand, state-of-the-art care is provided to very poor minority patients at Children's West and Children's East. On the other hand, looking more broadly at sickle cell disease, gaps in funding have slowed the development of improved treatments and produced an extreme range in the quality of clinical care across the country. Put simply, are disparities a local issue or a national issue?

At the national level, insurance has been shown to be a key factor in health care access differentials. After the age of sixty-five, when Americans become eligible for Medicare or nearly universal health coverage, racial health disparities narrow significantly.[39] But racial differences, while smaller, persist. In 1997, after about six months of field observations, I became convinced that health care access was only one piece of the disparities puzzle. Observing clinic encounters, it seemed that what happened to black patients after they accessed health care profoundly impacted health outcomes.[40] In particular, I witnessed how practitioners inadvertently discouraged black patients from returning for care and impeded patient access to further tests and treatments. Because insurance was, and in some cases still is, considered the primary culprit in disparities in health care, at the time I had difficulty finding articles describing postaccess issues. Since then, a number of studies have shown that primary care physicians and specialists in fact do send disproportionately more white patients than black patients on for further testing and treatment.[41] So what medical, cultural, personal, and institutional signifiers and structures trigger physicians to recommend preventative treatments, therapies, or tests for some patients and not others? And how, through the use of authorized discourses (scientific, institutional, extrainstitutional), do practitioners redefine these signifiers in order to expand or limit patient access? Even more confusing, are health disparities linked to health care? Put another way, are black patients receiving too little health care treatment, or are white patients receiving too much?

When it comes to locating blame for health inequities, there are a number of uncertainties that stand in the way of clarity: (1) uncertain discrimination in terms of the role racism plays in daily clinical interactions, (2) uncertain treatment efficacy in terms of the benefits of different types of therapies, and (3) uncertain suffering in terms of how to identify the value of health care interventions given the fact that people experience suffering so differently. I discovered that rather than paralyze physicians, these uncertainties allow doctors room to advocate for their patients through treatment protocols tailored to specific institutions. Transcending evidence-based medicine, these protocols are attentive to the physical realities of suffering, as well as the social realities of resource limitations and institutional culture. Sold as purely evidence-based, these protocols reduce physician discretion in the clinic by turning medical uncertainty into institutional certainties. The medical and social uncertainties still exist, but within the institutions of these pioneering hematologists, attending physicians and nurses become obligated to employ a particular set of practices that both treat the patient and change the way medical professionals see sickle cell patients. Patients went from being treated as perpetrators of their own suffering to victims of their disease.

In part I, "The Questions," I describe how the uncertainties mentioned here shape patient care. Following the descriptions of the less-than-optimal experiences of two sickle cell patients at CHW in chapters 1 and 2, chapter 3 examines the evidence-based solutions to equalizing treatment employed by sickle cell centers. Randomized studies cannot solely determine how to treat a sickle cell patient whose chronic conditions increase with age. At a fairly young age, patients may have a constellation of disabilities including strokes, necrosis of the hip, lung problems due to acute chest syndrome, or pulmonary hypertension. Chapter 3 describes how a physician's personal sense of duty to his or her patients informs a treatment hermeneutic. Chapters 4 and 5 ask if it is realistic to use health care disparities as a proxy for suffering. Suffering for chronically ill patients can be extreme, but so can suffering caused by poverty and incarceration. Given that health care decisions are never about a cure but about a series of trade-offs, chapter 6 explores why health care may not be the appropriate domain for tackling social inequality.

In part II, "Reforming the System," I describe the ways in which the sickle cell community intervenes to try to increase health care access and improve health outcomes. Chapter 7 considers the effectiveness of the sickle cell community's discourses of suffering as a strategy for developing practitioner empathy. I argue that discourses of suffering are useful because our health care system exists conceptually more in the domain of charity than in the domain of social justice. Charity exists only within structural inequality, and acts of charity typically redeem the donor without empowering the recipient. Social justice, in contrast, turns access to resources (a form of agency) into a right rather than a gift. Chapter 7 explores whether discourses of suffering are sufficient to ameliorate racial health and health care disparities.

Chapters 8 and 9 address novel approaches toward health and health care disparities. Chapter 8 examines the model of adolescent transitioning as a way to acculturate chronically ill patients to the culture of medicine. Chapter 9 describes a thought experiment that demonstrates that medical professionals develop treatment access based on their structural position within their institution and on what they consider to be a life worth living. Employing the conclusions of chapter 9, chapter 10 explores the holistic approaches to sickle cell patient care that many adult patients favor. This chapter examines whether a redistribution of health care resources and funding in the direction of alternative treatments might be the best form of social justice.

My argument about the relationship between justice and health differs from those of anthropologists Nancy Scheper-Hughes and Paul Farmer. In *Death without Weeping: The Violence of Everyday Life in Brazil,* a profoundly moving analysis of suffering in a poor community in northeastern Brazil, Scheper-Hughes argues that morality is prior to culture:

> Anthropologists (myself included) have tended to understand morality as always contingent on, and embedded within, specific cultural assumptions about human life. But there is another, an existential philosophical position that posits the inverse by suggesting that the ethical is always prior to culture because the ethical presupposes all sense and meaning and therefore makes culture possible. . . . the ethical as I am defining it here is "precultural" in that human existence always presupposes the presence of another. That I have been "thrown" into human existence at all presupposes a given, moral relationship to an original (m)other and she to me.[42]

In her call to speak truth to power, Scheper-Hughes asserts that cultural elaborations of suffering must not be treated with equal anthropological deference. Some cultural beliefs, she argues, reproduce suffering and therefore need to be exposed as a source of evil: "The search for meaning in suffering has allowed humans to blame themselves and others for their own sickness, pain, and death, to rationalize suffering as penance for sin, as a means to an end, as the price of reason, or as the path of martyrs and saints. . . . The justification of another human being's pain and suffering is, according to Levinas, the source of immorality."[43] She blames structures of oppression, inequality, and culture, or the "culture of silence," for continued suffering.[44] Without claiming an explicit connection to Marxist theory, Scheper-Hughes makes an argument that her subjects are falsely conscious.

Physician and anthropologist Paul Farmer articulates the relationship between justice and health slightly differently from Scheper-Hughes. Farmer argues that medical care is a human right because to cause human misery by denying access to standard medical treatments is a form of violence. He believes that health care, as a human rights issue, should be the primary focus because taking care of the health of the poor requires a redistribution of wealth and resources. Like dominoes, health care redistribution initiates the toppling of a series of social ills. According to Farmer, "Previously closed institutions have opened their doors to international collaboration designed to halt prison epidemics. This approach—pragmatic solidarity—is, in the end, leading to penal reform as well."[45] In addition, Farmer notes that people see health as an unquestioned need or right, different from abstract legal or theoretical rights that complicate the question of who are the aggressors and victims: "A focus on health alters human rights discussions in important and underexplored ways: the right to health is perhaps the least contested social right, and a large community of health providers—from physicians to community health workers—affords a still-untapped vein of enthusiasm and commitment."[46]

Farmer does not offer an ontological explanation as a call to action. Instead, he argues that there are very pragmatic reasons why wealthy people and nations should invest in the health and well-being of the poor, namely, to avoid becoming a casualty of an epidemic that knows no race or class borders. In this way Farmer locates the will to protect the health of others in a selfish will to avoid infection. By connecting the will to protect the health of the community to the desire for self-protection, Farmer makes a functionalist argument about the origins of human rights. The unquestioned moral stance about health, the untapped vein of commitment and enthusiasm, is rooted in pragmatism rather than empathy. The reason Farmer's argument vacillates between empathy and pragmatism is that he recognizes that there is no solid footing when it comes to the link between health and justice. All linkages are culturally elaborated understandings of rights supported by different notions of the way the world works. Indirectly Farmer acknowledges this by directing his argument to two different audiences, the neoliberals and the feel-good liberals.

My claim is not that there is a connection between justice and health; discourses connecting the two already exist. Notably, a number of scholars have argued that persistent racial health disparities are antithetical to American notions of equal opportunity. What I am interested in is the failure of these claims to galvanize a movement around reform. Other health care system concerns have inspired calls for radical change, but not concerns about unequal treatment. Rather than attributing this paralysis to bias, I argue that uncertainties make it difficult to locate the source of or solution to racial health inequalities.

*Uncertain Suffering* accepts the premise that there are connections between justice and health, but rather than definitively name them, I embrace uncertainty. This book confronts the fact that there is uncertainty about the presence or relevance of racism in the clinic; that there is uncertainty about treatment efficacy and the value of medical interventions over social interventions; and, finally, that there is tremendous uncertainty about how patients experience pain and disability, and therefore cultural and personal elaborations may be the only objective means for assessing suffering.[47]

Believing that context matters, I try to avoid making universal claims about suffering. Importantly, health care justice looks different in a country with an extremely high infant mortality rate than in a country with an average life expectancy of more than eighty years.[48] I start from the premise that health disparities are a problem because most Americans believe they are a problem. What I critique are the approaches to dealing with health disparities, which from my perspective reproduce the problem by failing to acknowledge the uncertainties.

Although I acknowledge numerous uncertainties, I do not treat health and health care inequities as a matter of perspective. They exist, although their shape and form remain unclear. While the contours of my object of study are hazy, I believe that understanding why these indeterminate forms exist matters.

My argument about the social relevance of unequal treatment comes not from me, but from the discourses already in circulation. In this respect I am not trying to impose a moral discourse on the medical community, but to observe and critique how they try to intervene. In this respect, my intervention is firmly situated in the disciplinary practice called cultural relativism.

Many people confuse cultural relativism with moral relativism. Moral relativism claims that all ethics are arbitrary and that there is no way to judge the absolute value of any set of beliefs or practices. Cultural relativism, a method of anthropological inquiry and engagement pioneered by Franz Boas, requires that the anthropologist not judge the cultural practices of one group against those of another. However, within cultures there exist dominant discourses and social practices, as well as resistance to those discourses and practices. Anthropologists do not simply legitimate the hegemonic discourses and practices of the powerful (moral relativism) but also try to understand those who struggle against those practices (cultural relativism).[49]

I do not believe that it is necessary to step outside the discourses under consideration in the health disparities literature or in the culture at large in order to author a metadiscourse about ontology or universal human rights. Racial health care disparities are not the result of a lack of acknowledgment that inequality and injustice exist. The issue is that so many moral universes and resource concerns are being negotiated that people have lost sight of the ideological underpinnings of racial inequality.

Racial inequalities are built around narratives about worthiness, and these narratives actually produce the outcomes they name. Presume a child is intellectually inferior, and after twelve years of schooling it is likely that both the teacher and the student will concur that he or she lacks intelligence. The uncertainties about a child's intelligence in kindergarten are made real by the time that child is a teenager. *Uncertain Suffering* explores the fact that a number of uncertainties contribute to our inability to definitively locate the origins of health disparities. Rather than consider these uncertainties a product of scientific or moral failings, this book explores how uncertainties actually open up possibilities for patient advocacy by naming suffering. By naming sickle cell patient suffering, the community opens up health care access to patients in pain. But I critique the community's overreliance on discourses of patient suffering in order to increase health care access. By legitimating only particular forms of patient suffering, as determined through evidence-based medicine, for example, health care professionals are again authorized to treat patients differently based on whether their suffering is viewed as real and therefore worthy of treatment.

## METHODS

I spoke with more than one hundred medical professionals, scientists, patients, advocates, and families at conferences, hospitals, sickle cell associations, and homes, conducting more than four hundred interviews in ten cities over a period of seven years. As a qualitative researcher, I wanted to focus on one disease and one community in order to understand how race works in the clinic; the experiences of sickle cell patients offer a window onto how race impacts treatment access. Because most sickle cell patients in the United States are black, I cannot compare the experiences of black sickle cell patients and white sickle cell patients. Nevertheless, a number of excellent quantitative studies document the differences in the treatment of blacks and whites within one disease category.[50] My qualitative study was never going to be able to match in size or in data collection what I consider important studies of unequal treatment. My interest was in the clinic as a performance space where scientific knowledge meets hegemonic discourses about race. My research focuses on how health and health care inequities are produced in the clinic, and how science is used to either open up or foreclose patient access.

I situate my analysis of health care disparities in the experiences of adolescent sickle cell patients who are transitioning to adult care and who embody uncertainty. I focus on the transition from pediatric to adult care because transitioning exposes a number of interesting presumptions that inform health care structure in the United States. I focus on blacks with sickle cell disease because their experiences in health care are closely tied to the social history and current status of blacks in the United States. I primarily use the term *black* rather than *African American* because many of the patients would classify themselves as Caribbean American or Ghanaian or Nigerian. Despite their self-identification, patient experiences in the clinic have more to do with race than with ethnicity, which is why *black* makes more sense as a descriptor.

By trying to understand the presumptions embedded in treatment protocols or standard narratives about sickle cell disease, my goal has been to understand how culturally we make meaning of disease within systems of inequality. I use the space of the clinic, broadly defined as a space dedicated to formal encounters between medical professionals and patients, and scientific association meetings as key sites for the production of meaning. I examine how patient dispositions toward health care are produced through patient-practitioner collaborations, and how these dispositions affect treatment choices on the part of both the patient and the practitioner. Finally, many of the disparities can be traced to the imagination. The breadth and quality of care a patient receives are often related to how chronically ill patients in collaboration with family members and providers create what I call *lifescapes*, hopeful narratives about what actions in the present will contribute to an imagined future. These narratives are tied materially to what medical sociologist Mary-Jo Good describes as the biotechnical embrace or the affective dimensions that determine high rates of social investment in biotechnology.[51] Conceptually, lifescapes and the biotechnical embrace speak to the role of the culture of hope in shaping health care resource allocation.

*Uncertain Suffering: Racial Healthcare Disparities and Sickle Cell Disease* addresses how race and medical uncertainty are entangled in the clinic and how this entanglement produces unequal treatment. In the end, all this uncertainty about the source of health disparities or how to ameliorate them does not excuse a rejection of the presence of unequal treatment, as if the ink blots in a Rorschach test are not there,[52] or a nihilistic response that rejects any moral grounding in what ultimately is a debate about what types of unequal suffering Americans are willing to accept. After discussing all the uncertainties, I try to recover what I consider a culturally relative foothold in debates about health care disparities and social justice.

PART I

# The Questions

# CHAPTER I

# Race and Uncertainty

Is it surprising that prisons resemble factories, schools,
barracks, hospitals, which all resemble prisons?

Michel Foucault, Discipline and Punish

Sickle-shaped hemoglobin can block blood flow to capillaries, essentially starving organs of oxygen. In addition to producing tremendous pain, repeated vascular occlusions often cause irreparable organ damage. Because of the association between pain and mobility, treating pain quickly and aggressively is considered by many hematologists to be a necessary standard of care. In an effort to authorize national treatment standards, a group of physicians working with the National Institutes of Health (NIH) published a monograph entitled *The Management of Sickle Cell Disease*. This document distills data from the latest scientific studies in order to present an evidence-based approach to sickle cell disease treatment. The chapter on pain presents the following protocol: "The goals for assessment of acute and chronic pain are to characterize a patient's pain and related experiences, provide a basis for therapeutic decisions, and document the efficacy of pain control. Because pain is subjective, assessment requires patients' self-reports, valid tools, and measurements repeated over time. Clinically, self-reports are supplemented by physical findings, laboratory data, and diagnostic procedures."[1]

The physicians, nurses, and social scientists who authored this chapter stress that when it comes to assessing pain, patients should be trusted. This manual encourages physicians and nurses to use the Wong-Baker Faces Pain Rating Scale to determine the intensity of a patient's pain. The scale graphically represents levels of pain from 0 "No Hurt"

(a smiling face) to 5 "Hurts Worst" (a sad face with tears), and patients
are asked to point to the image that best represents their level of pain.
The authors continue:

> Severe pain should be considered a medical emergency that prompts timely
> and aggressive management until the pain is tolerable. The following rec-
> ommendations are for treatment in the emergency room, day treatment
> center, or hospital if the patient is admitted directly. 1) Begin hydration.
> Total fluids should not exceed 1.5 times maintenance (including volume for
> drug infusions). Initial fluid should be 5 percent dextrose + half-normal
> saline + 20 mEq KCl/L, adjusted for serum chemistry results, 2) Assess the
> patient for the cause of pain and complication, 3) Rapidly assess pain
> intensity using a simple measurement tool.

Finally, they advise the following emergent care for acute episodes:

> The patient in acute pain at an emergency room or clinician's office usually
> has exhausted all homecare options. Failure of home or outpatient therapy
> signals the need for parenteral medications, which include strong opioids
> like morphine. If a patient is on long-term opioids at home, tolerance may
> have developed, so the new episode can be treated with a different opioid
> or with a higher dose of the same drug if it is the only one the patient toler-
> ates. In general, medications and loading doses should be selected after
> assessment of the patient's current condition and consideration of the
> patient's history.[2]

Despite the authority of this NIH publication, evidence-based protocols do not ensure treatment efficacy. Even if two physicians claim to
follow these NIH recommendations, it is highly unlikely that their treatment practices are identical. In fact, these objective recommendations
leave plenty of room for improvisation, or for the insertion of subjectivity into clinic care. Physicians and nurses can choose to privilege lab
tests over the Wong-Baker rating, or belabor a patient's history at the
expense of a rapid assessment. These divergent practices can have a
huge effect on treatment outcomes. Exploring the experiences of an
adolescent patient named Max, this chapter asks if this improvisation is
responsible for racial disparities in health care.

When I first met Max, in the winter of 1999, he was a couple months
shy of his eighteenth birthday, and the hospital staff was threatening to
punt him from Children's Hospital West to a local adult care hospital.
"Punting," a somewhat typical disciplinary tactic, involves transferring
unruly adolescent sickle cell patients to adult care early. Unruly can
mean that the patient is too dependent on strong pain medications and
therefore a difficult case to treat, or too annoying, a quality shared by
many chronically ill adolescent patients. Max was the prototypical

unruly black adolescent male who inspired fear, contempt, and loathing in the medical staff.

Max was also one of the unfortunate 20 percent of sickle cell patients with a severe form of the disease, meaning he was hospitalized more than three times a year. Even in the hospital, managing his pain was very difficult. The uncertain etiology of pain and the lack of tools to objectively measure pain meant that nurses and residents could ascribe whatever origins they wanted to his sickle cell crises. In varying degrees some argued that his pain was psychosomatic and others that it was pathophysiological. For Max, who was from the projects, demands for pain medication were often read as drug-seeking behavior rather than a response to legitimate suffering. Various members of the staff rallied to make sure that Max never stepped foot in the hospital again after his eighteenth birthday.

Max's story demonstrates that rather than try to identify a single source or even multiple sources for disparities in health care access, Americans need to look at the overlapping and self-referential stories we rely on to make sense of race and inequality. Stories about race and genes, IQ differences, social dysfunction, and individual failings are used to turn the blame for differential rates of incarceration, the educational achievement gap, and health disparities back onto the black community. These stories are often entangled in psychiatric and medical discourses, which because of their authority can be used to legitimate racial inequality in the clinic. But Max's story also implicates Max and his mother, Lena, who were unable to step outside the cultural narratives about race that diminished their agency both within and outside the clinic.

In order to record Max's story, we met in a hospital conference room with his social worker, Vanessa Rogers. Max had been admitted a week earlier for a painful crisis. The timing of this crisis could not have been worse. With Max now two weeks shy of his eighteenth birthday, the campaign to oust him was at its most fierce. Max, knowing that he had already lost the battle, was simply trying to make sense of his impending transfer.

Max had a coffee-and-cream complexion, and his manner, despite his reputation among nurses and doctors, was surprisingly gentle. His large, almond-shaped eyes, which crossed slightly, exuded naïveté. Max was dressed in pressed straight-cut white jean shorts that came down below his knees, a spotless white tank top that accentuated his sculpted upper body, and expensive white-on-white sneakers. He was hooked up to an intravenous morphine drip, and the medicine was clearly making him a bit groggy and itchy. Ms. Rogers, in her forties, resembled the quintessential black maternal figure, even though she was single and childless. She was dressed in a modest denim jumper that hid her large chest and hips, allowing her to retreat from the gaze of her colleagues.

Without much prompting, Max began describing a recent experience: "Me and Jesse basically have the same treatment. All the sickle cell kids basically have the same treatment. We all get either morphine or Dilaudid. We all get Benadryl to stop the itching. We all get hot packs to help. We got the same problem so we all know what each other is going through. Like I was in a lot of pain and the doctor kept on bugging me. Just 'Daaaa' all in my ear. And I'm sitting here crying. Tears coming out my eyes. I'm crying, telling him, 'Man, I don't know. I'm hurting. I need my medicine. Can you give me some medicine?' And the doctor still there just asking questions."

Max continued, "Jesse was my roommate at the time. Jesse said, 'Man, look. I'm going to tell you how you supposed to do it. You supposed to do this and this and that.' Telling the doctor, 'Look, you got to help him because he's sitting there hurting. Why you sitting there asking him questions? He just hurting more and more. He ain't getting no better. Why you asking questions? You can ask the questions later while you get his medicine now.'"

"I'm sitting there telling him, 'I need my medicine.' He's sitting there asking me all kind of other questions. 'Who lives in my house? What's my this and this and this? Who smokes in our house?' 'Why you got to know all that? I'm hurting. I need my medicine. You get me some medicine.'" While recounting the incident, Max both told the story and at the same time relived it.

Breaking from his reenactment, Max proceeded, "Then the doctor get all scared. He felt he got threatened and this kind of stuff. So he feel Jesse threatened him because Jesse telling him, 'Why you couldn't find all that other stuff out later. Just give the dude his medicine so you could find the questions out.'"

Wanting clarification, I inserted, "And the doctor said he felt threatened?"

Max responded, "Yeah, the doctor felt like both of us was threatening him. And I'm sitting here crying, tears running out my eyes. But I'm threatening him?"

I asked, "Is this a resident or an attending?"

Without skipping a beat, "It was a resident."

"So he made a report? And did somebody come to you and say . . ."

"I think it was even Vanessa. I think Vanessa was the one who even came up to us." Max tried to make eye contact with Vanessa, but Vanessa made a deliberate effort not to interrupt Max. Instead, she sat very quietly with her eyes cast down toward the table, hands in her lap. Finally realizing that Vanessa was not going to help him piece together his story, Max continued, "I don't remember who came up to us. But he said that we was in there threatening him about what we need to do. And I'm sitting here like, 'Threatening him?'" Max speaks as though he is truly bewildered. "Jesse know about me. I know about Jesse. Jesse is sitting here telling him what he needs to do for me since he obviously don't know what he needs to do for me. He sitting here asking all kind of questions. He could ask those stupid simple questions later." Max showed obvious derision for the protocols performed by residents as part of their training.

"My mom and Vanessa just talked [to them]. [They said,] 'Well from now on just don't say nothing. Just keep your mouth closed.' But if I see my homeboy is sitting here crying and the doctor he over there asking him questions about his family. . . . Even though Vanessa and them told me not to say nothing I'm still going to say something because that's my homeboy. I know how it feel to be in the same pain and they don't. So get the dude his medicine! Ask him the questions later."

So I ask the reader, What did you imagine while reading this excerpt? Did you believe that given the situation you might feel threatened like the resident? What aspects of the situation made you feel that way? Max's speech (Ebonics)? The fact that there were two black adolescents "ganging" up on a single (white?) resident? Did the fact that Max and Jesse were in a hospital room, possibly in hospital gowns, matter to your perception? Did you sympathize with Max's tears or reject them as manipulation? I ask these questions because at one level what is at play is the culture of the imagination. How race, age, suffering, gender, and citizenship are imagined plays a tremendous role in how health care is organized at the institutional level and practiced at the clinical level.

What strikes me about the white resident's interview with Max is the resident's inability to empathize with Max's suffering. By denying Max his pain medication, the resident was acting as a gatekeeper, protecting the hospital from what he considered an unwarranted use of narcotics. From the resident's perspective, Max's demands amounted to theft or an unwarranted (possibly perceived as unlawful) use of drugs. The resident had been taught that Max was a violent, manipulative, drug-seeking thug incapable of suffering. Hegemonic discourses about race and class impeded the resident's ability to empathize with the suffering of his patient. The resident's insistence that he ask basic and irrelevant personal questions before "diagnosing" Max could be read either as sadistic or as the act of a former medical student who has been trained to process patient information through a very narrow conceptual filter, what medical anthropologists call the medical gaze. So do we blame medical schools for choosing students who lack the empathy to collaborate with people who are unlike them, or do we blame medical schools for failing to teach students how to make protocols patient-centered?[3] Perhaps the blame rests with Max?

Max's history at CHW had been troubled. He had been accused of writing graffiti on bathroom walls, theft, and obstreperous behavior. Nurses and residents, who were overwhelmingly white, deemed his behavior threatening and disruptive, even criminal. The hospital used his eighteenth birthday, which occurred two weeks after the interview, as a justification for transferring him out of CHW.

During the interview Max described the pressure he felt from the staff: "Every time I come to the hospital they always pressing the issue about when I'm going to move [to adult care]. Dr. Hansen he brings it up a lot. They praying so hard that I hurry up and move until he wrote the number down and told me as soon as I get discharged to call him that day. It's on a big white piece of paper under my telephone so I can't forget it. That's how bad they want me out of here." I asked him if he was going to follow their orders. "No, I ain't calling them the same day. I'm calling like two or three days later just so I can get them mad. Just because I know what I'm supposed to do and when I am supposed to do it. You don't have to keep telling me. I mean they just pressing the issue to the limit."

I asked Max's social worker what the cutoff age is for pediatric care for chronically ill young adults with congenital diseases. Vanessa said that some patients can stay until they are twenty-five years old. Not wanting to appear too definitive, she qualified her answer by saying, "But it's not clear to me what the criteria are for that." Grinning, Max asserted, "And I should be one of those patients."

For chronically ill teenagers who have been receiving care in one hospital for most of their lives, the idea of having to switch hospitals is overwhelming. When I asked Max to put his fears into his own words, he replied, "Just for the simple fact that I've been coming here since I was one month old and I have never went to another hospital other than for either a checkup or an appointment at another hospital. They don't know nothing about me. I mean, [another doctor will] know everything about my problem, but he don't know me, my body. These doctors here know how to treat me."

Max provided an example: "When I come to the emergency here they take a long time, but when I get into the room they know exactly what to do and that's admit. They know that from the beginning. As soon as I walk through the doors and I'm telling them I'm hurting, they're calling up to the fourth floor and reserving a room for me. When I go to another hospital and I walk through the double doors and I tell them I'm hurting, it's gonna take me about twenty-four hours to get a room probably."

I asked him to describe a prior experience with another emergency room, and he responded, "I remember one time I came in an ambulance to an emergency room. That's when they had asked me, 'What kind of medicines are you taking?' I told them I was taking Vicodin. I was like, 'I been taking Vicodin up to two tablets every four to six hours, really every four hours, and it's not helping me.' So the doctor said, 'Okay.' So he walks out the room, writes up whatever they write up. Then the nurse come in with two Vicodins and a cup of water and telling me to take them. 'What are you going to give me two Vicodins for when I just told the doctor that it's not working. If it was working, I wouldn't be at this emergency room.'"

He described what it means for CHW staff to know how to treat his case: "Right here as soon as I come through the doors they already know this kid is going to be admitted. When I'm right there at the front desk signing in, the nurse walk by and she say, 'How you doing Max?' And I be like, 'Bad,' or like, 'Not good.' It's just they be like, 'You're hurting?' I be like, 'Yeah.' So I guess that's when she'll go back there and call the fourth floor to reserve a room. When I go in there waiting to see the doctor it only take the doctor about five minutes to check me out. And as soon as the doctor walk out, the nurses come in there with the IV stuff getting ready to stick me to help the pain crisis."

Wondering how he envisions the future, I asked, "Do you think if you went somewhere else, eventually they would start to know you?" He replied, "Eventually after a couple of years at most. But yeah, eventually. Because like Vanessa, a couple of months after she met me, she could already tell if I'm hurting, if I'm lying or if I'm telling the truth.

Because usually I be like, 'I'm doing fine,' but I really ain't doing fine. I'm really hurting. Now when Vanessa sees me she don't even got to say nothing, and she know I'm hurting. But she'll still ask me, 'Well, how you feel?' I be like, 'Fine.' And she'll look at me like, 'Yeah, right. Go on tell the truth.' That's when I'll just start laughing."[4]

Making sense of the significance of race in Max's experiences is difficult given that all the characters in his narrative are acting in what one might consider a reasonable manner. Dr. Hansen, who has worked with Max and his family for almost eighteen years, must protect the staff and his relationship with the staff. Therefore, Dr. Hansen's prodding to get Max to call another physician makes sense given his responsibility to protect the quality and efficiency of a working community. The emergency room at the other hospital, which has, ironically, many more African Americans on staff and is in a predominantly African American neighborhood, is unfamiliar with Max and therefore does not want to risk overprescribing pain medications. Finally, children's hospitals specialize in a particular developmental age-group and are not equipped to handle adult issues. Transferring patients after they reach a certain age makes sense given that the entire organization of a children's hospital, from the playrooms to the inventory of medications, is designed specifically to handle the health care needs of children. One could argue that Max's problems are developmental, or more accurately his own, and therefore the problem is not with the institution but with Max.

The idea that there was something pathologically wrong with Max rather than with the institution was validated by a psychiatrist who was called in to evaluate Max a month before his eighteenth birthday. She determined that Max was a "sociopath," exonerating the children's hospital from any moral or legal obligation to treat him. According to the fourth edition of the *Diagnostic and Statistical Manual of Mental Disorders,* someone with a personality disorder, including sociopathy, has the following symptoms:

> The symptoms of antisocial personality disorder include a longstanding pattern (after the age of 15) of disregard for the rights of others. There is a failure to conform to society's norms and expectations that often results in numerous arrests or legal involvement as well as a history of deceitfulness where the individual attempts to con people or use trickery for personal profit. Impulsiveness is often present, including angry outbursts, failure to consider consequences of behaviors, irritability, and/or physical assaults.
>
> Some argue that a major component of this disorder is the reduced ability to feel empathy for other people. This inability to see the hurts,

concerns, and other feelings of people often results in a disregard for these aspects of human interaction. Finally, irresponsible behavior often accompanies this disorder as well as a lack of remorse for wrongdoings.[5]

Running down the list of symptoms, I considered Max's case. Max had never been arrested, although at the time of the interview his brother was in juvenile detention; guilt by association was certainly operative not simply at the familial level but at the racial level as well. Many people questioned whether or not he had been deceitful, but there was never any proof. At times he was impulsive and showed anger, but he was aware of the repercussions of his behavior. For example, he planned to deliberately wait two days to call his new doctor just to make Dr. Hansen mad. Max demonstrated tremendous empathy toward people he respected, among them Vanessa Rogers, his mother, his girlfriend, his girlfriend's mother, and the physicians and nurses on the sickle cell clinic team. On the other hand, he did not hide his contempt for some residents and nurses on the wards. But was his contempt the result of past negative experiences, his adolescence, or both?

By taking care of his mother and never getting into trouble except at the hospital, Max played the role of the good son, in contrast to his brother. From the perspective of the psychiatrist, the particulars of Max's experiences and behavior outside the hospital were irrelevant. His disruptive (adolescent?) behavior meant he was unable to conform to societal norms, and therefore she labeled him a sociopath. On the advice of his social worker, Max's mother discharged him from Children's West before the diagnosis was placed in his chart. This happened just a week after I interviewed him in the conference room.

In this case, every actor employed discourses that have some scientific, social scientific, or administrative legitimacy—discourses that are authorized or orthodox, and those that exist in the realm of *doxa* or the taken for granted. The embedding of doxa, common sense, or what Clifford Geertz called "of-courseness" into scientific orthodoxy produces racialized discourses.[6] I use the term *racialized discourses* rather than *racist discourses* because perceptions of black people's inferiority or their threat to the social body have been sublimated into scientific and social scientific discourses about dysfunction or intellectual ability. They imply race but do not explicitly cite race. For example, the CHW psychiatrist willing to diagnose Max as a sociopath believes in the legitimacy of her profession, believes she is a competent diagnostician, and believes that her assessment is correct. What she failed to do was diagnose the institution.

In *Total Confinement: Madness and Reason in a Maximum Security Prison*, anthropologist Lorna Rhodes explores how a prison creates the conditions for "madness."[7] Prisoners resist deprivations imposed by the prison staff by acting out in ways that are then coded as psychotic. So, couldn't "reduced ability to feel empathy for other people" apply to institutions that fail to respond to suffering—something physician and anthropologist Paul Farmer describes as structural violence?[8] The psychiatrist ignored Max's background and gender and the hospital politics that brought her into the dispute. She overlooked the fact that the hospital had the power to hire and fire her. In the end her professional license legitimated her diagnosis, and her diagnosis secured her employment. The psychiatrist is not a racist, but all the mechanisms, from the discourse used to talk about poor blacks as dysfunctional to the sublimation of social categories into psychosocial categories, inadvertently produce racial disparities. Uncertainties in medicine and psychiatry are such that medical professionals can unburden institutions of responsibility for patients like Max through particular diagnoses or treatment decisions. Diagnosing Max as a sociopath relieved the staff and the institution of any legal or moral obligation to care for him. For African American adolescent teenagers, transferring them to adult care prematurely shifts the responsibility for managing the number one symptom, pain, from the institution to the patient.

To better understand Max, in the summer of 2001 I decided to interview his mother, Lena, at her home in the projects. Lena, a sturdy, dark-skinned woman in her late forties, was self-admittedly not afraid of anything or anyone. Raised in the same projects in which she now resides, over the years Lena has had to confront violence, poverty, and illness. She gave me a tour of all her previous homes. The tour required no walking on our part, just a finger to point to different one-story cinder block apartments. As prescribed by the project rules, whenever there was a change in the number of people living with her, Lena was required to move. She started in a two-bedroom apartment, then moved to a three-bedroom with the births of her daughter, Tasha, and Max, then a four-bedroom apartment with the birth of Max's brother, Reginald, and finally back to a two-bedroom now that Tasha was dead and Reginald was in prison. Tasha died at nine of sickle cell disease, and Reginald was accused of stealing a car with a group of teens. The second room was for Max, although he spent most of his time at his girlfriend's apartment or in the hospital.

We sat in Lena's small, meticulous living room on an overstuffed couch and chairs. Deeply introspective, Lena used language sparingly and preferred to respond to questions rather than initiate conversation. Sitting on glass end tables were pictures of all three of her children captured at various ages. Lena provided what seemed to be a very honest appraisal of her children. She defended her children but was also harshly critical of them at the same time: Max was overly dependent on his immature girl-friend, Reginald had thrown away his opportunities, and Tasha never smiled. Lena showed me a picture of the one time Tasha forced a smile; Lena laughed while closely reexamining the framed photo.

Unlike Max's sickle cell disease, Tasha's was uncomplicated, and she never spent a significant amount of time in the hospital. In fact, the day before she died Tasha spent the afternoon roller skating around the project courtyard. Lena said that Tasha fell, but she landed on a patch of grass and did not hit her head. By the evening, however, Tasha com-plained about a severe headache, and Lena gave her pain medication and sent her to bed. In the early morning, Lena heard moans coming from Tasha's room. When she went to check on her daughter, Lena noticed that the area around her mouth and nose was blue and purple. When asked, Tasha said that she could wait until morning to go to the doctor, but by six in the morning Tasha's moans were loud, and Lena noticed that the purple spot had grown. She called the neighbors, who drove Lena and Tasha to the hospital. By 9:16 in the morning Tasha was dead. The doctors never discovered the cause of her death but assumed it was related to sickle cell disease, possibly a reaction to the pain med-ication or perhaps a neurological event like a stroke.

Tasha died on a day when Max was being discharged from one of his numerous hospitalizations. The irony that the supposedly healthy child died and the sick one lived is not lost on anyone. The unexpectedness of Tasha's death contributes to Lena's proactive approach to Max's health care, but the uncertainties associated with the disease feed anxieties that Lena simply lives with. Max was only seven years old when Tasha died, but the permanence of his loss was something he grasped right away. Tasha was Max's best friend, and it took years and the assistance of a psychiatrist to help him cope with the loss.

Before we sat down to a Popeye's chicken lunch, which I purchased and Lena condemned as "not as good as my fried chicken," Lena described Max's experiences at Children's Hospital West. "When Max turned teenager, [staff] attitude changed. He got involved in a gang. He wasn't out there doing nothing wrong because he didn't have time, he was in the hospital. It's just the idea he's in it. When I found that out I got really nervous thinking guns and drugs and all that, and it wasn't."

I asked Lena what gang he joined. Trying to put his choice into context, she began by saying, "It's like this here: Bloods and Crips." I replied, "So it was a kind of a violent gang? What was it, Bloods or Crips?" Lena answered, "Blood. This area here is Blood."

Recognizing that being in a gang can mean many things, I tried to let her know that I was not passing judgment on Max because of his Blood affiliation. I asked, "Can you survive as a teenage male and not be in the Bloods here, or is it a choice?"

"I think it's a choice," she said without much deliberation. "I think Max chose it because he's sick, and that's his backup other than me. See? And he's not into drugs. He don't use a gun, he's not jacking and robbing and stealing. I think he really did it for the name, and to get along at school. I guess if you belong then you can deal with school better. But Max never was at school. He was always too sick. He go to school maybe a week out of three months. So, that was hard. School was really, really hard because he was never there. I got some report cards with nothing on it. 'Excessive absence,' that's it. So, he didn't get the education that he needed. Now I know it's the Unified School District's fault. They should have been responsible knowing they have a sick kid in their system. To get the help that he needed. They didn't. See, so. It was real hard for me, but, like I always say, 'only the strongest survive.' So, that's the way I deal with it."

Probing further, I asked, "So he joined a gang. You were worried at first, but you realized that he's never going to be really involved in . . ." Interrupting me, Lena shook her head, "No, he's not involved like that, no. But the change through the hospital. . . . A lot of things was happening in the hospital. Blaming him for things that he wasn't doing such as having company, and they going in the bathroom, and they writing on the walls. At one point they say that he was taking a controlled substance, and it was candy. But it was supposed to have been a controlled substance so they invited the police into that. But, I was right there to stop that one. When they analyzed it, it was candy. So, see, that made them, you know, even more separate. Every time Max was in there as a young teenager, something always happen. Nothing never happen until Max and Jesse were in the hospital together."

I interrupted and asked if they also kicked Jesse out. "Yeah. But that's how they get rid of them. I see that now. Because the first time it happened was to Rita's son, Jesse. They accused him of going in a nurse's purse, and flushing money down the toilet, and a whole bunch of stuff. They accused Max of stealing a pager out of a mother's purse. Ahh, I'm telling you it was something. I was wondering, because Max kept saying 'I want to get out of this hospital.' I'm saying, 'Son, I don't know where to take you, this is the best place for you.' 'I don't want to be here no more, they blaming everything on me' [Max said]." Lena admitted that Max played into staff fears by always using a red marker to doodle on his whiteboard. Lena also noted that while it intimidated some of the nurses and residents, it was a very tame form of resistance: "Nothing bad, but he always would come there with red clothes on, red shoes, red shirt, red everything [she laughs]. I think he was intimidating them with that."

Lena described Max as "heeding his heart," meaning his Blood affiliation was important to him and therefore he liked to flaunt it. Lena's fear was that since he became an adult, he had to be much more careful when it came to showing his loyalty. She was not concerned that Max would do something wrong, explaining, "I don't worry about him getting into no trouble or anything. Never been arrested or nothing. He's the laid-back one [she laughs]. He's not a violent Blood." Her concern was with how others, including physicians, saw Max.

Already knowing a bit from Vanessa about how Lena tried to exculpate Max during his teenage years at CHW, I wanted to hear from Lena about her efforts. I asked her if she tried to explain to the hospital staff that Max was not a threat. She replied, "They wasn't listening to nothing. They wanted Max and Jesse out in any way that they could. They did it really dirty. I always defend Max, but when he's wrong, I don't defend. I've seen a lot of stuff happening to my son that was not true. And I wasn't going to stand and let them do that. Like, when they say that he stole a pager. They brought security, they was gonna handcuff him and all that."

Clearly still very upset, Lena continued, "We had a roundtable discussion about it, and I told them, 'Look, you back off because you lying. My son ain't took no pager!' It's just the way that they was doing it, you can tell this is a setup here." Reenacting the moment Lena said, " 'I refuse to let y'all put that in his medical records. I want my apology to him and to me for making me come way out there on the bus to be at this meeting for nothing.' That's when I said I got to get him out. When Jesse would be there, oh boy! Every few minutes my phone was ringing. 'Max is doing this.' Max stayed on the phone more than anybody I've ever seen in my life, so how could he be doing so much? As long as there's a phone in that room, trust me, it's busy. So, how could he be doing so much? Where do he have time to go steal something? You know."

Lena recounted a meeting between Max and the nurses. Max wanted the nurses to know that he was in a gang but that that did not mean he was violent or threatening. Naively, Max thought that if he was truthful, the staff would develop greater empathy for him. Lena described how everyone oohed and aahed as he told his story. She said people commented afterward that Max didn't look like a gang member, which Lena considered disingenuous given Max's race and residence. Even if some people suspected before the meeting that Max was in a gang, the meeting, organized by Vanessa, marked a sea change in his treatment by hospital staff. Lena explained: "After that, everything started changing; doctors' attitude, everything. I've just refused to let them do my son like that until I was ready to transfer him out of there. So, he's out, I'm glad. Children's Hospital was wonderful to us. I learned a whole lot of stuff I never thought I'd need to learn about sickle cell, and different people. I'm glad that that hospital was there. If anybody ever have a kid who gets sick, that's where they need to go because they are going to find out what's wrong. They will correct it if it can be corrected."

In a situation where there is hostility toward a patient, is care compromised? In hospitals, antipathy for patients is not uncommon. Contempt is often distilled into pejoratives such as *gomer, dirtball,* and the more recent *ger,* short for *nigger,* used to label difficult black patients.[9] Some argue that pejorative terms offer a release valve. Physician Peter Dans lists the common justifications as "frustration and anger in managing certain patients, fostering group solidarity among caregivers under stress, and the alleged 'dehumanization' of medical training."[10] After interviewing graduating medical students in four cohorts, Dans observes that overall medical students do not find pejorative terms useful. Dans concludes that if such terms are being employed by medical staff, then institutional correctives are needed to foster better care for particular subgroups—an interesting conclusion because he is basically arguing that a feeling of impotence on the part of medical staff leads to frustration, which is then unleashed on patients.

I would argue that diagnosing Max as a sociopath was an instance where a pejorative label was instantiated, or made real using the authority of psychiatry. Pejorative labels are more than simply "not useful"; they can be used to legitimate the withdrawal of medical care and therefore contribute to racial health care disparities. In the case of Max, by labeling him mentally ill the hospital staff turned uncertainty about the relationship between his gang affiliation and his adolescent rebelliousness into a certain diagnosis. From the literature, we know that African

Americans are more frequently diagnosed as schizophrenic and less frequently diagnosed with mood disorders.[11] The fact that blacks are over-diagnosed as having severe mental problems that carry with them tremendous stigma (sociopathy and schizophrenia) means that we should question what these diagnoses are proxies for, as we should question what *ger* and *dirtball* are proxies for.

The relationship between medical staff antipathy and the quality of patient care seems probable, but it has yet to be proved. In fact, most of my informants, many of whom suspected racism, had nothing but positive things to say about the medical treatment at CHW. Lena was no different. I asked Lena if Max ever seemed to have problems with access to pain medications because of his run-ins with staff. She responded, "No, they didn't withhold it." Almost in the same breath Lena praised the medical staff and noted instances when Max almost lost his rights to unfettered treatment access: "They said the PCA pump . . . where he could push for his own pain medicine . . . said that he's stuck an object up in it and was getting extra morphine. I say, 'You show me how he did it.' They tried to show me how he pushed this [Lena demonstrates using her hands] up into that thing to make more morphine come down. And it didn't work. This thing won't even go that far up there. You see? So, I said, 'No, no, no, don't tell me that.' I said, 'Don't put that shit on my son's record because y'all lying now. You need a key to open that. He ain't jimmy no kind of lock. And this thing do not fit up in there.' Vanessa, everybody was in that room. That happened a couple of times. They said that he forced the machine to push extra medicine. That's when Max said, 'Y'all keep me on this stuff all the time anyway, and I don't like to be on it no way. So why did you think that I would try to be sneaking more?' And then it's gonna set off an alarm if you *do* get more. So, how could he be doing it?"

I asked her why they were accusing Max of stealing extra medicine. She saw it as part of a larger effort to punt him from pediatric care: "That's another way of making the record look bad to get him out of there. That's what it's all about, is to get him out of there. They didn't know how to transition him out to another hospital unless they did it in a dirty way. See, just before they put Max out, I checked him out so they didn't get that chance. I checked him out and put him at General Hospital. And from General Hospital he went to Western Medical Center and that's where he's at now."

There were no comprehensive sickle cell programs to transfer Max into that matched the quality of the one at CHW. There was a program at the county facility, but participation there entailed long waits, and it was almost impossible to develop a close relationship with a patient advocate like a doctor or nurse. Therefore, the question of Max's transfer situated itself as a health care access issue. A black female chaplain at Children's West argued at a meeting that transferring sickle cell patients out of pediatric care was an ethics issue because the hospital was effectively denying care to patients like Max. Sitting in on the meeting, I was struck that nobody except a few social workers understood the ethics argument, and most resented that their actions were framed as unethical. When I asked the two physicians why Max was transferred, the response was a cursory, "There were a number of reasons." Basically, most people involved felt that it was simply better to let Max go than to threaten the rapport between the sickle cell clinic and the ward staff.

While it would be easy to blame the institution and individuals within it for Max's loss of access to the best sickle cell program in the city, there was no single variable that could be identified in a statistically significant study.[12] One of the most interesting aspects of racialized discourses is ascription. In education, for example, race often determines which children are identified as "bright" and "energetic" and which are identified as troublemakers. Did the staff ascribe meaning and motive to Max's behavior based on his race? Given the subtlety of racism, many people in the sickle cell community grapple with questions about whether actions that seem to put them at a disadvantage are the result of racism or something else.

At a national level, the sickle cell community struggles with whether or not funding levels for the disease are commensurate with those for other diseases, and if not, is the disparity related to racism or to the fact that sickle cell falls somewhere between an orphan disease and a major disease? Sickle cell disease affects seventy thousand, mostly black, Americans. Cystic fibrosis, many in the community note, affects about thirty-six thousand, mostly white, Americans. The cystic fibrosis community, notably the Cystic Fibrosis Foundation, has vastly greater financial resources, but as one hematologist noted, this community has been politically proactive and has felt empowered enough to rate the quality of cystic fibrosis centers around the country. The sickle cell community has never been as proactive and has been reluctant to set high standards. A difficult question to answer is, are the access issues related to race, advocacy, or something else?

For Max, there were few instances in his experiences with staff that one could definitively call racist. The ways that race mattered in Max's case were indirect and nuanced, with gender and class seemingly playing a much larger role. Max's social worker, Vanessa, tried to encourage staff empathy by having Max tell his story of suffering. The narrative was incomprehensible to the staff given what they already "knew"—and I use quotes here deliberately—about Max. The cultural signifiers—gangs, Ebonics, dress, racial performances—overshadowed any counternarrative Max tried to construct about his own suffering.

Literature on the role of narrative and emplotment in clinical practice describes how patients and medical professionals develop a story about healing that then gets enacted. For example, an occupational therapist and a parent construct a narrative of great hope for a child injured by a stroke. Together the parent and therapist might develop a story about the child being "smart and full of potential" or demonstrating that "he desperately wants to run around and play with his brother." Depending on how the child's agency is narrated by those in power, additional therapies and interventions are likely to be prescribed. If the therapist and parent disagree on the narrative, then what happens? I argue that emplotment happens in very specific instances, generally when professionals and patients are able to share power. The medical staff at CHW saw Max as foreign, uncultured, a barbarian. The cultural signifiers Max used to narrate his suffering were simply incomprehensible to the hospital staff. Instead of trying to translate his story into signifiers they could understand, the staff simply replaced Max's descriptors of his suffering with racist, classist, and gendered tropes.

Max had no control over what amounted to a prewritten narrative about him. Not only could the staff not empathize with his suffering, but they concluded that he was the cause of tremendous suffering. Lena and Max's doctors and nurses were never going to share a vision about Max and his future or emplot themselves in a clinical narrative that encouraged rather than discouraged further medical intervention. What occurred was a war of signifiers in which Lena and Max were simply outgunned.

## HOBBLING TOWARD RACIAL EQUALITY

Chris Rock famously said, "If a friend calls you on the telephone and says they're lost on Martin Luther King Boulevard and they want to know what they should do, the best response is, 'Run!'"[13] Demographer Derek Alderman, in an analysis of streets named after Martin Luther King in the Southeast notes, "The average total per capita income for an MLK census tract is $7,999, which is significantly lower than the average city per capita income of $11,916."[14] The fact that most of the streets in the United States named for King run through some of the poorest black neighborhoods speaks volumes about the legacy of the civil rights movement. Echoing the disparities in census data, health disparities, the educational achievement gap, and income differentials are similar indicators that something deeply troubling is at work. These disparities pale in comparison to the rates of incarceration for black males, which are so high that it is hard not to analogize the prison to the plantation. Sociologist Loic Wacquant describes the transformation of slavery first into Jim Crow and then into what he describes as the most efficient "race making" machine yet, the current prison system. In a section Wacquant titles "The Resurgent Dangerousness of Blackness," he writes,

> Among the manifold effects of the wedding of ghetto and prison into an extended carceral mesh, perhaps the most consequential is the practical revification and official solidification of the centuries-old association of blackness with criminality and devious violence. The condemnation of Negrophobia in the public sphere has not extinguished the fear and contempt commonly felt by whites towards a group they continue to regard with suspicion and whose lower-class members they virtually identify with social disorder, sexual dissolution, school deterioration, welfare profiteering, neighbourhood decline, economic regression, and most significantly violent crime.[15]

French theorist Michel Foucault predicted that our brutal carceral system would be a historical footnote, replaced by a more sophisticated surveillance apparatus with the power to normalize behavior.[16] Clearly Foucault did not understand the power of race and class in the United States.

The motivating structures for racial differences, both imagined and instantiated, are housed deep within the American subconscious. The black body is seen as abject, and blackness associated with defilement. Julia Kristeva defines abjection as a product of internal loathing: "An extremely strong feeling which is at once somatic and symbolic, and which is above all a revolt of the person against an external menace."[17] Racial loathing represents itself in film, literature, and even politics, as we see in the case of white segregationist Senator Strom Thurman, who privately loved his black daughter while supporting laws to disfranchise the black community.[18] In Thurman's case, he repudiated his desire for two black women by supporting racist legislation. Abjection of self, in the case of Thurman, is turned into abjection of an entire race, a race associated with his desired daughter and mistress. Racism or aversive racism can be tied to desire or loathing, or the repudiation of a race based on the feeling that that race is in some way impure or tainted.

In *Medical Apartheid: The Dark History of Experimentation on Black Americans from Colonial Times to the Present,* Harriet Washington describes how racial abjection has produced what Giorgio Agamben describes as "states of exception" in medicine where the rules of bioethics are applied differently in the case of black and white subjects.[19] Anthropologist Mary Douglas, in *Purity and Danger,* describes the ways in which cultures organize their conceptual universe around categories of filth and purity. At an instrumental level, ideas of pollution influence behavior and threaten those who attempt to transgress the social order. At an expressive level, notions of pollution reinforce a sense of identity by linking social practice to moral order.[20] The instrumental and expressive functions of purity and danger are mutually reinforcing, since beliefs about what is good and right are mirrored structurally in a system that, for all intents and purposes, functions. It is important to note that because taboos are relational rather than essential, objects like race can occupy different conceptual domains depending on the context. This is why we can describe the connection between race and abjection even though the American public celebrates basketball player Michael Jordan or President Barack Obama. The extreme ways in which the public both embraces a handful of blacks and simultaneously excoriates the black community as a whole are a sign that race itself is overdetermined by its associations with binaries: purity/danger, good/evil, industrious/lazy, mammy/ho.

Almost fifty years after the first civil rights legislation passed in 1964, conversations about black inferiority, displaced into the smoky back rooms of corporations and college dorm rooms in the 1960s, have unabashedly reemerged from behind closed doors. The line marking where discourses on race end and racist discourses begin has shifted toward new extremes. What was once considered hate speech has become everyday public speech acts. People defend this speech by arguing that these opinions simply reflect reality, and that people who disagree are simply purveyors of "political correctness."[21]

The resilience of antiblack sentiment can be understood using Theodore Adorno's theory of negative dialectics.[22] Puzzled about the support for capitalism in the face of profound wealth inequality and worker exploitation, Adorno proposed that dialectics, or the constant negation of the object that Hegel and Marx argued propelled history forward, were undermined by dogmatism. History, therefore, is not the product of historical materialism, or the synthesis of the thesis and its antithesis, but the product of fragmentary miscalculations. Primal ideologies, taboos, and identities negate the dialectical negation. Put simply, people are able to live with contradictions and find ways to make sense of a fractured reality. This, concluded Adorno and other Marxian scholars, is why systems based upon a supposedly rational redistribution of wealth fail.

The failure of twentieth-century black liberation struggles has provoked a similar critical pause among critical race theorists. These legal scholars began unpacking the relationship between law and culture in an effort to understand race and retrenchment during Ronald Reagan's administration in the 1980s. Legal scholar Kimberle Crenshaw says that the field of critical legal studies (CLS) "also challenges the perception that the civil rights struggle represents a long, steady march toward social transformation."[23] Crenshaw argues that CLS scholars do not view legal rights discourse as necessarily compatible with the larger need for cultural and social transformation.

We need to ask how the War on Poverty in the late 1960s and 1970s turned into a war on poor blacks denigrated as "welfare queens" by President Ronald Reagan. There are more whites on welfare in the United States than blacks, but blacks have more typically been excoriated for taking advantage of the system. Reagan's fictitious welfare queen was described as owning a Cadillac, the stereotypical trophy car for blacks in the inner city. In the book *Losing Ground* (1984), Charles Murray concretized Reagan's iconic figure of the black welfare recipient. Without irony, Murray describes Aid to Families with Dependent Children (AFDC) as the bête noire of the welfare system. He writes that, "embarrassingly," AFDC was not going to the widows it was intended for but to women who had never been married. Then, without offering any proof, he opines, "The most flagrantly unrepentant seemed to be mostly black."[24]

With Ronald Reagan and the rise of the Moral Majority, the floodgates opened, and racism became not only acceptable but the necessary antidote to the liberal speech justifying unmeritocratic advantages for blacks. The result has been that in the last thirty years, the incarceration gap has risen sharply even though the arrest rate of whites and blacks has remained stable. The white-black gap in incarceration was one in five in 1985. In the first decade of the twenty-first century, the gap was around one in eight.[25]

Perceptions that the black body is polluted and subhuman (unless proven otherwise) spill over into domains beyond incarceration. Health care and health care policy are organized around caring for the health of the citizenry. Public health spending is rationalized based upon the need to protect innocent victims from needless suffering. But the high rates of felony convictions and the subsequent loss of the basic right to vote mean that a large percentage of blacks are marginal citizens. Also, higher rates of poverty in the black community mean that blacks are not seen as contributing to the pool of public health funds. Finally, discourses about how blacks are responsible for their own disfranchisement means many wonder if the black community deserves public assistance of any kind. Max, without realizing it, donned his costume and assumed the role of the undeserving black male thug. From the institution's point of view, his expulsion was a no-brainer; the antihero always gets his due.

In the end we are left with more questions than answers about the role of race in the reproduction of health disparities. As legal scholar Richard Thompson Ford argues in *Race Card: How Bluffing about Bias Makes Race Relations Worse*, it is possible to have racism without racists.[26] Institutional racism is a legacy of class-based discrimination, gender discrimination, the discourses emerging from sociobiology, and the production of a prison industrial complex. Many actors in the production of racism have no idea that the categories they employ and the unproblematized beliefs that they hold contribute to inequities. For example, the extraordinary rates of incarceration, the result of draconian laws and unequal sentencing, are contributing to racial segregation that mirrors in some places the black-white divide that existed during Jim Crow. This segregation is itself producing educational and health disparities. Discourses about being tough on crime and zero tolerance produce a lack of forgiveness and empathy, creating a sense that some people are deserving and some undeserving of social benefits. In the case of Max, there simply was no social imperative to take care of the health care needs of a poor black gangster from the projects.

# CHAPTER 2

# Sickle Cell Disease in the Clinic

In the fall of 1999, while conducting field research at Children's Hospital West, I visited a sickle cell teen support group. The meeting took place in the bowels of the hospital, where medical professionals, patients, and families meet to digest the suffering occurring on the floors above. We sat around the conference table. The nondescript room decorated in different shades of characterless beige easily contained our party of ten.

Included in the group was an articulate, handsome, light-skinned fourteen-year-old boy whose discomfort was measured by his constant shifting in his chair and scanning of the room. Another participant was an attractive chocolate brown twenty-four-year-old who had been, until the first of four major strokes, a gifted student. At the time of the meeting she functioned at the level of a ten-year-old and had to attend with her aunt and guardian. Also present was Sydney, a beautiful light-skinned girl and one of ten children in a devout Seventh-Day Adventist family. Given her angelic beauty and religiosity, I was taken aback by how tough she was. She used brutal honesty like a weapon and refused to engage in small talk with her peers. Also in attendance was Doug, a homeless man in his thirties. Doug was successfully juggling homelessness and parenting a one-year-old with sickle cell disease. Very sweet and talkative, he wanted to get a glimpse into his child's future. Doug brought up that he suffers from pain, and that since his daughter's diagnosis, he had attributed his pain to the fact that he has sickle cell trait. His comment was met with silence, further marking his outsider status.

Overseeing the event were the organizer, Vanessa Rogers, the black social worker for the hematology department, and Janice Friedman, a white psychologist from the oncology department. Finally, besides me, the group included LaTasha and her best friend, Tarika, who also had sickle cell but who was treated at a different hospital.

Trying to interview teenagers is difficult. Often they have very little to say to adults, particularly to relative strangers. LaTasha was different. She was outgoing, curious, and talkative. Dark-skinned with straightened hair, LaTasha had a wonderful personality, and although she was homely, she more than made up for her lack of beauty with what some would call her "ghettofabulous" style. During the meeting LaTasha revealed that she had had a devastating stroke, but that she was excited to be in nursing school and planning her future. The meeting elicited only superficial information about each teen, so when I went to California in the summer of 2001, I called LaTasha to ask her if we could meet. She told me she was in the hospital and invited me to visit her.

When I visited, LaTasha was wearing white pajamas as she sat in her bed watching television. Her former confidence and style were missing. She had tried to dye her hair blonde, but it had come out red. Her weight gain was noticeable, and resting on the food tray that hovered over her bed was a Styrofoam container of chicken brought in from the outside. She was so distracted that our two-hour conversation oscillated between her apologies for being ravenous, disparaging comments about the talk-show guests on a daytime talk show, spontaneous cries when her back pain overwhelmed her, and attempts to piece together for me a fractured narrative of her life. This interview and the three-hour interview the following day captured some key dilemmas confronting sickle cell patients and medical professionals in the hospital wards. The encounter reveals the medical difficulties involved with treating sickle cell disease; the ways in which race is simultaneously relevant and irrelevant in the clinic; the impediments to education and employment given the unpredictable nature of the disease; and the complicated dance performed between patients and physicians when it comes to medical consent for late adolescents who have reached the age of majority.

This chapter ethnographically reveals why transitioning adolescents from pediatric to adult care is such a big concern for the sickle cell community. LaTasha's lack of knowledge about her illnesses and treatments would clearly limit her ability to advocate for herself in an adult care setting. This lack of knowledge about basic biology and medicine was fairly consistent among the adolescents I observed, including adolescents who were known to be excellent students in school. Part of patient ignorance results from an acceptance of medical paternalism. Patients like to put their faith in physicians and nurses, much as homeowners put faith in a contractor. Most homeowners do not ask their contractor how electrical circuits work or how to create a waterproof seal around a shower. Similarly, adolescent patients consider medical knowledge the domain of the physicians and nurses who take care of them.

But the story is not simply a one-sided tale of patient abdication of responsibility. It must be noted that patient ignorance of medicine is often encouraged by medical experts. Most physicians and nurses do not want patients to question every procedure. Repeating what seems like basic information is tedious, and spending the time required to explain, for example, why a case of sepsis could lead to death reduces efficiency. In order to get detailed information about their case histories, sickle cell patients have to assume the role of the nosy pest. Patients are simply not encouraged to seek information.

Reinforcing this paternalism are adolescent transitioning programs like the one where I met LaTasha. These programs often deal with interpersonal concerns rather than hemoglobin counts or scientific literature on various treatments and conditions, including necrosis of the hip. Outside of teaching patients to hydrate, eat properly, and treat pain at home, few truly empower patients to understand the scientific aspects and medical uncertainties associated with their disease. These transitioning programs attempt to create more supple patients who leave their emotional baggage at home when they enter the hospital.

The main point of this chapter is to place the reader in the belly of the beast, so to speak, to ethnographically demonstrate how lack of knowledge and medical paternalism increase patients' anxieties and fears. When there is an absence of information, patients like LaTasha create stories to make sense of incomplete knowledge. Beyond noting the gaps in communication and the stress these gaps place on patients, this chapter draws readers into the world of sickle cell disease, secondary complications, treatments, and the personal stakes. I present the topics as they occurred chronologically except in a few instances where, for greater coherence, I combined information that was revealed at different times. I chose to present the interruptions and non sequiturs to give a sense of LaTasha's desperate need for distraction during her six-week-long hospitalization but also to note that even though sickle cell patients suffer, suffering does not happen in the absence of humor and silliness.

After greeting her with a hug, I turned on the tape recorder, knowing from our phone conversation how much she wanted to share. "So, tell me, what's going on? You're really scared, huh?"

As if no time had passed between our meetings, LaTasha responded immediately, "Because this is the second day that he's telling me that I could die."

"Who's telling you?" I asked for the record.

"Dr. Hanson keeps telling me that." Dr. Hanson was also Max's physician. A smoker and a bit irreverent, Dr. Hanson presents a certain emotional detachment from his patients. His lack of interest in playing the heroic MD was part of what, I believe, made him an excellent hematologist.

"Why is he saying that to you?" I asked.

"Every time he wants to do something, and I don't agree to it, he'll be like, 'Well, you must want to die because if you don't do this, then you could die.'" The tactic of instilling fear is one strategy for ensuring patient compliance, particularly when it comes to willful adolescent patients who are old enough to make their own medical decisions. LaTasha was twenty at the time of the interview and therefore above the age of consent for medical treatment.

Pushing her, I asked, "Like what didn't you want to do?"

"I didn't want to go to surgery today and get another line. But, look, what was the point when it's gonna get right back infected, you know? They're just gonna have to take it out again." A port, or line, is a device that is surgically implanted under the skin, providing permanent access to a vein via a catheter. Patients who no longer have what is termed peripheral venous access ("good veins") require lines. At times these lines become infected, which can lead to serious and sometimes fatal blood infections.

LaTasha had already been in the hospital for a month and a half. In addition to having a blood infection, she was experiencing an extended painful crisis. Her illnesses required that she be on three or four (she was not sure) antibiotics, oxygen, a powerful schedule II narcotic, and Benadryl to counter the effects of the narcotic. She was expected to be in the hospital for another two weeks. I asked her what her initial symptoms were, and she mentioned pain in her back, legs, and arms. Then she began eating and drifted from the topic of her illness, saying, "Sorry to be eating, but I'm hungry."

"No, go ahead. Vanessa and I just pigged out." I had taken LaTasha's former social worker, Vanessa Rogers, out to lunch at a Mexican restaurant. Six months before our meeting, Vanessa had switched from hematology to oncology, where the funding for patient programs is orders of magnitude greater than for sickle cell patients.

LaTasha responded, "Oh, Mexican food? I love Mexican food." Then I told her I would bring Mexican food for her the next time I visited. She put in her order: "Enchiladas, quesadillas, plenty of salad, burritos"— basically everything.

Trying to move the conversation back to her illness, I asked, "How do you feel being here so long?"

"My friends have been doing things without me. Partying, going to see all the movies, and just everything. And I'm stuck in here. They come to see me, but it's not the same because they can do what they want to do. I have to sit in the bed all day. I can walk around, go see Sydney and Allen, but it's just so boring here."

"How often do you have to come to the hospital?"

"Every two to three months." The frequency and length of her hospitalizations put her in the category of patients with severe disease. Patients who experience more than three painful episodes per year, about 20 percent, are placed in this category. It is important to note that the correlation between severity and mortality is weak, meaning the category is not a useful tool for gauging risk.

Very matter-of-factly, LaTasha said, "This is my home. My house is my home away from home."

"You were in school, right?"

"I went to nursing school," she answered. LaTasha's mother, a licensed vocational nurse (LVN), inspired LaTasha to try nursing school. It was difficult to understand why she would want to follow in her mother's footsteps. At the same time that LaTasha talked glowingly about wanting to become a nurse, she also lamented that her mother, who has high blood pressure, worked too hard. LaTasha's mother makes only ten dollars per hour and therefore must work double shifts. Her taxing schedule means she rarely has time to visit LaTasha in the hospital. LaTasha is the age of majority, so she no longer needs her mother to make medical decisions for her. Nevertheless, at numerous points during the interview it was obvious how much she still needed her mother to be her advocate. LaTasha's solution was to call her mother every time a physician asked her for permission to perform a procedure.

"You were so happy the last time I saw you. You felt really happy," I commented. "What's happened since then?"

"They dropped me because I missed so much school. And I told them, 'I can get sick at any moment.' But they still dropped me anyway, and I still have to pay for the time I was there."

"Will they let you go back?"

"They called me and told me I could go back, but I didn't want to go back because it would have been the same thing if I would have got sick again. Then they would have still kicked me out. So, there was no use for me to go back." Returning to her lunch, LaTasha interjected, "My favorite part is just the skin and this part. I don't really like the legs."

"Are you thinking about what you might do since you can't . . ."

"I want to go to Maxine Water's school for nursing." LaTasha was referring to the Maxine Waters Employment Preparation Center, which provides training to youth and adults who want to return to school. "I want to be a nurse that works on the floor with children. . . . I want to work in a sickle cell clinic."

Doctors and nurses have grown increasingly concerned about how little adolescent sickle cell patients know about their disease. Their lack of knowledge makes them vulnerable, particularly at a time when they are about to move from pediatric care to adult care. In adult care the services for patients are limited, and patients have to advocate for themselves. LaTasha was so apprehensive about adult care she let me know that she planned on staying in pediatric care until she turned twenty-five, which the hospital allows for chronically ill patients. So, I decided to find out how much LaTasha knows about her disease. I asked, "What do you think about sickle cell disease? What is it? I mean, what's going on?"

"It's a horrible disease. I know that, and I hate it."

"Your pain crises, do they come on at certain times? Do you have any. . . ?

"Anytime. I could be lying in my bed, or I could be at a party or at a club or something. It could come on at any time."

"Do you do anything at home first to try to get rid of it, or do you come straight to the hospital?"

"Hot baths, hot packs, medication . . . it doesn't help sometimes." When her home remedies failed, she sought help in the hospital, where she was prescribed hydromorphone, known by the brand name Dilaudid. "Morphine works better, but I'm allergic to morphine now."

"Do any of your brothers or sisters have it too?"

"They both have the trait, my brother and my sister." At the time LaTasha's brother was twenty-seven years old, and her sister was twenty-two.

"How do you feel about Children's West? Do you want to move on to another hospital, or do you want to stay here?"

"I'm only staying here because of Dr. Allen." Dr. Allen, a white man from the Midwest, was the head of the sickle cell program at CHW. "He's a very good sickle cell doctor. That's the only reason why I'm still here, or I would have left, how the nurses treat us." LaTasha's best friend, Tarika, who accompanied her to the teen support group, preferred her hospital because she never had a problem with the nurses. Essentially, Tarika chose the quality of interpersonal relationships at a lesser ranked hospital over the effectiveness of medical intervention at one of the top comprehensive sickle cell centers in the country.

"How do they treat you?"

"Not good all the time. I'm not going to say all of them, because we have some nice ones."

"Give me a story, good and bad."

"Well, there's not really a story, but it's just sometimes they're just rude and mean. If they're gonna be like that, they shouldn't work with kids." Both LaTasha and I became aware of LaTasha's roommate, a three-year-old cancer patient, who began to cry. "That's the only thing I don't like about being in the room with a little girl . . . a little patient."

"How come they don't put, like, you and Sydney together, or . . ."

"Well, she has a roommate. They do sometimes, but she's in there with Alex right now. She's probably going home before both of us. Or maybe me and Alex will share this room because I like this room. I'm not gonna change no more. Well, I hope they don't make me change because look in the bathroom." I got up and looked in the bathroom. "Go inside and look how big it is. We have a shower in there and everything. This is my favorite room."

Moving back to a conversation about her health, I asked, "Tell me about the time you had a stroke."

"In like ninety-five or ninety-six. I don't really remember having the stroke. I only remember I was unconscious when I had all that stuff. . . . The seizures, the strokes, everything. I don't remember any of that."

LaTasha was already in the hospital when she suffered a major stroke. It took her two years to recover, and she is amazed that she is not paralyzed like her friend who lost the use of her left side.

Soon after we started to talk about her stroke, LaTasha became distracted and repeatedly tried to page a nurse. "It takes so long to answer that call up. The nurses are all up there too. That really makes me mad. Someone could be in here having a stroke, or dying, or be done fell out of their bed on their head or something, and they take forever to answer it." Eventually the cancer patient's nurse walked into the room. LaTasha implored, "Could you tell my nurse if I can have my Benadryl, please?" LaTasha both asked for and demanded her Benadryl, a strategic move that may or may not have been intentional.

"Are you starting to itch?" I asked, knowing that many patients are allergic to their pain medication.

"Yeah," she responded.

I changed the subject to Melinda, a teen we had discussed on the phone. "So, what happened to Melinda?"

"She had to be carried out of the hospital, strapped down, because she was hitting nurses and doctors. . . . Well, how it started is, she was playacting like she wanted to kill herself. So a nurse had to stay in the room with her all day. And then she started getting mad because they know that she plays sick a lot, so they wasn't giving her IV pain medicine. They were just giving her pills and stuff, and she was mad because, you know, they wouldn't give her IV medicines. So, then she just went off. I wasn't here, but she just went off and she started hitting nurses and doctors. They had to give her, like, drugs to calm her down. And then they strapped her up and took her out of here to [another hospital]."

"So, is she allowed back, or she can't come back?"

"She can come back, but only with her family. She was cursing out her sister and stuff, and her sister's pregnant, her sister doesn't need that stress. Her sister had already lost one baby." I had met Melinda, who was seventeen, on other occasions. Melinda's mother had been a prostitute, and Melinda's father one of her clients. Her father was old when Melinda was born, and her mother was on drugs, so at nine years old Melinda went to live with her sister, who was eight years older. At the time of the interview, both of Melinda's parents were dead.

Melinda's face had a cubist quality with exaggerated features, none of which seemed to fit together. Melinda had no charm, was extremely needy, and seemed to suck the energy out of a room. She reminded me of the importance of continuity of care for sickle cell patients. I imagine that it must be difficult for a nurse or physician to muster sympathy for Melinda without having known her as a small, vulnerable child. Adolescent patients who are kicked out of pediatric care must develop relationships with adult medical providers, who often find it difficult to see them as children. In the adult care setting these patients are categorized as lacking self-efficacy, which basically means they are seen as demanding, immature, problematic patients.

LaTasha and I started talking about her friends with sickle cell, Sydney and Jamal. Then LaTasha became distracted by the television. "Look at her chest! She's only nineteen!" I had no idea what she was referring to even after glancing at the show. LaTasha explained, "This is a show about are they real or fake."

I mimicked her enthusiasm for the challenge: "They're fake . . . what do you think?"

"I have to see when she comes out. [pause] They are huge!"

"That's like size, what . . . F, G, H?" I laughed.

"I think they're real. She's too fat for that dress, though, I'm sorry."

We discovered that the young woman's breasts were real. LaTasha compared herself: "Mine are little. Well, not that little. I hate 'em. I wish they could be smaller. They're not as big as hers, but they're big." We spent some time watching more guests present their breasts for scrutiny. I had a hard time determining if LaTasha's constant switching between topics was related to her Dilaudid, her itching, her pain, or the fact that she was an adolescent. In any case, LaTasha demonstrated that it is impossible to focus exclusively on one's pain and suffering.

I decided that I should leave and try to catch her in a different mood the next day. After saying good-bye and reaffirming that I would be bringing Mexican food, I discovered how alone LaTasha was. As I was about to go she said, "But, I want you to stay here with me until they do this because I'm very scared."

"What are they doing?"

"This [a line] is about seven inches on my leg and they're pulling it out. And it hurts so bad. And that's why I need someone in here that's familiar."

My heart went out to her, but I knew that I would not be able to be her surrogate parent. Procedures like this were loosely scheduled, and the surgeon might not come until the early evening. I decided to get her to focus on the nurses she trusted who could help her get through this. "Okay, okay. So, who's your favorite nurse? Do you have any favorite nurses?"

"My favorite nurses are . . . Latoya, she's a night nurse. Tanya is a night nurse. Benelle, morning nurse . . . um . . . Lakeesha, she's a morning nurse. And then, my favorite RNs are . . . Anna, Beth, um, Carrie, Jodi, and Cheryl. Oh, and Elizabeth." Her favorite night and morning nurses, licensed vocational nurses, were black. Her favorite registered nurses were all white. There were in fact only a handful of black RNs at CHW.

I encouraged her to imagine the surgery, and I reminded her that because she was on Dilaudid, the procedure would not hurt as much. This was a small consolation given that sickle cell patients know that the pain medication does not erase the pain, only dulls their perception of it. LaTasha grew increasingly anxious and asked me if I could find her nurse, Claudia. LaTasha wanted to know when she could take her Benadryl and when the surgeon was coming. I went out and told the nurse at the nurse's station that LaTasha wanted to speak to Claudia.

After returning to the room, I asked LaTasha about her schooling. She told me that she decided to go to school after seeing a commercial for nursing school. Her mom was okay with her daughter's decision but was concerned that LaTasha would not finish the program since LaTasha was still working toward her GED.

Claudia, her nurse, eventually arrived and informed LaTasha that she was not due for more Benadryl until 4:00 P.M. LaTasha begged her to make it 3:30. They compromised and decided on 3:45. She also asked Claudia to tell the surgeon to come right away because she wanted me to be with her.

Claudia said, "They have to come in between surgeries. So, when they find a chance to come. . . . There's no way of telling you how long, because we don't know how long surgeries last."

LaTasha questioned Claudia further, "How come you guys can't take it out?"

"Because we're not trained to do it."

"The only thing you do is pull it out . . . I could do it myself." Often hospital logic escapes patients, particularly a patient like LaTasha who was weary of the control hospital protocols had over her life.

Claudia explained, "There could be complications if you don't do it right, and we don't want that."

With both humor and anger, LaTasha said, "I can do it myself, just bring me a gauze!" I laughed.

In a very professional tone, Claudia responded, "There's a little bit more to it than that. It seems simple, but it's really not that simple."

LaTasha finally relented and asked the nurse, "Would you bring me my fruit, please? Oh, I need a fork too, please."

In addition to her pain and itching, LaTasha also had a fever of 104 degrees from an infection caused by her port. Even so, she kept eating and asked, "Do you see how much I'm eating? I'm just eating, eating, eating." Finally she explained that she had had a birth control shot to relieve her bad menstrual cramps which often precipitated a painful crisis.

The hormones in the birth control medication caused her to feel ravenous. She continued, "I just eat all day, that's all I do. That's why I want
to get home, because I do stuff at home. But sitting here all day, I just
eat all day. Do you see I've been eating ever since you came? I can't help
it either. It's just I'm always hungry." CHW had a McDonald's in the hospital, which was always full of parents wanting to treat their sick children. Sometimes patients could get vouchers for McDonald's. LaTasha
joked, "You have to tell Vanessa that the five dollars for McDonald's
wasn't enough. And, you know, five dollars can get you a whole big meal,
plus supersize."

Then Jennifer, LaTasha's new social worker, walked by the room.
Jennifer was young, blonde, petite, cute, extremely inexperienced, and
quite a change from Vanessa, who was in her forties, matronly, and serious. Jennifer was a temporary employee until the sickle cell team found
Vanessa's replacement, preferably someone who was fully certified and
who wanted to work with sickle cell patients. LaTasha called to Jennifer,
"Hey, Jennifer, how are you?"

Jennifer responded disingenuously, "I'll be back in a little bit, okay?"

"All right," LaTasha said hopefully.

Bluntly, I asked, "Do you like her?"

"Yeah. I like Vanessa better, but she's younger so she's more down
with us, and stuff. I can talk to her more, because she's so much
younger."

The conversation returned to fake breasts, longings for Doritos and
cream cheese, and LaTasha's friends. The surgeon did not arrive after
two hours of waiting. I finally said good-bye.

The next day I reconnected with LaTasha. I prepared for my visit
by stopping at a Mexican food stand. When I arrived, LaTasha still
had an oxygen tube, which caused her to develop scabs in her nose.
Surprisingly, Melinda, the girl who was kicked out for hitting doctors
and nurses weeks before, was in LaTasha's room connected to an
intravenous drip. Melinda, now allowed back into the hospital, had
been admitted the night before. A nurse entered the room shortly
after I arrived and excused herself for having to take LaTasha's blood
pressure.

After the nurse left, I asked, "How much oxygen are they giving
you?"

"Two liters. I even have to have oxygen at home because when I sleep
I stop breathing. So I need the oxygen to keep me breathing while I'm
sleeping."

LaTasha's lungs had been permanently damaged by acute chest syndrome (ACS), a blockage of circulation in the lungs caused by sickling. ACS is a leading cause of death for sickle cell patients. Physicians with very little knowledge of sickle cell disease sometimes treat ACS with more oxygen. I followed a five-year-old, Bethany, whose lungs had been ravaged by this form of treatment when she was an infant. Out of desperation the physician finally called the Children's West team to find out what to do to save Bethany. The team informed Bethany's doctor that she needed a blood transfusion, which was the standard form of care. With a blood transfusion the concentration of sticky, crescent-shaped hemoglobin in her blood was reduced, which reestablished proper blood flow in her lungs. Bethany survived, and her mother moved her child to CHW's comprehensive sickle cell center.

About ACS, LaTasha said, "Yeah, it damaged my lungs." Then she turned to Melinda and offered her some of the Mexican food. "Here, Melinda, you can have this one. I love Mexican food, that's my favorite kind of . . . well, besides soul food, that's my favorite kind of food." This sparked a comparison of the best soul food restaurants. I mentioned Sylvia's in New York, and she mentioned Puff Daddy's restaurant, called Justin's.

LaTasha was no longer anxious about dying, the surgery to remove the line in her leg was over, her fever was lower, and she believed now that she was going to be in the hospital for only a few more days. Although the conversation moved between topics, LaTasha was more focused.

We discussed her recent decision to move out of her mother's house and live with her best friend, Tarika. She said that she simply felt it was time. "I'm an adult, I'm ready to just be . . . do my own thing, you know. When I'm on my own it's so cool. Me and my mom, we argue, but five minutes later, we're back friends, you know. Me and my mom are just so close. Yeah, my mom, she always says she wants me to move out, but she really doesn't want me to move out.

LaTasha's long-term plan was to live on her own for a year and then move back to Louisville, Kentucky, with her mother. LaTasha spent the first eight years of her life in Kentucky, and now that her family was, in her words, dying, her mother was anxious to reunite with the remaining members. Her mother's sister was drinking, and her mother wanted to return because, LaTasha said, her mother was a good influence on her aunt. LaTasha was hoping to have finished getting her LVN license by the time she moves.

Considering LaTasha's plan to get her own apartment, I asked, "Do you have a job?"

"Well, I get SSI, and they're going to give me housing, like low income. It goes by my job. . . . Like, by how much money I get a month. So then my rent will be like subsidized rent." I asked her what jobs she had held. She told me she once had a job feeding the patients at the same convalescent center where her mother worked.

I commented to Melinda that she looked like she was going to fall asleep. LaTasha responded for Melinda, "She's always like that when she first comes to the hospital. We all are because we're so drugged up that we just sleep."

LaTasha's comment motivated me to ask the unanswerable, "Can you describe the pain, or you just can't?"

"It's indescribable. The only people who understand are like," she pointed to Melinda, "she understands because she goes through it. But, like, for people who don't go through it, you can't explain it. I'm telling you it's worse than cramps. It's worse than smashing your finger in the car door. It's worse than hitting your knee on the edge of the table. It's worse than all of that. It's just excruciating. I can't explain it. It's just . . . It's like someone's taking a sledgehammer and just hitting you wherever the pain is. Mine is mostly in my back sometimes. It's like someone doing that [made a motion as if swinging a sledgehammer] to your back or your legs."

While LaTasha described the pain, a nurse came in and explained to Melinda that she needed to go back to her room. Again LaTasha answered for Melinda, "She's just sleepy, but she don't want to be in her room." Then she showed me an electronic police car given to her by people who deliver toys in the pediatric wards. I imagined these people who want to brighten the day of a sick child through charity are probably ambivalent about giving toys to a twenty-year-old adolescent on intravenous Dilaudid. LaTasha confirmed my presumption: "The officer said, 'Maybe you don't want this, but you can give it to one of your little sisters or brothers.' I said, 'No, I want it for myself.' He was like, 'Are you serious?' I was like, 'I might be twenty years old, but I still play with toys,' I love toys." LaTasha was unabashedly appreciative. Like all the adolescent patients I met, she was part adult and part child.

"Look what they gave me! Push the buttons, look what it does. It says, 'The route is in pursuit. We're in pursuit. We're en route um, car eighty-eight.'" I am horrified that these children, many of whom live in high-crime neighborhoods where police presence is high, would be given a toy that reenacts high-speed chases, a staple of urban life and local television news. "But mine is broken," LaTasha lamented. I silently mused about how this act of charity was self-redemptive for the giver and not at all empowering for the recipient.

"What do you do with these toys?"

"Give them to my little cousins and stuff."

Melinda finally spoke, "She probably go and give them to her godson."

"Yeah, or my godson. Like, when I get stuffed animals, I just give it to him, or my mom loves stuffed animals too. My mom has a loft at our house. You go up the ladder, just all stuffed animals there. Just full of stuffed animals. My gosh, there's so many."

We moved from a discussion of Beanie Babies to Jamal. Jamal was a twenty-year-old sickle cell patient and friend of LaTasha's who was hospitalized. During that time his girlfriend's two-year-old son, also receiving treatment on the same hematology/oncology floor, died of leukemia.

"He was two years. He had leukemia, but his whole system just shut down. He passed Saturday." Melinda corrected her. "What did I say, Saturday? Friday night. And he died in his sleep, though, that was good. So we know he didn't suffer."

After comparing the severity of her best friend Tarika's disease to her own, she slipped into a detailed discussion of her stroke. "Usually I'm here two weeks and I'm out. This has been an exception. But, I've been here for three months one time . . . no, four months one time. When I had my gallstone surgery, you know, when I got this big scar." She broke for a moment to mother Melinda, "Here, lay back, Melinda, lay back. . . ." Then she quickly resumed, "That time, I was here four months straight because I had strokes, seizures, oh, just everything. My kidneys shut down, my lungs collapsed, everything just went wrong."

"You know why it happened, though? Because a week before I came to the hospital . . . well, actually the Sunday before I went to the hospital . . . I went to church with my aunt and uncle. We were on our way home from church. . . . No, we were on our way *to* church, and I told them that I thought I was losing my faith in God. They told me to pray for a sign. I prayed for a sign while we were in church. You know when you go up to the altar in church? That next Monday my stomach was hurting, and I wasn't eating anything. So by Wednesday I hadn't eaten anything in two days. So my mom took me to IHOP, and I love pancakes. That was my first time ever going to IHOP. My mom knew I must have been sick because I didn't eat anything, and I love pancakes. So she brought me to the hospital. I don't even remember them giving me an X-ray. I just remember asking them for pain medicine, but they wouldn't give me none. I had to get the X-ray first. So, um, my mom told me that after that is when they saw I had gallstones. They finally gave me pain medicine. I went to sleep and didn't wake up until two, three, two and a half months later. I was in a coma and everything. And, when I was in a coma, that's when I saw God, and that was my sign. I knew it was my sign when I woke back up. I was telling my mom and my sister and my friends that I got my sign I was looking for. So, I know not to doubt anymore because I've seen God."

"Did you remember hearing voices at all when you were in your coma?"

"You know what, I had kind of woke up, and I remember seeing my sister and my best friend just next to my bed just crying. But I couldn't say anything. I couldn't speak or nothing. I tried, but it wouldn't let me say anything."

Again she broke to speak to Melinda: "Lay down. You want to go lay on the couch?"

Melinda answered, "No, I'm leaving now." Melinda made a gesture as though she was about to leave and then settled back onto LaTasha's bed.

LaTasha, in an aside, said, "I ain't going nowhere. I can't. I got an IV in my foot."

"So, two and a half months in ICU. Your mother must have been . . ."

"They had gave up on me. But my mom didn't want them to turn off the machines. They had gave up."

"They were going to turn the machines off? Why? What did they say?"

"Because I wasn't living by myself. I was just living with the machines. I wasn't breathing on my own. I had to have a tube in me for me to use the bathroom. I wasn't doing anything on my own. So, the doctors just gave up on me . . . and the nurses. So, my mom used to talk to the chaplains a lot, and the chaplains told my mom, 'Well, if it's time for her, then the Lord will take her.' But they were saying they don't think it was time for me. And when I woke up, my mom was so happy. And, let me tell you, I woke up the worst way. They had my legs up. They were putting a tube inside my privates.[1] Trust me, I hadn't had sex or anything, so you know that hurt. The tube was about this big." She represented the size by making a circle with her fingers. "They were putting it inside, and I woke up crying, screaming for my mom. They wouldn't get my mom. They said, 'Wait, and when we finish this, if you go ahead and let us do it, then we'll get your mom.' Finally my mom was so happy to see me awake. Oh, gosh. And I didn't even know where I was when I first woke up. Because this hospital looked so different. I was like, 'Where am I?' I thought I was at somebody else's hospital."

"You woke up being able to talk and everything."

"Yeah, I just woke up, as if I had been sleeping. I just woke up."

"And your mom, did she quit work during that time?"

"She couldn't work. The social workers were, like, paying our bills because my mom wouldn't leave me. And the Sickle Cell Foundation, they were paying some of our bills. She totally neglected my sister and my brother for that two and a half months. They understood, but she totally neglected them."

"Do you ever think of your life as extraordinary, like, 'Oh my gosh, this is . . .' or do you think of it as just . . .

"I'm living. But I don't do anything that's really extraordinary, so I don't really think of it like that."

"Do you ever want to have children?"

"Yeah. I got pregnant my first time having sex, I had a miscarriage. I had sex April 19 for the first time, a week and a day before my twentieth birthday. I used protection too, but it didn't help. But everybody says they think he did something to the condom because he wanted to have a baby really bad. Even my mom thinks he did something, and they're making me believe that he really did do something."

"Is he still your boyfriend?"

"No. No. We broke up because when I had the miscarriage he wasn't there for me at all. He called me a stupid bitch and everything when I had the miscarriage. Like it's my fault I had the miscarriage, you know. It's not my fault. The Lord . . . It wasn't meant for me to have a baby then."

"Would you have kept it?"

"Yeah, I don't believe in abortions."

"How did you meet him?"

"On the Party Line. It's like a lot of teenagers on there, they just call. Just call and talk to people. Some people are evil, where they're cussing people out. But sometimes you could meet a really nice person on there. I met him and I *thought* he was a really nice person but he wasn't. . . . I'm not going to say he wasn't because he was. In the beginning, he was. But after a while it was just like. . . . Gosh. I could tell that he was going to get abusive because he used to, like, grab me and pull on me. But I only saw him like twice a week. I didn't tell my mom or my brother because my brother would have kicked his butt. And my mom would have probably kicked his butt. So, my mom still doesn't know. And my brother, he still doesn't know because my brother still would beat him up to this day, knowing that he was doing that to me. He never hit me, but it was just grabbing me and pushing me and stuff like that. Like, when I didn't want to do things he wanted me to do or something. I can't believe I gave my virginity to him. I could have still had it. You know, that's something that you give to somebody special. He wasn't special enough. . . . Even though I don't regret it, he still wasn't special enough for it."

The conversation moved to a discussion of her best friend and how she did not have a boyfriend and how they tried to avoid dating gang-bangers and ex-convicts. In LaTasha's words, "I don't want to talk to no gangbanger because I am not trying to get killed."

Then the nurses came in and tried to get Melinda to return to her room. Melinda had been asked several times to move back to her room. Finally the nurses demanded Melinda move, saying, "Melinda . . . you need to go back to your own room. You can't sleep on other people's beds. Okay? And if your bed is not working, or if there is something wrong, we can get you another bed. But you cannot be in the same bed as LaTasha or with any other patient. That's just the hospital rules. Sorry."

LaTasha offered a compromise, "She can lay on the couch, though, can't she?"

Instead of answering LaTasha, the nurse asked Melinda, "Why don't you like your bed?"

Acting as Melinda's advocate, LaTasha said, "No, she just wants to be in here with me. There's nothing wrong with her bed. She just wants to be in here because she's not feeling good and she says I make her feel better."

"Well, that's what I worry about. If she's not feeling good and gets dizzy, the couch isn't probably the best thing. And she's falling asleep. You know what, Melinda, you really need to be in your bed with the bed rail up. I'm afraid you're going to fall out. I'm worried about you lying on the couch."

Forever maternal, LaTasha said to the nurse and then Melinda, "You've gotta put the rails down so she can get out. I'll come to your room as soon as we finish talking, okay Melinda?" LaTasha then asked the nurse to evaluate some dry skin on her cheek. Uncertain what it was, the nurse simply redirected the question back to LaTasha. LaTasha decided it was probably eczema even though she had never had it on her face. Then LaTasha asked the nurse to give her another syringe so that she could give herself more Dilaudid from her patient-controlled analgesia (PCA) pump.

While the nurse prepared the syringe, LaTasha offered this story: "This one girl was telling me that her boyfriend . . . she don't come to this hospital no more . . . but, she was saying her boyfriend had stole a key, and he used to take these and sell them. The syringes, he used to take them. I was like, 'You guys should not be doing that.' I had told my social worker. This was a while ago. But the girl never came back to this hospital, so they couldn't do anything about it. It was terrible. I was like 'Oh, my gosh.'" All of a sudden LaTasha sat up straight, put her hands on her lower back, and groaned, "I am hurting so bad!"

I waited until she resumed her slouched position and asked, "So that button, you press it and it comes out?"

"Yeah, every ten minutes I can push it. Could you give me that medicine and my soda so I could take it so she could leave me alone?"

While looking and smiling at the nurse, I asked LaTasha, "Is this one of your favorite nurses?"

"Yeah, she's one of them. She's cool." The nurse clearly enjoyed the compliment but did not stop working to thank LaTasha.

After the nurse left, I asked, "Did you tell your boyfriend you have sickle cell?"

"I tell every . . ." LaTasha stopped talking suddenly as soon as the PCA pump signaled that she could give herself another dose of medication. "Okay, see now I could push it. When you see it's empty at the bottom, that's when I can push it, when it says . . . watch, when I try to push it it's going to say 'patient lockout.' Well, after it finishes giving it to me, it's going to say 'patient lockout' down there. And then I can't push it until they get empty down there again."

"And where's your pain?"

"My back, my sides, which are my ribs. I just call them my sides. My legs, that's it right now."

"But, it's pretty much constant all the time?"

"Uh-huh. At night, it's really bad. Because I'm just laying here, and that's all. Like now, I'm talking to you, so it's feeling better. Or if I'm into the TV or in the playroom it's feeling better. But when I'm just laying here by myself, I can't call anyone because everybody's asleep. Then that's when it's really bad." Referring to the PCA, she explained,

"It gives me two milligrams. . . . Well, two thousand micrograms. . . . It makes me dizzy when I first get it."

There was a break in the conversation during which LaTasha seemed to be evaluating how she was feeling: "It helped a little. But I can do it every ten minutes. I can do it again at eleven ten." Mentioning the time reminded her of another schedule. "Oh, my stories are about to come on!" Television organized LaTasha's otherwise amorphous days. Resuming our conversation, LaTasha said, "At eleven ten I can do it again. Well, almost eleven ten. I mean twelve ten! I'm saying eleven ten."

"So, how does it make you feel better, like what does it . . ."

"Well, I don't know, it just stops the pain sometimes."

"Oh, it really stops the pain, it doesn't just make you feel, like, more relaxed or something?"

"Well, it doesn't *stop* the pain, it takes the edge off. Like, it's not hurting as bad as it was right before I pushed it. It takes the edge off. I'm not gonna say it stops the pain, but it helps. It makes a difference . . . a big difference."

Referring to the stipend that I gave her for participation in my research, she reminded herself, "I have to hide that money you gave me, because people will be going around stealing it. I have my purse in the bottom drawer. Could you get my purse, please? Put it in the yellow thing, please. And, you know what, I'm so happy that you gave me that money because I am so broke. They stole my money."

"Who stole your money?"

"We don't know. Somebody. They went around stealing people's money, and they've even been stealing food. You know it have to be somebody really fat to go around stealing somebody's food. And I told my mom, and she felt so bad because she gave me her last twenty bucks before she gets paid. And she has to spend mostly all her money on bills so she wasn't going to be able to give me any more money. So, that's a blessing that you came today and you gave me that money because I didn't have any money. And I don't like being here not having any money because sometimes, you know, I want to order me food, or go to the gift shop, or get me something from the vending machine or something. I have one of my friends go to the store for me or something. And I like having at least ten bucks while I'm here. At least. So, I'm really grateful for the money that you gave me."

"Well, I'm glad it helps. Thank you for being willing to talk to me, and tell me . . ."

"But, I would have even done it without the money, too. I just wanted you to know that."

The sickle cell clinic nurse-practitioner entered the room. Deborah, who always dressed in dark, attractive business attire and wore thick-rimmed designer glasses, was the unofficial head of the sickle cell team. Her knowledge of hematology was extensive, and she was always well versed in the latest journal article on sickle cell disease. In the years I followed the team, her knowledge seemed to match that of the physicians. Ultimately, what distinguished her was the fact that she took the nursing part of her title very seriously. She projected genuine warmth toward her patients, and she knew by heart the medical and personal details of each one.

Deborah smiled at me but then immediately turned to LaTasha and asked, "What are you doing in here?"

"They changed my room because Elaine was driving me crazy." She seemed to want to engage Deborah in an extensive discussion of eleven-year-old Elaine, who was always trying, according to LaTasha, to get into her business, but Deborah was too politically savvy to fall into that trap.

"Oh, okay." Deborah avoided taking sides without hurting LaTasha's feelings, said good-bye, and left the room.

LaTasha decided she wanted me to take her to the gift shop before I left. In order to do so, she needed a nurse to flush her IV and then close up the opening with a heplock. The entire procedure took fifteen minutes.

While waiting, I asked, "So, you think about the future?"

"Yeah, I think about the future a lot."

"Are you worried at all, or you're okay?"

"No, I'm okay with it. I just don't want my mom, my sister, or my brother or my godmother to die before me. But I also don't want them to suffer with me dying before them."

"You don't want them to die before you. . . . Why not?"

"Because I don't want to have to stay behind. I don't want to have to bury any of them."

"Yeah, but they want to die before you."

"I wish we all could just go at the same time."

"That would be interesting."

"Because I don't know what I would do without my mother, or my sister, or my brother. I could live without my godmom, but I couldn't live without my mom or sister or brother. I just couldn't. This [the pain medicine] is making me sleepy."

Knowing that some sickle cell patients die because the pain medication reduces their respiration and they simply stop breathing in their sleep, I asked, "Do you want to put the oxygen back on?"

"That's not gonna help. I probably need to go." She really wanted to get out of the room.

"Maybe go to sleep?"

"I must really be breathing out of whack, huh? My breathing must be really bad if you even told me to put my oxygen back on."

LaTasha then became distracted by her very cute three-year-old roommate in adorable slippers.

Thinking about what LaTasha might have been like when she was a baby, I asked, "Do you remember when you found out that you had sickle cell?"

"I was too young. I found out when I was a year because I had pneumonia five times in one year." I gasped. Continuing, she added, "And then they tested me for sickle cell. But now they test every black child for sickle cell, black and Hispanic.

"Five times in one year. And they never did a blood transfusion? Do you think that caused the lung damage, those early pneumonias, or was it later?"

"I don't know. I never even thought about it." LaTasha was an example of an adolescent patient who did not know enough about her disease to become her own advocate.

LaTasha started itching so much she started to focus on her need for Benadryl. She decided against more Benadryl, which would have put her to sleep, because she so desperately wanted to go to the gift shop to get a magazine in order to distract herself from her boredom.

As LaTasha was getting settled in her wheelchair, the nurse told her, "You're getting blood today."

Shocked, LaTasha said, "I'm getting blood!? Why? What's my blood count?"

"It's 6.4. And just because you're taking so many medicines, we don't want you to, like, have any problems. And we want to make sure that you're well hydrated. . . ."

A bit angry, LaTasha clarified, "No one told me that I was getting a transfusion."

Relieving herself of responsibility, the nurse said, "I just got the order."

"The doctor came by this morning. He didn't tell me. Do you know if he talked to my mom?"

"No, do you want him to before we give you the blood?"

"Yeah. She might not want me to have it."

"Oh, you think?"

"Even though I'm old enough to say if I want it or not, but . . ."

"Well, the reason is because a lot of the antibiotics you're getting now can cause damage to your organs if you have too much of a high concentration. If you're low on your hemoglobin, that's a higher risk of having problems with your organs, you know?"

"Yeah." The nurse left, and LaTasha tried to figure out how she felt about the blood transfusion. Finally, LaTasha called her mom. "Hi, Mommy. . . . No, that was them from the hospital because they want to give me blood, but I told them they got to call you first. . . . Okay, they said the reason why they want to give me blood is because they've given me so many antibiotics that it can mess me up. If my blood count is low. Oh. . . . Yeah. . . . It's the doctor. . . . Okay, look, call the nurse's station. Ask them to have you speak to the doctor. Ask to speak to Dr. Hansen, or any doctor that's taking care of me. . . . All right, I love you. . . . Okay, where you at? . . . Okay, I'm going to call you. . . . I'm going to page you in about fifteen, twenty minutes . . . huh? . . . Because I got to talk to you. . . . I know. Okay, I love you too." LaTasha hung up and matter-of-factly said, "My back is hurting." Referring to the heplock, she said, "I wish she would go ahead and hook me up."

Before going to the gift shop, LaTasha asked me to wheel her to the room of her friends. There were eleven sickle cell patients in the wards, although among those admitted LaTasha counted only Melinda, Sydney, Allen, and Jamal as her good friends. We entered Sydney's room and found her in extreme pain. Sydney let LaTasha know that she was not at all interested in talking. LaTasha was not put off by Sydney's rejection and told Sydney she would come back later. At the gift shop LaTasha commented about all the stars gracing the covers of the magazines: Eminem, Beyoncé, and others. After our short trip down to the gift shop, I returned her to her room and we said our good-byes.

How does one connect these data to health care disparities? Within this ethnography there are examples of nurses who do not connect the dots when it comes to patient needs, and a nurse-practitioner who does a fantastic job connecting the dots. There are patients like LaTasha, Sydney, and Jamal who are smart and able to work with the nurses and doctors, and then there are others like Melinda who feed into the nurses' stereotypes about sickle cell kids from the inner city. There are examples of both fettered and unfettered access to pain medication;

poor communication and good communication; competence and incompetence; patient maturity and immaturity; and licit and illicit behavior on the part of patients.

If we accept that LaTasha's experiences differ from those of white adolescent patients with chronic diseases, then we need to search for clues in the ethnographic data that might help us get a handle on what we even mean by health care inequities. If we want to try to improve the system, there are some questions we might ask, including: Is LaTasha treated "worse" than other patients because of her race, gender, class, and/or disease? How would we know? Should the hospital begin doing more to ensure that patients like LaTasha are not kicked out of educational programs? How directive or coercive should physicians be with late adolescents who resist treatments? How significant are individual moments with practitioners to the overall quality of LaTasha's care and health, given that she lives in poverty and meets abusive men through the Party Line?

It is helpful to recall the categories used in the literature to distill racial health and health care disparities: race/gene nexus (solution: ethnic pharmacogenomics), patient behavior (often described as culture), practitioner racism, and insurance. None of these categories seem to work as an explanatory model in the case of LaTasha, and even if we had a model that seemed promising, how do we compare LaTasha's health outcomes to those of other patients? (For example, was her coma the result of physician neglect?) Quantitative researchers would argue that a good social scientist could cleverly create independent variables, which could then be used to determine if LaTasha's health outcomes were compromised in any way. But some clever statistical approaches in the medical literature indicate that systems and unconscious bias produce disparities.[2] Other statistical approaches support the conclusion that disparities are not the product of systems and bias. The quantitative approach has produced no consensus but has only generated criticisms about different researchers' statistical methods and analyses.

The Children's West sickle cell team recognized that within their institution sickle cell patients were treated worse than their peers with other chronic conditions. They also noted that their patients were being denied access to treatment based on false presumptions and ignorance. Rather than weigh in on the debate about medical systems and staff bias, the CHW sickle cell team has used their failures as an opportunity to name a different approach to disparities. From their perspective, treatment access inequities are the result of lapses in evidence-based approaches to care. Their intervention is based on the belief that if their patients receive timely treatment using the latest evidence-based approaches to sickle cell care, then race and insurance become less crucial factors. Specifically, the CHW team institutionalizes a set of protocols identified in the National Institute of Medicine's book *The Management of Sickle Cell Disease,* which is a distillation of knowledge disseminated in the medical literature and discussed at national conferences.[3] The evidence-based approach to treatment attempted to eliminate staff subjectivity from patient treatment, and from the team's perspective, their approach was effective.

In the hands of other physicians, LaTasha might not have survived, and my interview with her demonstrated that she received the most advanced levels of medical care in the hospital, from the PCA pump to routine blood pressure checks. If this approach seems to work for sickle cell disease, perhaps it should be applied more broadly. But is strict adherence to evidence-based medicine enough to improve black-white disparities in life expectancy and morbidity generally? In the next chapter, I describe how evidence-based medicine does not eliminate medical uncertainty. This approach has the potential to reduce health care inequities, but these treatment protocols are themselves fraught with uncertainty.

# CHAPTER 3

# Health Care Access and Medical Uncertainty

How do Max and LaTasha's physicians know if their patients are receiving equitable health care? Even among people with the same disease, what constitutes a legitimate basis for determining health care equity? LaTasha's specific physical and psychosocial issues are different from Sydney's or Jamal's, and from those of the cancer patients who occupy the same floor. Physicians do not treat abstract patients, represented in the statistical literature in terms of sample size and probability; they treat individuals. To make sure that his sickle cell patients receive quality care, Dr. Allen, the head of the CHW sickle cell team, has operationalized evidence-based treatments particularly for pain management. He employs the authority of statistically significant findings even though he knows that standardized protocols take you only part of the way toward excellent health care. To understand the dance Dr. Allen must perform in order to improve his institution and improve individual patient care, one must first understand what evidence-based pain treatment is, and the role of uncertainty in physician discretion.

John Bonica published *The Management of Pain*, considered the bible on the topic, in 1953. A U.S. Army anesthesiologist at Tacoma General Hospital, Bonica was one of the first physicians to recognize pain medicine as a subspecialty. He formed the first multidisciplinary pain clinic in 1947 and was involved in developing the gate control theory of pain in the 1960s. Bonica, Ronald Melzack, and Patrick Wall are credited with producing early innovative theories on pain. Despite the recognition of pain as a subspecialty in the 1940s, it was not until 1973 that Bonica and several colleagues convened the International Association for the Study of Pain with the goal of developing a taxonomy for pain. There was a steady stream of publications on pain up through the 1980s, but in the 1990s nothing short of an avalanche of literature on pain and pain treatment blanketed a once sleepy subdiscipline.

Historically physicians have resisted treating pain. In the late eighteenth century in Philadelphia, Dr. Benjamin Rush taught his students that painful treatments were needed to cure American diseases that were tougher, he thought, than European diseases. Violent diseases, Rush argued, require painful remedies. Ideas about stoicism found an affinity with ideas about asceticism and individualism to produce a disdain for pain relief. Perhaps as a way to rationalize the suffering they inflicted on patients prior to the discovery of anesthesia, until the mid-1800s surgeons maintained that their Hippocratic obligation was to save lives rather than to alleviate suffering. In the nineteenth century that changed. In describing the "Age of Pain," historian Martin Pernick says, "In the mid-1800s, a growing number of practitioners turned toward a utilitarian professionalism," which he argues allowed greater risk taking in pain relief. Pernick attributes this change in attitude to the "sentimental romanticism of literature and the arts, the benevolent humanitarianism of social reformers, the calculating mentality of the new medical statisticians, and the perfectionist naturalism of rival medical sects."[1] A materialist might attribute these changes to the discovery of diethyl ether, nitrous oxide, and chloroform in the 1840s. In either case, it is clear that new medical discoveries were filtered through emerging cultural notions of physician duty.

It was not until the 1950s and 1960s that narcotic use was associated with amorality, addiction, and antisocial behavior. Medical pain treatment became conceptually entangled with illicit drug use, and so physicians chose to limit narcotic use to avoid possible patient addiction. That attitude began to shift in the 1980s, when daytime talk shows emerged as a fertile ground for new discourses on the body. These discourses reframed the social import of diseases and in many cases cast patients as the victims of evil. Even alcoholism and other behavioral diseases were traced to traumatic childhoods or biology. The message was clear: individuals needed to be more understanding of the ill, and the scientific community needed to end their suffering. At some point the new openness about issues like chronic illness and pain fell into lockstep with the science of pain management. In the 1990s, along with a growing sense that ill people should not be forced to endure unnecessary pain, new pharmaceuticals for pain treatment were introduced, including the very controversial OxyContin.

In spite of a growing consensus that began in the 1980s that pain, particularly for cancer, should be treated aggressively, almost thirty years later sickle cell patients remain the exception. Presumptions that blacks use drugs at significantly higher rates than other racial and ethnic groups support a kind of hypersurveillance of sickle cell patients. Therefore, in the case of a genetic disease with a known etiology and established treatment protocols, physician discretion still plays a key role in patient access to medications. As medical legal scholar M. Gregg Bloche argues, "Pervasive uncertainty and disagreement, about both the efficacy of most medical interventions and the valuation of favorable and disappointing clinical outcomes, leave ample room for discretionary judgments that produce racial disparities." Rather than accept physician discretion as a given, Bloche argues that through legal governance and institutional design, disparities in treatment can be reduced. Bloche proposes "cost-control that is rule-based when empirically feasible; financial rewards for patient satisfaction, health promotion, and favorable outcomes; and efforts to encourage stable doctor-patient relationships and resist market segmentation along race-correlated lines."[2]

According to Bloche, these legal and institutional correctives have the power to influence the choices physicians make but do not have the power to affect attitudes. He notes that "myriad presuppositions, stereotypes, and other psychological barriers to empathy and understanding influence clinical judgment in ways that are beyond the reach of organizational and legal arrangements."[3] What the physicians I worked with discovered is that institutional structures and arrangements can indeed have a profound effect on personal attitudes, including physician and nurse empathy. This chapter explores the efforts on the part of the sickle cell community to change medical staff attitudes toward sickle cell patients by operationalizing evidence-based treatment protocols that draw attention to patient suffering.

The movement within the American medical community to create consensus began in earnest in 1977 when the National Institutes of Health developed the Consensus Development Program, designed as "the focal point for evidence-based assessments of medical practice and state-of-the-science on behalf of the medical community and the public."[4] By pooling data from the statistical literature, evidence-based medicine attempts to standardize treatment for various illnesses throughout the United States. By operationalizing evidence-based treatment procedures, the sickle cell community hopes to reduce physician discretion and increase the consistency of health care across the country. In an interview with Dr. Allen, he explained why he believed sickle cell patients receive worse care than, for example, cystic fibrosis patients: "One of the problems with sickle patients, I believe, is health care professionals make a connection between African Americans using drugs and existing stereotypes; and that coupled with [health care professionals'] lack of knowledge about sickle cell disease . . ."[5] Dr. Allen's experiences with racial disparities in pain treatment were consistent with the literature, past and present.[6] To overcome these prejudices and improve health care access for his sickle cell patients, Dr. Allen rationalizes treatment through the deployment of cultural notions about good and evil in the guise of biomedical science. These discourses attempt to shift attention away from issues of race and toward issues of suffering.[7] Discourses of suffering have significantly more social capital than discourses of race, and Dr. Allen uses them to close what he perceives as a racial health care treatment disparity within his institution.

Following patients with sickle cell disease at Children's West, I became intrigued with the clinic's method for securing patient access through the deployment of novel understandings about sickle cell patients and sickle cell disease. The clinic team spent most of its time tending to outpatients but also oversaw the care of their hospitalized patients. This division between clinic and wards meant that the sickle cell team had to rely on residents, nurses, and attending physicians to diagnose and treat their patients. In the emergency department as well, patients were often treated by nonclinic staff. Thus in two instances, in the wards and in the emergency department, the clinic team had limited control over treatment practices.

What the clinic team learned through their patients was that residents and nurses were leery of adolescent sickle cell patients. The staff presumed that their poor, black adolescent patients who professed to be in extreme pain were really drug seeking. As a result, patients were often denied access to pain medications, or their pain was insufficiently treated. The sickle cell team intervened by demanding that the emergency room staff follow an explicit protocol when a patient enters with a painful crisis. The protocol included the quick and aggressive treatment of pain based on the theory that pain is real, that a patient is the best judge of his pain, and that delaying pain medication causes secondary complications. The sickle cell team also developed individualized patient pain profiles, which were placed prominently in each medical chart. They did this so that the staff did not spend time second-guessing the veracity of a patient's claim about the type and dosage of medication required.

Routinizing pain treatment in order to take staff subjectivity out of the treatment equation improved the quality of care in the emergency department and on the wards. The patients reported more positive experiences with staff, and the team was pleased with the quality of the care. At that point in my research I did not question the clinic's approach to pain. I trusted my informants that sickle cell pain was entirely a pathophysiological event requiring immediate and aggressive treatment. Any other treatment approach, I concluded after spending three years with CHW's sickle cell team, was due to ignorance, racism, or both.

From my observations it seemed that the barriers to equitable health care access rest in medical staff education regarding cutting-edge sickle cell treatments. With the proper scientific knowledge, I assumed, racist staff would at least be forced to submit themselves to the protocols known to work. I was to learn later, however, that uncertainties in medicine complicate the relationship between knowledge and treatment. Uncertainties in medicine allow medical professionals to fill in missing scientific information using nonscientific discourses, notably classism, sexism, and racism. I was to learn that even the most seemingly straightforward "scientific" approach to sickle cell treatment is informed by social and political *doxa*, or unquestioned cultural presumptions about the way the world works.

In *Outline of a Theory of Practice*, Pierre Bourdieu describes *doxa* as "systems of classification which reproduce, in their own specific logic, the objective classes, i.e. the divisions by sex, age, or position in the relations of production, make their specific contribution to the reproduction of the power relations of which they are the product, by securing the misrecognition, and hence the recognition, of the arbitrariness on which they are based: in the extreme case, that is to say, when there is a quasi-perfect correspondence between the objective order and the subjective principles of organization, . . . the natural and social world appears as self-evident."[8] By classifying some suffering as natural and other suffering as cultural, discourses of suffering attempt to make treatment logics seem self-evident. Denying health care or providing health care is seen not as a political decision but as a rational act emerging from an objective appreciation of physical suffering.

A significant body of literature describes how culture informs the questions asked by scientists, the approach taken to answering those questions, and how the data are interpreted.[9] I found it surprising not that culture informs science but that basic protocols for sickle cell care could be neglected, ignored, or challenged by individuals who simply want to cast patients as perpetrators rather than victims of suffering. It seemed obvious while at CHW that many health care disparities were the result of practitioner ignorance of evidence-based approaches to care.

After switching research field sites, I was forced to challenge my rather two-dimensional perspective of the relationship between access and medical staff education. The sickle cell clinic at Children's Hospital East, which is run by Dr. Peter Achebe, introduced myriad complicating questions about the role of institutional culture in structuring patient access. The experience also offered me an interesting perspective on how medical uncertainty affords physicians room to create different treatment protocols that may not be equal but are nevertheless efficacious in different ways. As philosopher Annemarie Mol and surgeon Bernard Elsman argue, disease detection, if done correctly, reveals nature, but treatment design is the product of culture.[10] By shifting the criteria used to determine treatment success, both institutions found ways to meet their goals. Children's West determined whether or not its patients were empowered by judging short-term outcomes: Did the patient receive fast and effective care? In contrast, Children's East used long-term outcomes: Did the patient finish high school? Is the patient doing well in college? Is the patient successfully employed?

The CHE clinic focused on long-term outcomes. For this clinic, run by black physicians, nurses, and social workers, pain was not understood as simply a pathophysiological event.[11] These professionals did not deny that pain was real, but they did argue that aggressive treatment of all pain can create dependence on powerful medications.[12] Physical and/or psychological dependence on analgesics is different from addiction, but for chronically ill patients, long-term use of powerful pain medications introduces a number of physical and psychosocial complications. The CHE team felt that less dependence on powerful narcotics opened up more life opportunities, including education and career development. The benefits of self-sufficiency, they felt, would more than make up for the short-term gains of pain relief. This did not mean that they denied patients powerful analgesics when these were truly necessary; it meant that they conditioned their patients to endure more pain before seeking medical help.

The comparison of the sites demonstrated to me that physicians shape health care access by their moral determinations about what constitutes a life worth living and their unique sense of duty to their patients, institution, and profession.[13] Similarly, embedded in any treatment calculus is a physician's understanding of a patient's duty to his or her own well-being.[14] All these physician assumptions are entangled in their protocols and preventative treatment strategies, what I call a treatment hermeneutic, which at an important level determines patient access. As Latour and Woolgar note in *Laboratory Life: The Social Construction of Scientific Facts,* scientific knowledge is produced through action, not simply ideas.[15]

But are different institutional correctives and individual physician treatment hermeneutics responsible for racial disparities in health, as Bloche argues? In the case of sickle cell disease, how successful are these institutionally different approaches at equalizing health outcomes? Immediately one sees the difficulty of trying to compare outcomes between diseases; sickle cell is, after all, a genetic disease that in the United States affects primarily blacks, who, as a group, share a particular constellation of economic and social issues. But even comparing a population affected by the same disease, it is difficult to evaluate the outcomes at different institutions, between various demographic groups, or even between individual patients. In terms of finding a way to eliminate racial health disparities, how do we make the transition from individual health care issues to institutional culture and regional politics in order to equalize treatment outcomes between various ethnic and racial groups? Interestingly, the different treatment approaches at CHW and CHE facilitated patient access and improved care, which challenges the presumed relationship between evidence-based medicine and commensurate outcomes.

Evidence-based medicine looks like the perfect solution, but it has been around for thirty years, and racial health disparities have not changed significantly during that time. So we need to ask, What counts as evidence in medicine given that the measures used to judge success may be incommensurate?[16] How are subjectivity and reality collapsed in randomized clinical trials? And how do uncertainty and physician discretion continue to work their way into the clinic despite the easy accessibility of evidence-based knowledge?

In the rush to create equal access and standardize care, the role of uncertainty in medicine is ignored because it contradicts our notion that medicine is a highly rational and exact science.[17] This uncertainty leads to different approaches to illness orchestrated in part by patients and physicians who have their own personal definitions of health and well-being. Ultimately these different approaches may lead to different outcomes.

While the state, as Foucault argues, has a stake in the "health of the social body as a whole," I argue that physicians and patients are uncertain state subjects.[18] What the state wants and what patients and physicians want with respect to health are rooted not in one philosophical tradition or epistemology but in several. The disabilities rights movement, conservative religious organizations, disease advocacy groups, the NIH, and individual patients all have a different sense of which bodies the state should support and which bodies should remain marginalized. They base their perspectives on everything from religious exegesis to demographics to different understandings of the social good.

There are many ways in which to shroud medical uncertainty in an aura of certainty. In the next section I will highlight two conceptual oversights in the scientific literature and scientific discourses—time and ethics—that ratify certain forms of suffering but obscure patient experience. Instead of arguing that the scientific community promotes a monolithic approach to time or ethics, I argue that the mere mention of either is enough to signify scientific authority. Neither, however, has any objective value or even consistent conceptual meaning.[19]

TIME AND ETHICS

The calculus about whether or not one is cured or whether or not one suffers is influenced by cultural perceptions about time. To be cured of cancer, for example, means that a person is cancer-free five years after an initial diagnosis. A cancer treatment is therefore considered a success even if the person dies six years after initial diagnosis. Similarly, the quality of that suffering is interpreted based upon the patient's age—an eighty-year-old versus an eight-year-old. Also, if a patient survived a cancer diagnosis for fifteen or twenty years before succumbing, then we often interpret the quality of his or her suffering differently than if a person survived for only one year.

In terms of deciding treatment efficacy, the length of a randomized clinical trial is determined prior to the study. Initially, the long-term effects of treatment are rarely at issue when making ethical decisions about the effectiveness of a drug during a phase III trial, and for ethical reasons a study will often be stopped if the short-term benefits of the treatment appear substantial. But are the length of the drug trial and the apparent benefits objectively determined, or are they informed by cultural and personal perspectives of time and ethics? For example, Dr. Achebe expressed grave reservations about giving babies hydroxyurea for a drug trial called Baby HUG. Hydroxyurea is a chemotherapy agent that affects fast-growing cells. Because the human brain grows very quickly in young children, Dr. Achebe felt that the potential long-term cognitive damage did not warrant the trial. Other researchers disagreed and argued that because hydroxyurea reduces the risk of stroke in very young children, preventing severe damage ethically trumped the theoretical potential of subtle brain injury. Dr. Achebe believed that babies at risk for stroke, as determined by a noninvasive early transcranial Doppler test, should be put on chronic transfusion therapy, which he believes is the safest and best treatment. But chronic transfusion therapy costs significantly more than hydroxyurea in both money and physician time. On either side of the debate, time (measuring success in the short term or long term) and ethics (parent, physician, and institutional commitment to patient well-being) are framed differently.

This debate about the ethical value of Baby HUG demonstrates that medical science is not a monolith. In *The Archaeology of Knowledge*, Foucault positions the relationship between knowledge and power as unambiguous; power informs knowledge.[20] But power, I argue, is itself ambiguous in the sense that, at least in the United States, a diverse array of powerful discursive traditions and communities authorize different forms of knowledge. In the case of medicine, some physicians find truth in a community-based approach to health and well-being; others find truth in pure research and medical interventions. In either case, a particular set of epistemologies inform a set of practices that can, at times, be contradictory.

Epistemologies are employed based upon context and their relative strategic value given the structures of relations of power. For example, the sickle cell clinic at Children's West promotes the discourse that pain is pathophysiological in order to open up access to analgesics for patients who enter the emergency room suffering from a painful crisis. The sickle cell team does so, however, primarily within the walls of their institution. These same physicians, when speaking to colleagues outside their institution, speak differently about the etiology of pain because they face a different set of audience expectations and professional repercussions. Put differently, scientific knowledge has several forms of agency. Uncertainty in biomedicine leaves room for a physician to creatively insert his or her political voice into local debates about what constitutes ethical health care practice. Physicians in one instance might apply rules of universalism, in another particularism, in another the idea of social equality, in another fiscal utilitarianism. These shifting frames, I argue, are obscured by a set of institutional and professional mandates that pretend to push medicine toward greater purity, meaning uniformity (evidence-based medicine) and democracy.

The move toward evidence-based medicine is so strong that it puts people who dissent from the status quo in an awkward position professionally with respect to grant funding and legitimization. In 2004, for example, Dr. Andrew Mosholder's presentation to the Food and Drug Administration (FDA) was canceled after he refused to back down from his conclusion that antidepressants increase suicidal thoughts in some children. Just months later, Mosholder's ideas were celebrated after evidence emerged that his conclusions may be correct. Only two years later, many parents of depressed children have publicly challenged these findings, saying that the drugs saved their children and therefore should be made readily available. Again, the statistical literature does not represent the experiences of individuals, making it harder to determine which rules to mandate.

After a number of drug scandals the FDA has felt pressure to transform its culture of medical paternalism and to embrace doubt and uncertainty.[21] In fact, the FDA may finally be coming to terms with the limits of its power to determine acceptable risk and may be embracing the notion that a truly informed patient determines his or her own risk. The outcome of a meeting to evaluate the approval process for rosiglitazone, a drug for patients with type 2 diabetes mellitus, shows a growing awareness that the approval system is underfunded and incapable of performing adequate scientific reviews of new drugs. But rather than argue that the system needs to return to the days of greater paternalism, critics of the system are finding new ways to honor medical uncertainty while also trying to protect consumers from false information and hope.

Rosiglitazone, for example, was found in clinical trials (most of which lasted only six months) to increase glycemic control, meaning that it helped maintain healthy blood sugar levels. Diabetes quadruples a patient's risk for macrovascular disease, but scientists do not understand the relationship between blood sugar levels and diseases such as atherosclerosis. Nevertheless, the FDA accepted the biochemical surrogate in place of clinical outcomes as a measure of efficacy and approved the drug. Following a randomized study of patient outcomes, it was determined that the use of rosiglitazone increased the risk of myocardial ischemia in patients taking the drug relative to patients in the control group.[22] Some patients on the drug died suddenly, and there was increased risk of angina and myocardial infarction.[23]

Members of two committees met in the summer of 2007 to discuss the regulatory issues surrounding the approval of rosiglitazone. The

Endocrinologic and Metabolic Drugs Advisory Committee and the Drug Safety and Risk Management Advisory Committee of the FDA made a number of recommendations summarized in a *New England Journal of Medicine* article by one of the committee members: "Ultimately, the committee voted to recommend not that rosiglitazone be removed from the market but rather that label warnings and extensive educational efforts be instituted immediately. The committee also requested further studies, but disconcertingly, none of the several proposed analyses of the ongoing clinical trials is likely to define an absolute risk for myocardial ischemic events in patients with diabetes who are taking this drug."[24]

The case of rosiglitazone highlights three themes. First, the six-month trials were determined by money and politics, not by scientific objectivity or ethics. The researchers could have chosen six days, six months, or six years given that the length of a given research study has no effect on P values. Because statistical significance is not affected by time, subjective understandings of efficacy (e.g., long-term vs. short-term outcomes) disappear from scientific results. Time ("Following a six-month study . . .") is essentially a rhetorical device subject to the interpretations of the reader. Second, the use of biochemical surrogates is related to the inability of the frequentist approach, deductive studies that produce P values, to deal with medical uncertainty and biological complexity. In the case of rosiglitazone, biochemical surrogates (glycated hemoglobin levels) were used because they are measurable and therefore quantifiable in short-term studies. Trying to understand the complex relationship between glucose levels and macrovascular diseases could take years, would be scientifically messy, and could lead to more medical uncertainty. Third, the case of rosiglitazone points to a need to reconsider which scientific knowledge is counted as fact and which scientific knowledge is marginalized. In the case of medicine, the experiential clinical knowledge of physicians may be more valuable than a statistically significant research study, but the medical community has yet to seriously consider how to ratify and deploy experiential knowledge. Importantly, clinical knowledge may be more beneficial to reducing racial health care disparities than the distribution of the latest wonder drug or, worse, "ethnic" wonder drug.

Before addressing the important relationship between physician agency and representations of time and ethics in biomedical research, let me first describe the major treatments and therapies for sickle cell disease in order to unpack what is at stake. Chronic transfusions, hydroxyurea, and bone marrow transplantation all involve different patient risks, health care resources, physician and patient commitments, and long-term expectations. Table 1 shows the types of information

## TABLE 1. A COMPARISON OF DIFFERENT SICKLE CELL TREATMENTS

| | Chronic Blood Transfusion Therapy | Hydroxyurea Therapy | Bone Marrow Transplant |
|---|---|---|---|
| *What is it?* | Patients receive simple or partial exchange transfusions, or erythrocytapheresis. | This chemotherapy agent increases production of fetal hemoglobin, which reduces sickling. | Hematopoietic (and nonmyeloablative) transplants replace bone marrow that produces hemoglobin that sickles with marrow that produces normal hemoglobin. |
| *What does it do?* | Transfusions reduce the concentration of sickled hemoglobin in the blood, thereby reducing complications caused by the disease, including organ damage. Reduces risk of stroke. | Decreases frequency and duration of painful vaso-occlusive crises and thereby reduces complications, including the most deadly, acute chest syndrome (ACS). | Patient has new bone marrow, which expresses normal hemoglobin, or with nonmyeloablative the bone marrow expresses a mix of sickled and normal hemoglobin. |
| *Benefits* | Reduces number of priapisms, which can lead to male infertility and leg ulcers. Improves pregnancy outcomes. Increases life expectancy and quality of life. | Decreases leg ulcers, aseptic necrosis of bone, priapisms, and stroke. Increases life expectancy, and quality of life. | Increases life expectancy and quality of life if treatment is successful. |
| *Eligible patients* | Patients with severe anemia, ACS, heart failure, dyspnea, hypotension, severe fatigue. For patients who have had a stroke, chronic transfusion therapy is recommended. | Patients who experience painful crises, perhaps 3 to 5 per year. | Patients under 16 who have had a stroke, recurrent ACS and painful crises, abnormal neuropsychologic function, lung disease, sickle nephropathy, osteonecrosis in multiple joints. Patients whose insurance will cover the procedure. |
| *Ineligible patients* | Patients with mild symptoms and complications, those who cannot comply with daily Desferal treatments, and who have developed severe alloimmunities. | Heterozygotes with sickle beta thalassemia or hemoglobin sickle cell disease. Those with allergies to hydroxyurea, those wanting to get pregnant, those who do not perform regular follow-ups. | Those whose insurance will not cover the procedure. Generally patients over 16, patients without a HLA donor, who have acute hepatitis, cirrhosis, renal impairment, sickle lung disease. Criteria continue to change. |

SOURCES: Samuel Charache, Michael L. Terrin, Richard. D. Moore, George J. Dover, Franca B. Barton, Susan V. Eckert, Robert P. McMahon, and Duane Bonds, "The Effects of Hydroxyurea on the Frequency of Painful Crises in Sickle Cell Anemia," *New England Journal of Medicine* 332 (1995): 1317–22; Mark Walters, "Management and Therapy of Sickle Cell Disease: Hematopoietic Cell Transplantation," http://sickle.bmt.harvard.edu/sickle_bmt.html (January 3, 2001); Elliott Vichinsky, "Transfusion Therapy in Sickle Cell Disease," http://sickle.bwh.harvard.edu/transfusion.html (January 4, 2001); National Heart, Lung, and Blood Institute, *Sickle Cell Research for Treatment and Cure*, NIH Publication no. 02-5214 (Bethesda, Md.: National Institutes of Health, September 2002).

patients and physicians must process to decide which of these three therapies to use. Clearly, treatment decisions require a complex evaluation of risk, and physicians present these risks differently based upon a particular set of assumptions.[25]

## TIME AND THE P VALUE

The annual scientific meetings sponsored by the NIH and the Sickle Cell Disease Association of America are organized to develop treatment consensus. Providers share the latest breakthroughs in sickle cell management, what one might call emerging best practices, in order to standardize the delivery of care for sickle cell patients across the country. The panels range from scientific sessions dealing with endothelial cell proliferation to psychosocial panels dealing with adolescent transitioning to adult care. These meetings are the place where discourses about the disease and the treatment are ratified. Prominent individuals are featured in invited sessions or are asked to participate in closed sessions with key individuals from the NIH. As a result, scientific discourses become attached to individuals who possess charisma, social capital, and access to resources. In many respects, scientific meetings are the birthplace of scientific hegemony.

In 2002, at the thirtieth anniversary of the National Sickle Cell Disease Program (NSCDP) and the Sickle Cell Disease Association of America(SCDAA), a panel was convened on the advantages and limitations of three therapy/treatment options: hydroxyurea, stem cell transplantation, and chronic blood transfusions. The panel, organized by Children's Hospital of Philadelphia, was the brainchild of Dr. Kwaku Ohene-Fremporg, one of the leaders in the sickle cell community. Each topic was handled by two physicians; one discussed the advantages and the other the limitations of a specific therapy. The physicians' papers were followed by a presentation by a registered nurse, who discussed family and psychosocial issues.

As an introduction to his paper, Dr. Elliott Vichinsky, a known polemicist with respect to chronic blood transfusion therapy, challenged a developing consensus within the medical community about the relative merits of hydroxyurea and bone marrow transplantation over transfusions.[26] He asked, "Can we have a debate? Is there another side?"[27] Given the pressure to develop national guidelines, Dr. Vichinsky's question is extremely important. Is dissension possible in such a climate? The annual sickle cell meetings present an opportunity to develop medical treatment consensus around national treatment mandates, which, Vichinsky noted, can often overwhelm legitimate debate. While he lamented the suppression of dissent from the emerging status quo, he nevertheless has been able to deploy his own set of guidelines regarding transfusion therapy outlined in *The Management of Sickle Cell Disease*.[28]

After opening his panel with the two questions, Vichinsky listed all the symptoms ameliorated by blood transfusion therapy and then stated that "patients can live sixty-plus years on transfusion therapy." Following his inventory of the beneficial aspects of transfusion therapy, he noted the side effects—alloimmunization, infection in HIV, iron overload—and then he explained how these side effects can be avoided or reduced. Dr. Vichinsky closed his talk by addressing how safe Desferal is and how noncompliance is the result of "services not being offered to keep compliance." He blamed lack of compliance on the dearth of patient-friendly programs that reward patients who show marked decreases in their iron overload. He ended with a bold statement about how blood transfusions offer the greatest number of "quality-of-life" years. According to his estimates, blood transfusion patients experience around nineteen quality-of-life years as opposed to those treated with hydroxyurea, which offers around seventeen years, and bone marrow transplant, which offers sixteen quality-of-life years.

Following Vichinsky's talk, Dr. Alan Cohen began his presentation by saying, "The greatest spokesperson for the disadvantages of blood transfusion therapy is [Cohen projects a PowerPoint picture of Vichinksy] Elliott Vichinsky." The room, packed with more than two hundred medical professionals, patients, and family members, erupted into laughter. Cohen touched immediately upon the holographic nature of biomedical research where viewed from one angle one gets a very different impression of suffering and risk than when viewed at a different angle. Instead of starting his presentation with the benefits of transfusion therapy, Cohen began by expounding on the complications that Vichinsky already presented. Using virtually the same statistics as Vichinsky, Cohen argued that the risk of transfusion-transmitted infections, such as HIV, is high. While Vichinsky presented alloimmunization, iron overload, and infection as avoidable, Cohen presented them as dire. Cohen asserted that the annual cost for transfusion therapy, about $50,000 per patient, is institutionally prohibitive and counsels that the "level of optimism needs to be tempered." Cohen ended by saying that although transfusions have been shown to reduce strokes in patients, only a third of the patients who were asked to participate in what is known as the Stroke Prevention Trial in Sickle Cell Anemia (STOP) study refused because they did not want to be on chronic transfusion therapy.

For years, chronic blood transfusions were considered the best treatment, and Dr. Vichinsky, a leader in the field of transfusion therapy, was called upon to create national standards. In a dinner interview with one of the pioneers in sickle cell patient care, this physician mentioned how disappointed she was with Vichinsky. At a Mexican cantina next to the NIH, she described with a mixture of sadness and frustration that Vichinsky never produced statistically robust results in his early studies of blood transfusion therapy. Until the STOP study, there had been no large-scale systematic study of the benefits and limitations of blood transfusion therapy. Physicians knew only anecdotally that transfusion therapy was effective.

The simultaneous insider/outsider status Vichinsky occupies today speaks to the rapidity with which medical discoveries shift in and out of favor, how criteria for scientific proof changes, and how professionals are under constant pressure to relegitimate their professional status. Many physicians had observed before the STOP study that blood transfusion therapy worked well for patients. It reduced complications and increased longevity. But these observations made by clinicians over the years are now considered anecdotal as the evidence-based ethic puts greater and greater pressure on physicians to statistically prove efficacy. The absence of statistically significant P values in Dr. Vichinsky's data has made it difficult for some physicians to interpret for themselves whether or not transfusion therapy is efficacious. The evidence-based emphasis on the P value has changed the criteria by which physicians determine truth from one of seeing is believing to interpreting data is believing. The valorization of the P value has substantially changed the clinical gaze.

We must take Dr. Vichinsky's question, "So what agency do physicians have to present a different side?" less as a lamentation and more as a call to rethink what counts as evidence in evidence-based medicine. Given that evidence-based medicine, as currently articulated in the scientific literature, deals poorly with biological complexity, how relevant is it to racial health disparities? Racial health disparities, after all, are the result of the interplay of complex systems both biological and structural, and seem to emerge at the node of various hegemonies.

Speaking to a physician at Children's Hospital West, I described my ethnographic methods, to which he said, "As long as you can get

a statistically significant P value." At the Sickle Cell Association meeting, standing next to two doctors in front of a poster presentation, I
heard one doctor read aloud the presentation title: " 'A classification
system for acute chest syndrome in children with sickle cell disease.' "
Then he snickers and says, "How statistically significant is that!? What
kind of P value did they get?" What is a P value, and what power does
it have to determine scientific legitimacy? A P value, or probability value,
of less than .05 determines if a scientific observation is statistically significant. Researchers mistakenly think that a P value of .05 means that
a drug should be successful in treating 95 percent of cases. Instead,
R. A. Fischer, who proposed the P value in the 1920s, intended for the
measure to be used as part of a meta-analysis that combines the statistical outcome of one study with the statistical outcome of other studies.[29] The P value fallacy, as Goodman calls it, is the use of single studies
to test the probability of an event, which then becomes the sole basis of
scientific truth claims.

Goodman objects to the artificial hierarchy situating deductive inference methods above inductive methods: "Enumerating the frequency of
symptoms (observations) given the known presence of a disease (hypothesis) is a deductive process and can be done by a medical student with a
good medical textbook. Much harder is the inductive art of differential
diagnosis: specifying the likelihood of different diseases on the basis of a
patient's signs, symptoms, and laboratory results. The deductions are
more certain and 'objective' but less useful than the inductions."[30] In
identifying how the P value became in one sense fetishized, Goodman
says, "It is a complex story, but the basic theme is that therapeutic
reformers in academic medicine and the government, along with medical
researchers and journal editors, found it enormously useful to have a
quantitative methodology that ostensibly generated conclusions independent of the person performing the experiment. It was believed that
because the methods were 'objective,' they necessarily produced reliable,
'scientific' conclusions that could serve as the bases for therapeutic decisions and government policy."[31] Goodman's solution is to use a Bayesian
approach, which encourages the researcher to determine a series of
potential hypotheses. This requires weighing evidence from prior
research and identifying epistemological uncertainties a priori. The
response in the medical community to this statistical approach combin-
ing inductive and deductive methods is one of derision.

Anthropologist Joe Dumit noted that the Bayesian approach for drug
trials exposes so much uncertainty that results become endlessly debatable

and indeterminate.[32] Goodman, on the other hand, is concerned that the P value is so malleable as to be incoherent. What researchers have, therefore, is a choice between indeterminacy and malleability. Doubt, for example, is easily reasoned away. According to Goodman, "If a P value of 0.12 is found for an a priori unsuspected difference, an author often says that the groups are 'equivalent' or that there is 'no difference.' But the same P value found for an expected difference results in the use of words such as 'trend' or 'suggestion,' a claim that the study was 'not significant because of small sample size,' or an intensive search for alternative explanations. On the other hand, an unexpected result with a P value of 0.01 may be declared a statistical fluke arising from data dredging or perhaps uncontrolled confounding."[33] A researcher's prior knowledge and expectations (unsuspected vs. unexpected) affect how the results are interpreted. The creative manipulation of variables and results in order to achieve a P value of less than .05 has and continues to lead to the tragic approval of dangerous medicines.[34] At the same time, physicians and other medical professionals are staking professional claims and receiving funding by developing studies that, they insist, will produce a statistically significant P value.

As an agnostic with respect to the legitimacy of either the frequentist approach or the Bayesian approach, I want to present the P value as a methodological point of entry where researchers can advance particular social, economic, and personal agendas. From a pain treatment study using seventeen patient visits, to a study titled "The Inclusion of Community Resources for Parents of Newly Diagnosed Infants with Sickle Cell Disease," at my first Sickle Cell Association meeting, I was overwhelmed by the number of short-term, long-term, psychosocial, biomedical, small-scale, and large-scale studies that all claimed to be part of the same methodological species. My favorite was a study described in a paper entitled "The Spiritual Needs of Sickle Cell Families." In the abstract the authors write:

Our plan is to identify the families' spiritual beliefs during comprehensive visits. . . . Appropriate families are supported on the role and power of prayer. If needed, quiet areas are reserved including a hospital chapel. A 24-hour multi-faith hotline is available with representatives from each denomination. . . . For example, five families with seriously ill children report a marked improvement in quality of life after their religious beliefs were incorporated in their medical plan. The use of prayer to help cope with chronic illness is a positive tool for selective families and should be respected and encouraged. *Long-term follow-up on objective outcome variables is proceeding with the goal to prove our hypothesis that spiritual beliefs decreases [sic] morbidity and improves quality of life.*[35]

It seems a shame that anthropologists have spent so much time deconstructing the notion that religious beliefs are categorically distinct from other beliefs only to see them being repackaged to test a null hypothesis; nevertheless, this attempt to quantify the relationship between affective states and treatment efficacy is a creative response to professional pressures for legitimization. More exacting criteria for truth verification would limit the expressive potential that currently resides in the P value. Opening up hospital space for spiritual reflection is neither nefarious nor located within any one epistemological domain. Rather, the introduction of spirituality into a hospital setting, regardless of the method used to legitimate it, could be motivated by ideas of embodiment and transcendence, multiculturalism, even neuroscientific understandings of the mind-body relationship.

The instability of the P value allows physicians to assert creative social agendas while simultaneously producing a simulacrum of scientific reality and medical beneficence. Jean Baudrillard argues in "Simulacra and Simulations" that "simulation is no longer that of a territory, a referential being or a substance. It is the generation of models of a real without origin or reality: a hyperreal."[36] The statistical methods used to generate the P value require simulation and, notably, trials of two months, one year, even three years represent a lifetime, as if the curative potential of a drug will remain constant over time and not produce secondary complications. In studies that use the frequentist approach, time can be compressed, elongated, or made finite in order for researchers to extract the results they want. Researchers present findings as though the length of the study was imposed by nature, a kind of biological time. In reality, however, the length of these studies is based on fiscal calendars, market pressures, politics, and patient and institutional pressures. The hydroxyurea study, for example, is presented on a Web site that presents an overview of evidence-based research as ethically progressive because "the Independent Oversight Committee, charged by the National Heart, Lung, and Blood Institute (NHLBI) to guard the welfare of the patients, terminated the study on January 31, 1995 because the patients on the hydroxyurea (HU) arm had significantly fewer episodes of vaso-occlusive painful crises, fewer hospitalizations, and fewer episodes of acute chest syndrome. The initial results were reported in the New England Journal of Medicine, May 18, 1995.

*Hydroxyurea is the first agent that can prevent above-mentioned com-
plications for sickle cell anemia.*"[37] What strikes me about the ethical
decision to stop the study is the absence of data regarding the long-term
consequences of hydroxyurea, a chemotherapy agent. The therapy
reduced painful crises and acute chest syndrome, but other advantages
and disadvantages, neither suspected nor expected, remained uncoded
and unquantified. The study recorded "the efficacy of hydroxyurea in
reducing the frequency of painful crises in adults," and because the
drug performed as anticipated, it was deemed ethical to stop the study
early.[38] The hydroxyurea research showed that there was a 44 percent
decrease in the annual rate of painful crises with a P value of less than
.001. What if the researchers had applied the Bayesian function and set
up prior predictive values for several possible outcomes? They might
have tested for myelotoxicity caused by the hydroxyurea or hematopoietic depression, or even drawn out the study for nine years to test
whether the drug increased the likelihood of developing leukemia. In
2004 one of my thirteen-year-old campers at sickle cell camp said that
hydroxyurea caused her avascular necrosis of the hip. Disbelieving, I
asked Dr. Achebe, who told me that some physicians are investigating a
connection between long-term hydroxyurea use and avascular necrosis.
The connection has not been established, but again the idea that stopping the hydroxyurea study early constituted best ethical practice only
makes sense if one considers time a monolith. I am not arguing that
hydroxyurea is dangerous or ineffective; rather, what strikes me about
this study are the methods used to determine treatment efficacy, and the
ways in which the discourse of ethics authorized the legitimacy of a
twenty-one-month study.

   The effort to accelerate the introduction of new pharmaceutical
agents into the marketplace was encouraged, in part, by the protest
group Act Up which in the 1980s challenged the U.S. government and
the FDA to be more forthcoming with new treatments for HIV and
AIDS. When Act Up first became prominent, no treatments were available to slow the progression of AIDS, and the movement was predicated
on the idea that even an experimental treatment was better than none.
With chronic illnesses, however, the time pressures are significantly different. What strikes me is that these differences do not inform a different ethical stance with respect to the length of a study. The elision of
time as a relevant variable in biomedical statistics again opens up room
for methodological creativity, but at the same time its absence alters
representations of risk. Anthropologist Carol Greenhouse says, "Time

is not about, or not first about, personal or collective experiences of change but about cultural formulations of agency and their compatibility or incompatibility within specific institutional forms. 'Agency' names cultural propositions about how the universe works."[39]

While biomedical therapies and cures work in what I will call "probability or P time," patients and physicians work in "clinical time," "personal time," and "social time." With respect to P time, the ways in which time is represented in peer-reviewed medical articles speaks to how, as Greenhouse notes, institutions formulate agency and authorize a temporal reality. Following a fairly rigid formula, these articles present the research problem, hypothesis, methodology, data, and results. The conclusion is validated by the reiteration of the statistical significance of the findings, generally expressed as a P value, which linguistically transforms information into biomedical facts.[40] The use of time to make ethical claims about agency relates to the ways in which claims about suffering are embedded in research methods. The P value allows medical professionals to put forth a diversity of social, economic, and personal agendas because time has no particular reference or value in biomedical research other than to support a teleology.

Evidence-based approaches to the care of Max and LaTasha have worked. Both patients are alive and relatively healthy even though they both are classified as having severe disease. But in neither instance is Max or LaTasha thriving as an individual. Could the ways in which cure and treatment are defined have an effect on their psychosocial outcomes? Is focusing on short-term amelioration of symptoms keeping the medical community from developing holistic treatments that take into account the life trajectory of chronically ill patients? Perhaps time has an ethical component that could become part of what we consider evidence in evidence-based medicine.

# CHAPTER 4

# The Affective Dimensions
# of Pain

In Gananath Obeyesekere's investigation of the emergence of three karmic eschatologies, he notes that for Buddhists there is a "logical contradiction in the explanation of suffering" that cannot be reconciled.[1] Notably, is suffering the result of the inherent weaknesses of the gods, or is karma less deterministic than thought? Obeyesekere represents these tensions not as dialectics but as aporias that threaten the integrity of the doctrine. The response to this contradiction has been for authorities of Buddhism to authorize discourses regarding the structural and agentive entities responsible for suffering, namely, karma or the gods. Within American medicine there is a similar drive to name the structures and agents responsible for suffering because the paradoxes threaten the integrity of the whole.

How, then, does medicine construct the ontology of suffering? In biomedical studies, suffering, like time, is an unstable referent that frames the hypothesis's meaning and value. In the case of hydroxyurea, a sickle cell pain crisis is presumed to be the number one cause of patient suffering. Therefore, the side effects or resulting inconveniences are dismissed as insignificant compared to the imagined suffering caused by a crisis. In this respect, the hypothesis names what suffering matters. On the Sickle Cell Disease Association of America Web site, a page touting the benefits of hydroxyurea ("Short-term side effects must be carefully monitored and long-term effects are still unknown") ends with a list of "potential savings from use of hydroxyurea."

- Total number of severe pain episodes in patients: 13,520
- Assuming that 50 percent of episodes result in hospitalization: 6,760
- Estimated total number of hospital days for these patients: 33,800
- Assuming cost per day: $800
- Total hospitalization costs for these patients: $27,040,000
- Potential savings in one year: $13,520,000

These data show little empathy for the patients. Missing from this article are descriptions about how hydroxyurea reduces patient suffering. What the reader learns instead is that hydroxyurea relieves a hospital's financial burden.

The confusion over whose suffering is relieved by hydroxyurea was made clear in another panel on pain management at the Sickle Cell Association meetings in 2002. The case presented to the experts was that of a fourteen-year-old boy who had had a "difficult clinical course," including renal damage and avascular necrosis of the hip. The result of avascular necrosis is osteoarthritis and debilitating pain, but he was too young to receive a hip replacement. He was on long-acting OxyContin as opposed to another analgesic because of his renal damage, and the nurses presenting the case said they were concerned about addiction. They also said that the boy had already been moved into adult care, to which a black hematologist, Dr. Wally Smith, commented, "Institutions punt patients when pain management gets too difficult," a reference to the practice of discharging pediatric patients and placing them in adult care prematurely. Even with all his health and social issues, this fourteen-year-old refused hydroxyurea. How could this boy's risk calculus differ from that presented in the literature on hydroxyurea? Put simply, what does the boy know that we do not?

The answer lies, I believe, in the hydroxyurea study's narrow definition of efficacy. According to the study's authors, if the number of painful crises were reduced in the assigned group of a double-blind, randomized clinical trial, then hydroxyurea would be considered effective. Painful crises are the hallmark of sickle cell disease, and patients in extreme pain require strong, hospital-administered analgesics. Painful episodes can lead to or are sometimes caused by a sometimes fatal condition known as acute chest syndrome, which if severe enough requires a blood transfusion. The study showed a decrease, by about half, of

painful crises (2.5 vs. 4.5 incidents per year for those assigned hydroxyurea vs. those assigned placebo), ACS (25 vs. 51 cases per year), and
transfusions (48 vs. 73 cases per year). It therefore located patient suffering in the number of severe painful crises, and by inference interpreted ethical action as the reduction of painful crises. But what if sickle
cell patients do not locate their suffering in the number of hospital
admissions for painful crises and do not fear ACS or prefer transfusions? The study coded suffering according to measures that may or
may not be meaningful to patients.

Away from public and professional scrutiny, many physicians
acknowledge medical uncertainty even if they preach adherence to one
disease/treatment paradigm. My interview with Dr. Lawrence Taylor
exemplifies this public-private split. In 2004, Taylor and I met in his
small office in Children's Hospital North (CHN), located in a poor
neighborhood in a midsize urban center. He was wearing a white lab
coat over dark slacks and a dress shirt. Taylor, who is white and in his
midthirties, had been recruited to direct the hospital's new adult center.
He had short, light brown hair and looked younger than his years, but
he was clearly worn out by his duties. Before switching to Children's
North two years prior to our interview, Taylor had worked at Stanford.
Unlike Stanford, CHN is in a racially mixed neighborhood with many
lower-middle-class and poor blacks and Asians. His devotion to his profession and his patients was clear, represented most clearly by the fact
that in his first year of clinical work he received no take-home pay. He
did receive a salary for his teaching, but he knows firsthand how poorly
reimbursed hematologists who specialize in sickle cell disease are.

Dr. Taylor had the energy, enthusiasm, and idealism necessary to
work in a subspecialty with little funding and with a patient population
that is typically lower-middle-class or poor.[2] During the interview I
asked him about how physicians deal with the paradox that sickle cell
pain is often characterized as psychosomatic, yet the same people who
subscribe to the idea that patient pain is often not "real" still accept the
hydroxyurea studies that show that the drug reduced the number of
painful episodes.

Dr. Taylor eagerly addressed my question with a question of his own:
"Do you read [Ludwig] Wittgenstein? I can tell you were tracking on philosophy." Dr. Taylor spoke so rapidly I did not have time to answer his
question, although if I did I would have told him that my research had
inspired an engagement with Friedrich Nietzsche and his challenge to the
politics of pity. In the mode of teacher educating a student, Taylor argued,

"If you think about whatever biologic theory of how consciousness and feelings should work, we don't even have a model. We don't even have an idea what a model should look like. Philosophy probably does have a lot to say there and, not to go too far, but Wittgenstein has this very intriguing view that even your perception of pain society has placed in you." Most anthropologists would agree in part arguing that culture provides idioms for expressing pain that may or may not have physiological origins.[3] Taylor continued, "Even your description, everyone says, 'Pain is real.' I'm the first one to tell you, but actually, that may not even be true. And it's also interesting to see how similar all these problem patients are." By problem patients, he was referring to patients who come back repeatedly and who claim that their pain treatment is ineffective.

Dr. Taylor continued to show himself to be more of a committed cultural constructivist than his interviewer. He said, "I don't know how many hours we've spent talking about the types of pain, occasions, intensity and it's very interesting because it's hard to find any consistent pattern of response. So, I try to explain it to patients, 'Well, not all pain responds.' There's a lot of nonnarcotic response to pain. It just doesn't respond to narcotics." At times Taylor seemed to dissociate the pain from the patient, turning the pain into the disembodied subject ("it") being treated. "And, you know, it's a very hard concept because, you know, I have a patient named Natalie who is one of our more difficult patients and moderately functional." Taylor described Natalie as a patient who has been openly hostile in the hospital because she felt that her pain was inadequately treated. "But, again, her only association with care is that narcotics make her nearly toxic and loopy. And that's what she thinks is pain care."

Most sickle cell physicians and nurses would tell me that the percentage of difficult patients in their care is small, generally less than 10 percent. But the amount of energy and time they consume makes their numbers seem greater. While extremely difficult, these patients push physicians to articulate the limits of care, which inspires discussions of best practices and ethics.

Continuing his description of Natalie, Taylor said, "I was told by another doctor, [Natalie] was literally escorted by the police out of [the hospital]. She was so abusive because they weren't giving her meds. You know, she'd scream at me so many times. She just needs more and more and more and more, and she's just so dysfunctional. But yet, there's no connection." When physicians lose their authority over their patients because they cannot deliver the promise of biomedicine to ameliorate suffering, labels such as dysfunctional are employed. The cause of Natalie's suffering is her dysfunction and not the limits of biomedicine or the culture of the institution.

Dr. Taylor drifted between a thesis that suggests the causes of suffering are unknowable and a description of Natalie situated firmly in the pragmatics of patient care. He discounted Natalie's belief that loopiness is pain relief. Instead, he and the other physicians limit her access to narcotics because her response to the drugs does not in their estimation warrant continued use. For many physicians, such as Dr. Taylor, grappling with uncertainty is interesting at a theoretical level, but embracing uncertainty at an administrative level seems like an impossibility.

Dr. Carl Davis, an adult physician at a county hospital in Southern California, discussed the same issues in an interview I conducted with him at his office in 2004. He has what I consider an interesting perspective on patients, treatment, choice, and suffering. Dr. Davis works in a state-of-the-art fifty-bed cancer treatment center. While the cancer treatment center is adjacent to the county hospital, the hospital and the center are worlds apart. The facility is a fairly new white marble and limestone building serving, according to Davis, some of the richest old-money whites in the area. Being a hematologist, Dr. Davis sees some cancer patients, but he focuses his research and clinical work around sickle cell disease. Dr. Davis has a gray Afro and large, rectangular, metal-rimmed glasses and typically dresses in either khakis or jeans. A strapping man in excellent physical condition, he has an exuberant spring in his walk and a sharp wit. Even though he often speaks cynically about misplaced idealism, Dr. Davis is an echo of the 1970s black power movement. He has demonstrated over the years an unparalleled commitment to the sickle cell community and the black community in his city. In addition to his scientific expertise, his longevity in the sickle cell community makes him an excellent historian. With Dr. Davis, I addressed the same issue about pain and hydroxyurea that I had with Dr. Taylor: "The people who argue that pain is psychosocial also say, 'Hydroxyurea reduces painful episodes.' It seems like you can't hold those same facts in your head at the same time."

Challenging me, Dr. Davis asked, "Why?"

"They contradict," I responded.

Dr. Davis's answer differed from Dr. Taylor's in form but not in content. "No. That's because people don't understand the placebo effect." Again I was told that pain and idioms of pain are cultural and psychological constructs that produce "real" clinical findings.

Pushing back, I asked, "You think there's a placebo effect with hydroxyurea?"

Clarifying his position, Dr. Davis said, "No, it has true physiologic effects which are clearly beneficial to the pathophysiology of the disease. But you have to remember that any time you do something to the patient, there is a placebo effect. And that can be as simple as talking to the patient. I've seen it in action."

Just to make sure we both are using the term *placebo effect* in the same way, I asked, "So, if you just develop this thing called . . . we'll just name it toralene . . ." Dr. Davis laughed and called me "the drug doctor." After acknowledging his joke, I continued, "And you take it, and you tell a patient, 'You know, this is going to reduce your painful episodes . . .' You think that it's going to reduce it?"

Adamant, Dr. Davis provided a scientific explanation: "If the patient believes them, it will reduce their perception of the pain. If we can go into the nerves and measure the degree of the painful stimulants, no. That hasn't changed. It's like up here has changed [points to head]. You dampen down the perception. We've all had this . . . you run into the doorway, the leg hurts like hell. You get distracted, it don't hurt no more."

I delicately asked him to apply his thesis to the politics of sickle cell care: "So, maybe do you think that in pediatric care you're sort of socializing patients to need these heavier narcotics, or . . ."

Not afraid of controversy Dr. Davis responded with gusto, "Of course, pediatricians are terrible at how they train patients to interact with their illness."

"In what way?"

"They develop all this dependence on the medical system. It's like mothering. And then the patient turns eighteen, and then they toss him out." Gesturing with a pointed thumb over his shoulder, he mimicked a pediatric hematologist, "'You're on your own now!' So, people are now beginning to recognize that that's not a good way to deal with patients. They are developing these transition programs because they haven't taught the teenager, 'You're responsible for getting up in the morning, and getting your homework done and drinking your fluids, and making sure you don't do the things that you know are going to cause you to have pain. Instead of depending on us to bail your butt out every time.'"

For clarification I said, "So, when your kid falls down, instead of going, 'Oh, are you okay,' you go, 'Oh, what fun,' you can actually change some of those perceptions around . . ."

"You can change people's way of dealing with things."

Dr. Davis believes strongly that in order for patients to benefit from treatment they must be socialized to respond to the health care system and sickle cell therapies in ways that are consistent with the culture of medicine. This is essentially an admission that there is an affective dimension to health care that requires that patients identify a cure the way medical professionals identify a cure, and that requires patients to expect from biomedicine what doctors are capable of delivering.

Returning to the initial dilemma, I pointed out, "But you say the pain is real."

"The pain's real. How you react to the pain is more important to how bad the pain is. See, diabetes is a good example. You empower the patient to manage their insulin and their blood sugar, right? And you see patients who do beautifully. Glucose is always one hundred, and they're very rigid with checking those finger sticks and adjusting the dose depending upon what they're doing, and so forth and so on. And then you see patients who can't handle it. That's a supratentorial problem. A disease problem."

Needing more clarity, I asked, "Is there real somatic injury that's causing this pain, or you just don't know?"

"Sure, sure. It's ischemia, lack of blood flow in the bone marrow. So, there's no physical findings because it's inside the bones and you can't see it or feel it. And, it's not usually bad enough to cause inflammation, but it's detectable by an ordinary physical exam. You can detect it on an MRI. A thousand bucks a test to show that the patient is really having ischemia."

Referring to the literature stating that if a sickle cell patient has a blood concentration of less than 30 percent sickle hemoglobin, then he should have no pain, I asked, "If the sickle hemoglobin is 30 percent or less, do you think that they are experiencing pain?"

Dr. Davis dismissed that conclusion: "Of course! Of course, because the cells can still get hung up in the microcirculation. The frequency is going to be much less, but it's not cured."

I encouraged him to address the politics of pain management by asking him to acknowledge the fact that some institutions will not provide pain medication if the concentration of sickle hemoglobin is less than 30 percent.

Shaking his head, he said, "I know, yeah, I know because they think you can't possibly . . ."

Interrupting, I stated, "But you can have a stroke when you have less than 30 percent."

Dr. Davis then brought up the existential question of pain and the medical issue of pain management to bear on how knowledge is politicized in the medical community. "See, but if you have a stroke there's an obvious physical finding. You see if you have bone marrow ischemia, and you have this edema that's pressing against the bone. Now, we all know that if you have leukemia or some kind of malignancy growing inside the bone, that pressure causes pain. We know it causes pain. [Many physicians] won't accept that sickle cell disease causes the same pain."

Aside from the affective dimensions of pain and pain treatment, there is what he identified as real suffering. Dr. Davis combined a discussion of the objective measures of pain with his straightforward assessment of how medical professionals continue to dismiss the legitimacy of sickle cell pain. He unself-consciously wove together his scientific understanding of sickle cell disease pain with treatment politics.

After discussing the uncertainties with respect to hydroxyurea and perceptions of pain, I asked Dr. Davis whether he encourages any one therapy over another. I began by asking him about the panel at the thirtieth anniversary comparing the various therapies. His response: "There is no therapy in medicine that is 100 percent effective. None."

Reminding him of the panel, I offered, "Well, [Vichinsky at the association meeting] was saying that blood transfusion therapy [provided] nineteen quality-of-life years versus sixteen quality . . ."

Smiling, he asked me, "Right, right, okay. Is it worth it?"

Throwing the issue back at him, I offered, "I don't know. I don't know if you can quantify quality-of-life years."

"Yes, you can. Yes, you can." Given his earlier discussion of the placebo effect and the influence that culture and education have on perceptions of pain, I was surprised by his answer. "But if the difference is this big [uses his fingers to indicate a very small difference], is the time and trouble of the treatment worth this difference? If the difference is big, then the time and trouble is probably going to be worth it. [The benefit of] chelation for [iron] overload is that it prevents you from dying. But, you know, even the patients don't want to do it even though they know. I mean transfusing two units usually takes about five hours plus travel time and waiting, okay. You're talking about all day. So, patients will vote with their feet."

"He [Vichinsky] thinks that if you build in enough incentives—"

Dismissive of Dr. Vichinsky's claims, Dr. Davis interrupted, "Yeah, yeah, I'm sure. Now, what are those incentives going to be? You may have to go out and get the patients and bring them in. Sure, all things are possible if you're willing to put forth enough effort to get them done. But, in a very practical sense, when you give patients treatments that are too onerous, they quit coming." Dr. Davis then provided a wonderful overview of the patient variables that make mandating one approach to sickle cell disease ridiculous. "You're talking about a disease where 20 percent of the patients are responsible for 85 percent of the medical cost. The majority of patients, certainly adult patients with sickle cell anemia, are mild to moderate. They don't even need hydroxyurea, you know. Hospitalized once a year, maybe. See, so, if you go to the hospital for five days, once a year, are you going to take a drug that means you're going to have to come to the clinic every two weeks to get your blood checked? That's twenty-six outpatient [visits] per year versus five inpatient visits. You're a reasonably intelligent young woman, right?" I was not sure how to answer his question. "And you have to give up your reproductive potential because we don't know if this is going to hurt your developing fetus. Are you going to take this drug? No way! How many hospital days is worth the twenty-six outpatient visits?"

"I don't know. I don't know."

Wedded to his quantitative approach to quality of life, he answered, "It turns out it's about fifty, somewhere between twelve and fifty. The patients will say, 'Yeah, I'll come about every two weeks, until you get this damn dose adjusted.' But, if it's less than that, they're not going to come, or they're not going to fill that prescription. And they may tell you, 'Okay,' but they don't follow through. See, that's patients' out. If they don't really like what you're saying, but you're not listening to their objection, then they just simply take the prescription and walk out the door, and miss their next appointment."

"So, how do you figure out what a patient is going to feel comfortable with?"

"Listen to what the patient is saying. Yeah, they'll tell you, if you're willing to be receptive."

"So, you don't feel any kind of commitment to any particular treatment, it's basically whatever the—"

"What do you need? You are an individual. I don't treat you like you're one of a hundred people. You're an individual. What's best for you? Because you're working or going to school. How do I help you have the maximum quality of life when I can't cure you of this disease?" Dr. Davis's response puts him in the category of a "patient-centered" physician, and every adult patient who I spoke with who works with him praises him. At the same time, Davis is not a warm-and-fuzzy physician.

What makes him so respected is his ability to let go of any notion that he is saving his patients. Medicine for him facilitates life, but he does not believe that medical knowledge should determine how one lives his or her life.

"So, what do your patients—"

Anticipating my question, he interjected, "So, we have like hardly anybody, I think we have only one patient on chronic transfusion."

"And, the other ones?"

"And we have a fair number that are on hydroxyurea. But, in our consultative practice we actually advise more patients you don't need hydroxyurea."

Curious, I asked, "What do you tell them? Just take folic acid and drink lots of water and rest . . ."

Continuing to fill the silence, he said, "And, you know, get your proper rest and as soon as you have pain, come in quick so we can be aggressive with the treatment. . . . And then we can try to abort the events, or shorten their duration."

"So, you're like Dr. Benjamin at Montefiore?" Dr. Lennette Benjamin has been at the forefront of the science of pain treatment for sickle cell patients. Her research is cited in *The Management of Sickle Cell Disease*, the National Institutes of Health's evidence-based manual for how to manage sickle cell disease. Instead of treating sickle cell pain as necessarily a symptom of an underlying condition, Dr. Benjamin treats sickle cell pain as the disease. Complications or secondary conditions, she argues, result from poorly managed pain. Her method, therefore, is to treat sickle cell pain aggressively and fast, and the value of her approach is reflected in lowered hospitalization rates and millions of dollars saved at Montefiore Medical Center since the inauguration of the sickle cell day hospital in 1989).[4]

"Yeah. That's the best. Unfortunately, we don't have the proper support to do that perfectly. I think that for a vast majority of patients, that's a much more effective and much better quality-of-life issue."

To push the discussion further, I brought up a case study discussed at a sickle cell association meeting: "It's interesting [at a] pain panel where they were talking about a fourteen-year-old boy who's, you know, he just sounds like a wreck. . . . And he refuses hydroxyurea, and I'm thinking he must still see this future for himself." I was interested in Dr. Davis's response because the nurses and physicians who worked with the patient considered this adolescent to be completely irrational and difficult, and eventually punted him to adult care.

"He has a reason. What's his reason? Nobody listens to him because they're convinced [that they are right]. The trouble with Vichinsky is— at least his public posture, now I don't know what he's like with the patient on a one-on-one interview. . . . The trouble with his public posture is he admits there are no other possibilities. There's only one highway here, and you need to be on it. But I suspect a lot of that is public posture."

Curious about where his limits are in terms of patient-directed care, I asked, "So you think the patient can figure out their own risks?"

"No, no . . . you have to educate them. I see patients that some doctors put them on hydroxyurea and didn't tell them about the pregnancy risk. So, I have to tell them."

"So, if you give them the risk information, then you think the patient's capable of making their own decisions?"

"Yeah, aren't they? You don't have to be a genius to know, okay, you're living this disease, I'm not, all right. You're the one who's in the hospital, you're, you know, dealing with nurses, some of whom are supportive and some of whom treat you like crap, okay. So, is this worth that? Patients can make a value judgment if they have the proper information. You may not *agree* with their value judgments because they may not tell you all of the things that go into their equation."

In contrast to the self-assured Dr. Davis, Dr. Taylor was clearly still trying to figure out how to respond to people who lead unfamiliar lives and how, in the haze of medical uncertainty, to deliver care. Taylor has a somewhat different perspective about his patients and about his role as a physician than Dr. Davis. Given that both interviews demonstrate how deeply social, personal, and political understandings of efficacy are, how does one universalize a treatment protocol?

Dr. Davis, believing that agentive patients choose their own suffering, rejected the notion that doctors should preach the advantages of one therapy over another. But it would be wrong to characterize Davis's approach as free of coercion. He encouraged his adult patients to be as independent of the clinic and hospital as possible and, therefore, discouraged blood transfusion therapy or any therapy that involved large sacrifices of time. Davis retained a fierce loyalty to his ideals, which included increasing patient health care access, but years of experience as a clinician, researcher, and patient advocate tempered his idealism, and now, some would argue, his pragmatism verged on cynicism. He simply did not believe it was his moral duty to save his patients (or families) from themselves, which is how some physicians, particularly pediatricians, approach patient care. Similarly, he did not want his career as a physician to be the sum total of his identity, and he found physicians who talk incessantly about their work overly sincere. At the same time, Davis was one of the foremost specialists in his field. He organized events, conducted research, and ran one of the best adult programs in the country. When I spoke with a number of his patients, they always noted how much they appreciated how he communicates.

At an association meeting in 2004, I interviewed one of Dr. Davis's patients, Martha, who in her late thirties has severe hypertension and requires oxygen. I could not help wondering, if Martha had been on chronic transfusion therapy, would she be healthier? Rather than resent her declining health, Martha expressed no regrets, and she did not ascribe blame to Dr. Davis. During the interview, Martha was sitting next to Ella, who was a very healthy sickle cell patient in her late twenties. Ella, in contrast, was at the meeting to gather information in order to challenge her physician. Ella felt coerced into complying with chronic transfusion therapy. She felt that receiving blood from men or women who were not in their childbearing years, as she was, might be negatively affecting her. Martha and Ella presented a paradox. Martha, who perhaps had reason to suspect the quality of her care, was satisfied whereas Ella, who was extremely healthy and the mother of three children, was completely unsatisfied, even angry.

This interview was clearly anecdotal, and, importantly, Dr. Davis's patients do not seem to have a reduced life expectancy because of how he delegates agency to his patients. Even on an anecdotal level, however, the contrast between Martha and Ella is important because it demonstrates that by embracing medical uncertainty and stepping away from ascribing moral value to patient treatment decisions, Dr. Davis empowers patients. Neither Davis nor his patients can predict where any treatment decision will ultimately lead in terms of health outcomes. What Davis appreciates is that unimaginable suffering for one person is acceptable suffering for another, and legitimate patient empowerment— unfettered health care access and excellent clinical care—removes the issue of blame. Questions about racism, or even reduced life expectancy, lose their salience when patients are able to own their health care choices and are not penalized for those choices.

Ultimately the issue of pain and uncertainty must be addressed, according to both Dr. Taylor and Dr. Davis, in patient socialization. Patients must not only comply with treatment but also must develop a

particular affective response to treatment. Patients receiving hydroxyurea need to accept that the treatment works and then adjust their
response to unanticipated pain accordingly, and patients whose pain
responds differently to the available narcotics must reduce their expectations of biomedicine. Patients and practitioners develop an implicit
treatment contract based on how a physician embraces biotechnology
and what a patient's expectations and hopes for the future are. Each
patient-practitioner dyad nuances their expectations of biomedicine differently. Some physicians want their patients to be as independent of
them as possible, and they encourage their clients to expect less rather
than more of biomedicine. Other physicians want their patients to
follow the latest treatment advice and encourage experimentation in the
hopes that new evidence-based approaches offer the best chance for a
long life. Patients adapt their understandings of their disease and expectations about a pain-free and morbidity-free life based in large part on
how physicians articulate the value of medicine.

The sickle cell community encourages the socialization of patients
into the culture of medicine, but the more typical approach is to educate
physicians about the cultural differences of their patients. Medical students are being trained in what is called cultural competency, which has
been, from the perspective of many who have tried to teach medical students about culture, an abysmal failure. Patients do a much better job
adapting to the culture of medicine than physicians do adapting to a
patient's culture. The culture of medicine is simply so powerful and
hegemonic, that when a patient is considered noncompliant based on
cultural reasons, then those cultural beliefs are cast as irrational.
Cultural competency simply rearticulates the hierarchy between
rational knowledge (medicine) and irrational beliefs (culture).

The problems with how "culture" is deployed instrumentally within
medicine was exemplified in one of the most contentious panels at the
thirtieth-anniversary meeting. A program director from the National
Heart, Lung, and Blood Institute held a discussion entitled "Meeting
the Unmet Needs of Adult Patients with Sickle Cell Disease." She
wanted the audience to develop quantifiable cultural competence scales
and quality-of-life measures. The audience was very cooperative at first,
answering questions about sexuality, rehabilitation services, work, and
personal disruptions caused by the disease. Then the audience began to
introduce personal narratives that strayed from the intended goals of
the group facilitator. One woman described how she refuses to go to
emergency rooms because the last time she went she overheard the

doctor tell another doctor that he thought she was crazy because she was not acting like a patient in pain even though she was claiming to be in pain. She said that if she becomes sick on the weekend, she now waits until Monday to see a hematologist. Another talked about feeling as though his physician undermedicates him. Another talked about Dr. Samir Ballas's article on how patients can feel abandoned by their doctors. Dr. Davis critiqued the direction of the conversation, saying that physicians need incentives to learn about sickle cell disease. The patient population is small, and so it is partly incumbent upon the sickle cell community, he argued, to disseminate information about the disease to physicians. In a somewhat confrontational tone, he said, "Look, where are the incentives to read all these articles on sickle cell disease when you only have two patients?" Some people in the audience were shocked, and the executive director of a regional sickle cell association said in an aside, "I'm glad he's not my doctor." Another member of this association said, "He took the Hippocratic oath. He needs to go." A physician in the audience said, "It saddens me that doctors need incentives. I'm doing it for love." Dr. Davis asked for the microphone, and a woman in the audience said, "Don't give him the microphone," to which another woman replied, "Now, don't attack one of the family."

The NIH program director tried to force the discussion back into developing codes for cultural competence by reiterating, in increasing volume, "What do you want your physician to know?" Again the audience members had a difficult time confining themselves to hackneyed notions of culture that could be represented in variables that could be taught to physicians, who in turn might treat their sickle cell patients better.

The concerns and experiences shared by the audience had very little to do with physician cultural competence. Audience concerns included physician ignorance of the disease and how to treat it, and lack of respect for the patient. For many in the audience, cultural competence is just a euphemism for racial tolerance, and so the attempt to locate treatment disparities in an abstract, quantitative variable identified as "culture" stifled a complex and nuanced discussion of the origins of unequal treatment. The program director continued to try to control the audience with the threat that if they did not cooperate, she would be powerless to help them. She followed up this reprimand with an oft-repeated "I'm on your side." She wanted the audience to realize that unless they could put "quality of life" and "cultural competence" into easy, digestible codes, then the NIH could not develop evidence-based approaches to improving care.

Many scientists within the medical community have essentially disabled themselves from articulating a relationship between health and social justice by relying on endlessly reductive scientific and social scientific data in order to determine their role as health care providers. A piece of data is statistically significant when it obfuscates its relevance to a moral "So what?" question. This means that the impetus behind a study must be naturalized, turned into a simple observation of a biological process, in order to remove any doubt about the legitimacy of the research question. The medical community relies on P values to determine everything from whether to open up a nondenominational prayer space in a hospital to whether chronically ill adolescents should be helped to transition from pediatric to adult care. One result of what I consider an overreliance on statistically significant results is that medical professionals lose sight of the value and meaning of health care as they are forced to prove over and over again that health care should be patient-focused.

Religion confronts death through explicit meaning-making, medicine through cost-benefit analyses embedded with implicit values and meanings. There are benefits to the medical system's reliance on this secular utilitarianism, but it also means that what we are saying about suffering is hidden from view by numbers. Statistically, suffering can be represented as reduced life expectancy, but the number of years one lives is not necessarily an adequate measure of suffering. Members of the sickle cell community have been trying to improve the usefulness of life expectancy by trying to quantify "quality-of-life years," but as I show, the quantitative measures do not mediate the divide between biomedical information and meaning. Using statistics to determine health care policy is a way of debating without articulating a point of view, ultimately sheltering those who use statistics from serious questions about health care's role in social engineering.

Most studies of access construct the patient as a rational actor limited by medical costs and physician availability and responsiveness. Within the literature, the agentive patient is one who utilizes health care in a timely manner, thereby ensuring the best possible health outcome.[5] With the elimination of obstacles to clinic care, patients are assumed to become the willing subjects of proper medical treatments and therapies. Physicians, in this model, treat patients according to understandings of risk taught to them in medical school; then, with the new focus on multiculturalism, the physician steps back from his or her personal biases and allows the patients to make an "informed" decision. Medical professionals with diverse views about suffering and risk are encouraged to suppress their biases in the interest of upholding a patient's right to self-determination.[6] This model of the ideal patient and physician elides issues of power, authority, and uncertainty, and it is this cultureless paradigm of social action that informs the ideal patient-physician collaboration. While I am critical of how narrowly this model defines ethical (read cultural) action, I recognize that embodied in this ethic is a hopefulness that equal health care, or more specifically equal health outcomes, is the next step toward a more enlightened democracy. The question, then, for someone interested in health care access is, Is there room to acknowledge the existence of plural medicines and plural outcomes without blinding ourselves to health care inequality and injustice?

CHAPTER 5

# Uncertain Efficacy

Within medicine, treatment success is couched as efficacy, and efficacy can be articulated a number of ways. For example, doctors can focus on short-term rather than long-term success, or they can prize more medical intervention and a longer life over less medical intervention and a shorter life. In *American Medicine: The Quest for Competence*, Mary-Jo Good reflects on the discourses of efficacy embedded in standards of care. She describes the movements in the 1980s, within the medical community, to manage risk and reduce malpractice lawsuits. Far from being purely rational and scientific, medical standards of care are steeped in cultural ideas about what constitutes health and well-being, which, Good argues, impact the quality and boundaries of health care. "What we conceptualize as good medicine—*what we think medicine should care about*—from the utilization of new biomedical knowledge and techniques to the crafting of therapeutic narratives for patients, has far-reaching consequences for our society's investment in designing, producing, and marketing therapeutics, as well as in the organization of health care."[1]

Given the local variation between the treatment priorities at Children's West and Children's East, I became curious about variations in understandings about sickle cell treatment efficacy at the national level. The areas of greatest uncertainty in medicine, and pain and chronic illness are two, are the places where prejudice, disguised in medical jargon, can flourish. At the national meeting in 2002 marking the thirtieth anniversary of the Sickle Cell Disease Association of America (SCDAA) and the National Sickle Cell Disease Program (NSCDP), the opening forum described earlier dealt with both the advantages and the limitations of the three primary therapies: hydroxyurea (a chemotherapy agent), stem cell transplantation, and blood transfusion. Tensions between various physicians were palpable as advocates of one therapy challenged advocates of other therapies. I was fascinated to learn that what I had observed at two local facilities was just the tip of a larger national debate about what constitutes a life worth living. In their debates over which treatments are better, physicians referred to "quality-of-life years," a measure based on the presumption that we can objectively weigh the value of a life. Again, are we assigning numbers to intangible qualities of life? Poor blacks living in violent inner-city neighborhoods are considered to have a lesser quality of life than people living in stable middle-class and upper-middle-class homes. Does this presumption color perceptions of treatment efficacy and diagnosis? For example, do physicians more often assume that stress is the cause of their black patients' symptoms and therefore reject the efficacy of medical intervention? If so, what are the repercussions? The same could be said about sickle cell patient suffering. Do some medical professionals, including social workers and psychologists, believe that patient pain is affected by the quality of a patient's life? As a result of this assumption, which forms of access to pain medication are sickle cell patients denied based upon their life circumstances?

At the same thirtieth anniversary, I also became intrigued by how money shaped the efficacy debates. The National Institutes of Health influences discourses about patient suffering and treatment efficacy by choosing to fund research into, for example, bone marrow transplantation rather than psychosocial research to study the long-term effects of silent strokes. NIH's power over and influence on local institutions was elegantly elaborated during an interview at Children's Hospital North. CHN's team psychologist Marilyn Trask described how her pediatric facility was forced to absorb adult patients after the local adult program closed in 2000. As a result, the center began to see numerous long-term issues for sickle cell patients and its thinking about treatment priorities shifted.

I visited Trask at her office in a building across the street from the hospital. Trask, in her early forties, is well known in the sickle cell community. At association meetings she has led an effort to bring the scientists together with the social scientists in order to make the scientific

efforts more patient focused and the psychosocial programs more attentive to the science. Describing what her team discovered after the adult
patients joined their center, Trask said, "We were able to get a much
clearer picture of what our interventions and our treatments . . . how
they sort of play out over the course of a person's life. I think the sickle
cell centers around the country tend to be either pediatric or adult
focused whereas our program now is very much focused on both."

Every five years the NIH's National Heart, Lung, and Blood Institute
accepts proposals from sickle cell centers across the United States.
NHLBI funds ten of these programs, which are then designated comprehensive sickle cell centers. The grant is extremely competitive, and in
order to receive the funding, centers must prove that they are equipped
to dispense cutting-edge clinical care. They must also propose novel
research projects, which often require center cooperation in data collection in order to generate what are considered significant results.
Trask's institution, a leading sickle cell center that has been designated a
Comprehensive Sickle Cell Center for more than two decades, proposed
a project based on its new understanding of the relationship between
pediatric care and adult outcomes.

Describing her center's proposal, Trask said, "One of the projects
that we proposed was looking at the adult brain. Basically we're thinking that people are continuing to suffer with subtle brain injury over the
course of their life. Some of the poor outcomes in adulthood are general
organ failure, but also subtle brain injury. So we set up to work with
[our local university] where they'll be doing brain imaging with the
adults."

Trask went on to describe the selection process: "All the centers com-
peted, and only ten were awarded. So, that was the first step that we
actually got the award. And then there's a decision made about the proposed network projects, and in fact [our center director] just asked us to
rank the projects that were proposed so that he can take that information back to another meeting to decide which ones will be the network
projects. So, another [project] is a multicenter bone marrow transplant
study. In fact, that has a higher priority than the adult neuropsych project from the reviewer's perspective, not necessarily from quality of life.
The focus on a cure is certainly the drive of medicine, whereas the focus
on quality of life is a struggle to keep at the forefront." When deciding which research to fund, the NIH articulates which forms of suffering are remediable and which are not, and which ones should take
precedence.

## UNCERTAIN DISCRIMINATION

The NIH's role in setting research priorities goes back to 1972, when sickle cell disease was finally recognized by the U.S. government. Since the Sickle Cell Anemia Control Act of 1972, the NIH has directly and indirectly put more than $1 billion into sickle cell research and treatment. The initial goal was to find a cure for the disease, but more than thirty years later, a cure for the vast majority of patients is not on the horizon. The sickle cell community appreciates the large amounts of funding from the NHLBI, but at the same time individuals in the community wonder if the NIH could do more. There was suspicion among some of my informants that race plays a role in what they perceive as disproportionate funding for other diseases, and many worry that sickle cell disease will never be taken seriously. In fact, some were upset that sickle cell disease was not listed as a targeted illness in Healthy People 2010, the program initiated by President Clinton in 1998 to end racial health disparities. Many of the people in the sickle cell community seem to be of two minds. On the one hand, the average life expectancy for a sickle cell patient has risen from around twenty to around forty-five in the more than thirty years since the NIH began funding the sickle cell program. Based on that success, many believe that levels of funding are adequate. On the other hand, two of the three major treatments for sickle cell disease, hydroxyurea and bone marrow transplantation, were originally designed to treat cancer. The fact that no treatment has ever been produced specifically for sickle cell disease makes some in the community wonder if they are receiving their fair share of research funding, or if funding is being allocated appropriately. Lack of clarity about the value of the various treatments and about the appropriateness of funding levels and priorities has translated into uncertainty about the salience of race or racism in the struggle to improve sickle cell patient access and care.

Given these uncertainties, it is highly unlikely that a sickle cell movement similar to the one in the early 1970s will develop. Keith Wailoo, in an examination of the history of sickle cell disease in the United States, notes the increased attention the disease received on the heels of the Voting Rights Act of 1965. As Wailoo notes, "In the early 1970s, sickle cell anemia had appeared on the national political scene as a case in point of long-ignored 'pain and suffering' among African Americans."[2] In 1972, the disease was the focus of several congressional hearings, and patients were sympathetically portrayed in M.A.S.H., Marcus Welby, M.D., and a television film, A Warm December.[3] The metaphoric connection between social and physical suffering did not emerge spontaneously. For several years prior to the passage of the Sickle Cell Act, the Black Panther Party used sickle cell disease as a symbol of the relationship between institutionalized racism and black suffering. The Black Panther Party successfully tied white redemption for slavery, Jim Crow, lynchings, and racial injustice to a commitment to alleviate the suffering of sickle cell patients. Recognizing the symbolic value of supporting sickle cell research, the Nixon administration shifted funding within the NIH to support a new sickle cell program. Nixon's strategy to increase expenditures for trendy diseases like cancer and sickle cell came at the expense of funding for other diseases such as heart disease.[4]

Nixon's symbolic corrective neither protected him from impeachment nor closed the racial gap in health outcomes. In stark terms, the black:white mortality ratio for males increased from 1.45:1 in 1979 to 1.59:1 by 1998, and for females increased from 1.50:1 in 1979 to 1.52:1 in 1998. On average, whites continue to live about six years longer than blacks. As Levine et al. conclude in "Black-White Inequalities in Mortality and Life Expectancy, 1933–1999: Implications for Healthy People 2010": "Use of the year 2000 standard population produced a poorer prognosis, in part, because it suggests that the US was substantially closer to racial equality in 1945 than it was by the end of the century. In contrast, the data based on the 1940 standard suggests that these racial inequalities were much the same in 1945 and 1998 in the US."

The authors continue by condemning the manipulation of statistics in order to imply that health equity goals set by Healthy People are being met:

> At best, it would be illusory to consider national public health programs a success based on other indicators as long as inequalities in mortality and life expectancy fail to improve. To do so would imply that all indicators are equally important or that it is somehow acceptable for black Americans to die at higher rates or live shorter lives, so long as a sufficient number of positive signals can be obtained from other indicators. Unfortunately, this is how the highlights for the final evaluation of Healthy People 2000 are framed: "At the end of the decade, the most recent data indicate that 68 objectives (21 percent) met the year 2000 targets and an additional 129 (41 percent) showed movement toward the targets. . . ." . . . Both the magnitude of and increases in these "excess" deaths suggest the need for fundamental changes in the ways that medical and public health practitioners are trained, compensated, and evaluated; the need for further research on the translation of prevention studies into practice; and the need for meaningful evaluation of federally funded research in terms of its impact on the inequality trends.[5]

Racial health care disparities have not significantly improved since the Sickle Cell Anemia Control Act of 1972, yet a broad-based social movement equating inadequate health care with social, economic, and political disfranchisement is nowhere to be found. According to a review of more than one hundred recent studies, significant disparities in diagnosis and treatment exist for cardiovascular care, cancer, cerebrovascular disease, renal transplantation, and HIV/AIDS. African Americans carry a higher morbidity and mortality burden for asthma and share a similar diabetes burden with Latinos and Native Americans. Finally, African Americans have reduced access to pain medications, rehabilitative services, mental health services, and maternal and child health care.[6] Two factors contribute to the absence of demands for radical reform: First, blacks are now in positions of power in medicine and in politics, and those who are bothered by the treatment inequities presume that they can reform the system from within. Second, largely symbolic mediating structures mitigate the institutional contradictions of health care and flatten demands for social justice.

One of these mediating structures includes disease lobbies, which since the 1970s have increasingly used congressional testimonies to generate support. These testimonies follow a familiar narrative structure. Advocates evoke the story of Job by casting patients as innocent, powerless, and afflicted by unjust suffering.[7] In this instance the advocacy group puts their faith in democracy and capitalism to redeem their suffering.[8]

Congressional reporter Judith Johnson describes how lobbying groups evoke urgency for their cause. She writes, "Those active in the lobbying efforts include groups which support research on AIDS, heart disease, breast cancer, prostate cancer, Parkinson's disease, Alzheimer's disease, diabetes, and others. Advocacy groups have generated a vast and sometimes confusing array of charts and tables comparing disease-specific research funding with statistics on morbidity, mortality, and health care costs in order to advance the cause of their disease over others."[9]

Kristine Napier, in "The Politics of Pathology," questions the value of disease lobbies given that basic scientific research, rather than research directed toward a specific disease, has produced some of the most significant health care discoveries. Napier notes, "Research on horseshoe crabs produced a way to diagnose life-threatening gram-negative bacterial infections in humans. Snake venom studies led to the development of drugs that save heart attack and stroke victims. A discovery made by dental researchers led to a major treatment advance for diabetes sufferers."[10] Importantly, there is uncertainty about the relationship between the allocation of scientific funding and the efficient amelioration of suffering.

The performative requirements of such lobbying make strident demands for piecemeal reforms and social justice mutually exclusive. During these testimonies, advocates and legislators assume the role of victim or spectator, avoiding at all costs identification as perpetrators. In the 1980s, for example, Act Up bypassed the performative space of Congress and demanded greater public accountability of the Food and Drug Administration (FDA) through civil disobedience. Gay men who initially led Act Up were cast as participants in their own suffering and therefore could not assume the role of Job. Notably, promiscuous gay men and IV drug users do not make good poster subjects. To this day, iconography to sell the value of AIDS research includes children and mothers whom we assume were infected by deceitful spouses or blood transfusions.

While the narratives of suffering, guilt, and blame are easily tied to tropes of good, evil, and American apocalypticism, basically stories we can all relate to, how these public outpourings ultimately affect research funding is more complex.[11] If one uses the number of deaths per year as a criterion, AIDS does receive a disproportionate share of research funding. In a slightly different example, each year there are almost four times as many lung cancer deaths (160,000) as breast cancer deaths (44,000), yet breast cancer research and treatment receives more than twice as much funding ($457.9 million) as lung cancer research ($161.3 million).[12] Is AIDS, which is associated with sex and drugs, given more funding because it is a new epidemic and therefore everyone is at risk, including good-looking gay actors and innocent children? Do we consider lung cancer patients victims of their own bad habit? Do we imagine all breast cancer patients to be young moms struck down in the prime of life? An analysis of news media, health care advocacy, and disease shows that the attention various diseases garner is based on both the population affected and the number of people affected. The authors state that AIDS is the exception: "One of the more consistent findings to emerge from our analyses is that the ratio of black mortality to white mortality tends to be negatively associated with news coverage, a finding that holds true for both the full and the restricted samples. In other words, the greater the disease burden for blacks relative to whites, the less attention allocated to that disease."[13]

Researchers have attempted to find a correlation between media attention, advocacy, and NIH funding but have thus far been unsuccessful. It is clear that disease burden does not correlate with levels of funding, so what criteria are used? In response to two congressional testimonies, the Institute of Medicine (IOM) published a report entitled *Scientific Opportunities and Public Needs: Improving Priority Setting and Public Input at the National Institutes of Health*. The report states that Senate appropriations for specific diseases declined from $785 million in 1993 to $133 million in 1998, although the number of specific items in appropriation bills rose from 193 to 201 in the Senate and from 115 to 150 in the House.[14] This indicates that appropriations were used symbolically to indicate sympathy and support rather than instrumentally to direct the NIH.

The IOM report lists specific criteria used to determine priorities, including "1. scientific quality of the research, 2. potential for scientific progress (the existence of promising pathways and qualified investigators), 3. portfolio diversification along the broad and expanding frontiers of research, and 4. adequate support of infrastructure (human capital, equipment and instrumentation, and facilities)."[15] The problem with this list is that from an outsider's perspective the criteria seem to be controlled more by a powerful group of insiders than by public interests.

In an attempt to find a rational and objective pattern in NIH spending, Gross, Anderson, and Powe in 1999 published a report in which they state that NIH funding correlates with "disability-adjusted life-years."[16] They argue that the burden of disease is not simply the number of people afflicted but the economic costs to society, mortality, prevalence, and incidence. Then they show that the dollars spent by the NIH correlate well with disability-adjusted life-years (DALYs), a measure of number of years of life lost to disability and early death that is calculated by comparing early morbidity and mortality to national life expectancy estimates. But Arthur Kleinman and Joan Kleinman caution in *Social Suffering* that DALYs are a culturally constructed metric: "The index is unable to map cultural, ethnic, and gender differences. Indeed, it assumes homogeneity in the evaluation and response to illness experiences, which belies an enormous amount of anthropological, historical, and clinical evidence of substantial differences in each of these domains."[17] For me, what is interesting about the correlation between NIH funding and DALYs is that our beliefs about unnecessary suffering, viewed in terms of loss of productivity, correlate with what we spend to mitigate that suffering. Put simply, we treat the suffering that bothers us.

Legal scholar Rebecca Dresser in "Government Priorities for Biomedical Research: What Does Justice Require?" asks why NIH funding is related to only one disease burden measure. She concludes the following: (1) The information on the exact relationship between NIH funding and disease burden is inadequate; (2) it is difficult to quantify unfairness given that prior funding and different research opportunities play a role; AIDS, or more specifically research on immunology, falls into that category; (3) the NIH is not the only funding source for medical research; perhaps other sources of funding would explain some of the appropriation choices; and (4) disease burden measures are based on different value judgments about quality of life and whose life is more important. Dresser summarizes her conclusions as follows: "Thus, one's position on the fairness of NIH allocation will to some degree reflect one's position on these values issues. In sum, like the debate over allocating health-care resources, the debate over research priority setting cannot be settled solely by reference to distributive justice considerations."[18] Given all the uncertainty around funding priorities in medicine, questions about whether or not race plays a role in how funds are allocated remain open to myriad interpretations.

The quantitative aspects of distribution remain in question, but qualitatively the introduction of congressional hearings has made some citizens feel that they have the power to shape health care reform, and the sickle cell community has benefited from being able to sell its story of suffering to the public. But is this new form of representation really equalizing the distribution of health care and ensuring access for blacks generally? Or is it simply reproducing health care inequities? Political scientist Murray Edelman, in *The Symbolic Uses of Politics,* describes how political action is both instrumental and expressive. He argues, "The achievement of a political goal by an interested group leads to claims for more of the same kind of benefit and not to contentment. Only through symbolic reassurances that 'the state' recognizes the claims and status of the group as legitimate is quiescence brought about, and the reassurance must be periodically renewed."[19] Rather than promote real health care reform, by which I mean a more equitable distribution of risk and illness, congressional hearings seem to quell radical demands for changes in our health care system. Congressional public theater pits one desperate "disease-of-the-month club" against another as they vie for a greater piece of the $27.9 billion per year NIH pie.[20] The target for reform becomes funding distribution instead of, for example, challenges to pharmaceutical companies that benefit financially from publicly funded research, or challenges to for-profit insurance companies that benefit from limiting access to care.[21]

## BLAME AND RESPONSIBILITY

Besides the question of what research deserves what funding, there is the basic question of what moral responsibility the public has to relieve suffering. For example, basing funding priorities on the number of people who die each year from a disease may be just as ethical as basing funding on social reparations. After all, it is difficult to predict the possible applications of any medical research. So when it comes to choosing between two excellent research proposals, deciding which to fund in order to produce the most benefit for society is, in some respects, a roll of the dice. Sickle cell disease funding is a form of social justice for blacks as breast cancer funding is for women, whose health issues continue to receive less attention than men's.

The largest impediments to disembedding discourses of suffering from health care distribution are American cultural beliefs about sacrifice and free will. To make vast inequalities in wealth consistent with our myth of democratic access to opportunity, wealth and suffering must be woven into self-narratives in order to make personal success palatable. Those born into wealth must be born again through a degree from a prestigious university or service to the community. The baptismal waters of hard work or earnest social contribution cleanse wealth and power from the taint of serendipity or, worse, leisure. As Max Weber demonstrates in *The Protestant Ethic and the Spirit of Capitalism*, those who work efficiently and who are able to accumulate wealth are perceived as having salvation: "In fact, the summum bonum of this ethic, the earning of more and more money, combined with the strict avoidance of all spontaneous enjoyment of life, is above all completely devoid of any eudaemonistic, not to say hedonistic, admixture. It is thought of so purely as an end in itself, that from the point of view of the happiness of, or utility to, the single individual, it appears entirely transcendental and absolutely irrational."[22]

Health care is a form of wealth, and the roles of sacrifice and suffering are just as important with respect to rights to health care as they are with respect to accumulated wealth. Employer-sponsored health insurance was established in Germany in the nineteenth century, but in the United States the first serious attempt to connect health insurance and work began with the drafting of a bill in 1915, during the Progressive

Era. The bill was sponsored by the American Association for Labor Legislation (AALL), an organization of economists who believed that stronger labor laws that buffer workers from income fluctuations ensure worker loyalty. The AALL anticipated that employment security would make workers less likely to call for radical labor reforms.[23] If the bill had passed, it would have required that laborers earning $100 or less per month receive medical care and income protection.[24] It was not until the 1940s that the American Medical Association (AMA) finally conceded to voluntary health insurance amid fears that legislation for compulsory medicine, or socialized medicine, would pass. By 1952, health insurance had been purchased by more than half of the U.S. population; however, the majority of the poor remained uninsured. The president of the AMA justified this class-based health care disparity by arguing: "Since one out of every four persons in the United States has a motor car, one out of two a radio, and since our people find funds available for such substances as liquors and tobacco in amounts almost as great as the total bill for medical care, one cannot but refer to the priorities and to the lack of suitable education which makes people choose to spend their money for such items rather than for the securing of medical care."[25]

After compulsory health insurance lost credibility following the election of Republican Dwight D. Eisenhower in 1952, the president of the AMA noted that the triumph of voluntary over compulsory health insurance meant that the issue of employer-sponsored insurance had been resolved in a "truly American way."[26]

The connection between hard work, temperance, rationality, and the right to health care was clearly established in debates leading up to the institutionalization of voluntary insurance. Even today, one cannot miss these conceptual entanglements. A Web site produced by the Health Research and Educational Trust designed to facilitate data collection on racial and ethnic treatment disparities lists quotations from a November 5, 2003, meeting. Nine members of the National Advisory Panel and Consortium for Eliminating Health Care Disparities through Community are quoted on why they believe collecting race and ethnicity data from patients is a crucial step toward ending health care disparities. One says, "If we have a population where there are a lot of disparities, then that population is not available for the work force. This is not a population that functions well. . . . [This issue is] not just about physical health but about the health of society." Another member is quoted as saying, "The major purchasers of health care are also employers of the diverse working population. If I'm New York City MTA (Metropolitan Transportation Authority), 10 percent of my employees are minority. Then I'm certainly going to want to have a plan that's available to my employees . . . [one] that I know will make sure that they get into work every day."[27] In my own research, I heard a physician mock the parents of his hematology and oncology patients by asking, "Do any of my patients' parents work?" He received gales of laughter for this comment.

Not only are work and insurance important signifiers of one's status as a contributor toward the social good; in the clinic the body becomes an essential metaphor symbolizing the quality of that person's sacrifice and suffering as well. To be physically fit is to be morally fit; to not depend on health care is to be appropriately independent and self-sacrificing. Health care access for the children of the poor and the working poor, Medicaid and the State Children's Health Insurance Program (SCHIP), is more comprehensive because the rights of children are not yet contingent on sacrifice or suffering. But those expectations change as children grow older. In many states, at the age of five children of the working poor lose SCHIP because parent income eligibility requirements change. Through physical fitness, employment, independence, and submission to authority, patients and patient families have some control over how their bodies are read in the clinic, but race, gender, class, and age limit individual agency. Presumptions about lack of intelligence, laziness, degeneracy, and psychosocial dysfunction often persist despite one's best efforts to prove otherwise.[28]

The requirement of patient innocence is particularly noticeable within the less lucrative areas of medicine (e.g., treatment of sickle cell disease) where sympathy translates into resource allocation and health care access. The sickle cell community has used discourses of patient suffering to win congressional support, but that support focuses narrowly on suffering caused by the pathophysiology of the disease. Other types of suffering that contribute to a disproportionate disease burden in the black community have been so flagrantly ignored that the rescue discourses that cast legislators who support sickle cell disease as heroes to the black community can at times seem rather ironic. Getting sickle cell research and treatment on the national health care agenda in 1972 and again in 2003 has without a doubt been beneficial to patients with the disease. But by relying on tropes of patient innocence and victimization, the sickle cell community has not radically changed how Americans conceptualize the relationship between citizenship and health care.

Genocidal discourses that portray individuals as representing extremes of good and evil share features with health care funding discourses that require patients to prove that they are worthy. A health care system that relies on tropes of innocence and victimhood is, I contend, untrustworthy. Everyone is in danger of being cast out of the role of victim, thrust into the role of perpetrator, and ultimately denied health care as one is denied one's humanity in the case of genocide. Sickle cell patients routinely get shut out of care because, particularly in emergency departments, they are cast as contributors to their own suffering. The sickle cell community attempts to rescue them through the deployment of counternarratives, but these counternarratives rely on tropes of patient innocence. One of the ways to recast sickle cell patients as victims is to stress the pathophysiology (biology) of sickle cell pain, the hallmark feature of the disease. Innocence and nature in this case are collapsed and set in stark contrast with the typical association between mind and culture (dysfunction, manipulation, myth, ignorance).

Selling sickle cell pain as entirely natural and beyond the control of the patient works strategically in the policy arena. Within the community, however, practitioners have tremendous doubts about the relationship between the mind and the body when it comes to sickle cell pain. Primarily the community recognizes that treatment choice is a choice between evils. Who suffers more, the twenty-five-year-old patient with unbridled access to powerful opioids who never finished high school and lives in poverty, or the patient who has learned to endure chronic pain and has a full-time job after finishing college? How one answers that question says more about the person providing the answer than about what is or is not real when it comes to suffering.

I did not fully appreciate the uncertainty of suffering until I was well into this project. Having recognized it, I realized that to truly understand health care disparities I had to do something radical and difficult. I had to begin to challenge presumptions about suffering and ask if health care disparities even matter. Why do we presume that a decreased life expectancy means increased suffering? Relatedly, why do we attempt to manage health care disparities within medicine if a life worth living and long life do not necessarily correlate? Why do we believe that groups identified by race, ethnicity, gender, or class deserve the same average life expectancy? Unexpectedly, my research on health care access developed into a study of discourses of suffering embedded in medical discourses, and what that says about how we position ourselves as spectators, participants, and victims of suffering.

## CLINIC CULTURE, HEALTH CARE DISPARITIES, AND THE IMAGINATION

Every physician addresses uncertainties about suffering, race, and medicine according to a personal moral calculus that collapses questions of meaning and disease management. Disease/treatment paradigms at the clinical level are based on particular understandings of the mind-body relationship, the efficacy of treatments, acceptable and unacceptable forms of suffering, the duty of patients and medical professionals to disease management, and a philosophy about what patients should expect in terms of quality of life. By operationalizing a particular treatment protocol, treatment paradigms eradicate medical uncertainty at an institutional level even if privately they still acknowledge medical uncertainty.

Strikingly, in my research the disease/treatment models were not as important to patient health care access, patient outcomes, or a patient's sense of his or her quality of life as was the commitment on the part of a hematologist to providing comprehensive sickle cell care. Whether or not a physician encouraged his or her patients to try to avoid using powerful narcotics, or encouraged chronic transfusion therapies over hydroxyurea, the paradigm was far less important to treatment success than how physicians structurally organized patient care to be consistent with their treatment hermeneutic and how successfully they socialized their patients to manage their disease according to that hermeneutic. In my research there were examples of successful approaches to sickle patient care that differ philosophically and medically; what they all shared was that they were promoted by physicians committed to opening up health care access to patients they believe were deserving of care.

Despite the complexity of my data, my conclusions are fairly straightforward. First, addressing racial health care disparities requires a recognition that suffering in the black community extends well beyond reduced life expectancy. Any serious commitment to ending health care disparities requires significant social investment in prison reform, education, employment, universal health insurance, and the environment. Second, health care funding should go toward comprehensive clinics and treatment centers in poor neighborhoods run by exceptionally well-trained physicians who have a real commitment to improving patient care. Finally, creating national treatment standards using evidence-based medicine represents one approach to care, but statistical significance should not blind health care to the treatment advantages found in alternative medicine or in community-based health associations.

The strategic use of what Hannah Arendt calls the "politics of pity," or how we choose to alleviate natural violence and mitigate suffering, is not an indictment of the groups that manipulate discourses of pity for their own benefit. Medical historian Charles Rosenberg argues that questions about who suffers result from boundary tensions, "that is, the existence of an implicit yet socially meaningful boundary between agency and the guilt-reducing randomness of somatic illness. How much are we responsible for our own pain and suffering? In an era of chronic disease, such questions remain unsettling."[29]

The problem of suffering (or evil) has an important intellectual history dating back to the doctrine of karma, Zoroastrian dualism, Plato (427–347 B.C.E.), and the Old Testament.[30] In terms of karma, anthropologist Gananath Obeyesekere describes the dilemma: "If the gods are powerful enough to ameliorate human suffering, then karma is not the deterministic doctrine it is claimed to be; if karma governs human suffering, then the gods cannot be powerful or capable of subverting it."[31] In the *Timaeus*, Plato describes God as one who created humans with the capacity for good and evil. For those who refuse to live righteously, suffering, Plato argues, is self-inflicted. Following Plato, the philosopher Epicurus (341–270 B.C.E.) posed a trilemma not to disprove the existence of God (or gods) but to consider how to respond to evil. He asked, "Is he [God] willing to prevent evil, but not able? then is he impotent. Is he able, but not willing? then is he malevolent. Is he both able and willing? whence then is evil?"[32] The problem he discovered was not that evil existed and that the gods allowed such suffering, but that evil upsets us.

Religious and philosophical explanations for suffering, or theodicy, took on new importance during the Enlightenment following the publication of Thomas Hobbes's *Leviathan* (1651). The German philosopher Odo Marquand marks the simultaneous rise of life expectancy and the rise of theodicy. When 40 percent of children in Europe died before the age of fifteen and day-to-day survival was in question, one did not have time to question the meaning of suffering. Utilitarianism, for example, which purports that people maximize their happiness, presumes that people have some sense that they can control their destinies and that they will be alive to reap the benefits of delayed gratification. It makes sense that utilitarianism developed in the nineteenth century with the rise of modern medicine and industrialization.

Theodicies are built around particular philosophies of human nature. Enlightenment theorists who considered the role of the state in mitigating suffering similarly employed philosophies about suffering and human nature in order to determine the rights and responsibilities of the state to the people and the people to the state. Religion scholar Mark Larrimore notes in *The Problem of Evil*: "A skeptic and materialist, Hobbes argued that human vulnerability and the uncertainty of all human knowledge make necessary the establishment of states whose sovereigns have virtually unlimited power to set the terms for the lives of their citizens."[33] Social contract theorists including John Locke, Thomas Hobbes, and Jeremy Bentham presumed that people are self-interested and that political order requires balancing the interests of the state against the selfish interests of individuals. Plebiscitary democracy, as espoused by Thomas Jefferson, Jean-Jacques Rousseau, and Thomas Paine, presumes that people are naturally good, and therefore the state does not have to protect itself against the will of the majority.[34]

With respect to our current health care policy, is there a consistent philosophy about the role of the state in mitigating suffering? The government at a superficial level protects the public from pharmaceutical companies selling ineffective or unsafe drugs, but it allows these companies to price effective drugs out of the reach of those who need them. Pharmaceutical companies are also given permission to usurp the oversight authority of the FDA because they have the right to test the efficacy and dangers of their own drugs. Similarly, insurance companies are regulated to some extent, but they are free to drop clients in order to maximize their profits. Finally, the government allows individuals to assume risk by not purchasing insurance under the utilitarian notion that people act rationally to maximize their happiness, but it requires hospitals to accept emergency admits. Thousands of policy choices are built around how we identify the victims, perpetrators, and spectators of suffering, but there is no consistency. It seems that our health care policy borrows from utilitarianism, Jeffersonian democracy theory, even Plato: a self-serving compilation of theories dragged into service to bolster one interest group or another. For example, our democracy rejects Hobbes's belief about the authoritarian state, but increasingly we are giving insurance companies the power to determine how we suffer.

Reviewing the literature on suffering and the role of the state, I have been able to identify a piece of the racial health care disparities puzzle. Theodicies shape health care agendas and treatment protocols. This market/public good calculus can be unsettling when the balance tips toward protecting markets and the public is forced to witness suffering at the hands of unsympathetic insurance companies and money-hungry hospitals. Michael Moore's documentary film *Sicko,* for example, intensified the debate around universal health care because it provided the public an opportunity to witness how health insurance causes suffering. Congressional testimonies similarly are meant to tip public sympathy away from protecting markets and systems and toward protecting individuals.

Utilitarians James Mill and his son John Stuart Mill recognized that moral reform of the rich and free education for all were necessary correctives to a system that could become, as the originator of utilitarianism, Jeremy Bentham, hoped and others feared, a panopticon, with the powerless caught in the controlling web of the powerful.[35] Like schooling which contributes to the circulation of the elite, discourses of suffering act as a corrective to a health care system that might otherwise be built around an almost completely self-interested market calculus. The result, unfortunately, is piecemeal, disease-of-the-week reform that only confuses the relationship between health care, health, and social justice.

What I consider the reactionary discourses of the politics of pity ("Invest research dollars into this disease because look at how my loved one has suffered") stand in as an answer to the "so what?" question. Because these discourses of blame are often decontextualized, they are insufficient to address the complexities of suffering. The most significant insufficiency is the lack of acknowledgment that people die, that suffering is subjective, and that putting more resources toward medicine, research, tests, and drugs is not always the most effective way to ameliorate suffering.

My concern is that entities controlling perceptions of suffering are also controlling access to health care. Imagine if the decision to educate children required a consensus about whether or not a particular group of children deserved an education. In a community forum, a person might argue, "Well, her parents want her to have an education." Another might respond, "But her parents are so poor they don't pay taxes, so does she deserve an education?" The right to an education is guaranteed, which takes the issue of access off the table, but as many readers will note, the quality of that education is tied to local taxes and parental income. For many, worthiness as a criterion for determining which children should receive a quality education seems as absurd as using suffering as a criterion for determining access to health care. Nevertheless, health care practitioners who work in less lucrative fields must employ the politics of pity in order to beg for research and treatment funding. The sickle cell community, which effectively employed the politics of pity in the early 1970s, continues to have to deploy discourses of suffering to receive adequate funding for the disease. But, I argue, disparities in health care will not be eliminated by the use of the politics of pity because these counterdiscourses have a flip side. By naming who suffers, who does not, and who is to blame, they are built on the same logics as genocidal discourses. While most of the discourses of suffering never develop into genocidal discourses, they blind people to the suffering of others by claiming that one group's victimization is more significant, profound, and worthy of concern than another group's. So, is there a way to improve health care outcomes without naming suffering yet still remain attentive to unequal treatment and health disparities? This was the question I was left with after discovering that the discourses of suffering that drew me into this study of sickle cell disease were strategic rather than revolutionary. Ultimately, I chose to abandon the comfort of my presuppositions about racial health disparities in order to be attentive to how these discourses engaged issues of rights, states, and what it means to be human.

CHAPTER 6

# Uncertain Suffering

The issue for me was the value of morality. . . . The issue was,
strangely enough, the value of the "unegoistic" instincts,
the instincts of pity, self-denial, and self-sacrifice which
Schopenhauer had so persistently painted in golden colours,
deified and etheralised, that eventually they appeared to him,
as if were, high and dry, as "intrinsic values in themselves,"
on the strength of which he uttered both to life and to
himself his own negation. But against *these* very instincts,
there voiced itself in my soul a more and more fundamental
mistrust, a skepticism that dug ever deeper and deeper: and
in this very instinct I saw the great danger of mankind, its
most sublime temptation and seduction—seduction to what?
to nothingness? . . . I realised that the morality of pity which
spread wider and wider, and whose grip infected even
philosophers with its disease, was the most sinister symptom
of our modern European civilization.

Friedrich Nietzsche, The Genealogy of Morals

Stepping outside of entrenched narratives of suffering and social responsibility, as philosopher Friedrich Nietzsche (1844–1900) did, is radical
and threatening. For disease advocacy groups, including the sickle cell
disease community, withholding pity for patients is considered heartless
and unscrupulous. Besides placing a social burden on the spectators of
suffering, standard narratives of suffering offer patients a way to identify with their disease, and help determine the objects to be studied and
treated. On the other hand, they also harden our gaze and limit our ability to recognize the diverse and complex origins of suffering. *Unequal
Treatment,* for example, does an excellent job proving that racial disparities in health care access and health outcomes exist, but it deals only
superficially with the question of why racial health care disparities persist.[1] Part of the reason, I believe, is that the available statistical data are
complex and often contradictory. For example, the statistical data show
that blacks are less likely to be referred for cardiac catheterization by
both white and black doctors.[2] Does that mean that racism is or is not

a factor? Perhaps white patients are overtreated? The literature on racial health disparities is fraught with such conceptual dead ends, making it difficult to articulate anything definitive about who or what is to blame. I was finally able to begin to understand the origins of the disparities after changing my question slightly. Instead of asking, Why do racial health disparities exist? I began to ask, Why does the black body continue to be treated as less capable of suffering and more capable of causing suffering?

This question demanded that I look beyond health care disparities to education, where there is a racial achievement gap; to income and wealth, where disparities by race persist; and to imprisonment, where the rates of incarceration for blacks far surpass those for any other group. The issue of disparities in medical care is thought to matter differently in the medical setting because it is assumed that sick people are victims of disease and therefore are thought to suffer. Or are they?

Ideas about suffering are culturally constructed, thereby providing an interesting site for anthropological study. Culturally accepted notions of who is a victim and who suffers are not stable across time. Conceptualizations of suffering are dependent on notions of causation, accountability, innocence, agency, rationality, and selfhood, all of which change relative to the age, race, wealth, gender, and assumed intelligence of the sufferer. This of course means that recasting sick people not as victims but as perpetrators is a possible strategy for denying them care. Because the identification of who suffers is always contested, the sickle cell community (particularly the medical professionals, advocates, patients, and families who attend sickle cell association or NIH meetings) must continually recast sickle cell patient suffering in order to make its elimination seem meaningful and relevant to the public interest.

Eva, who was introduced at the beginning of the book, revealed during an interview the problems with hegemonic social constructions of suffering. The hallmark feature of sickle cell disease is pain, which is caused by microvascular occlusions, or veins blocked by sticky sickle-shaped blood cells that cut off the flow of oxygen to parts of the body.[3] The result is hypoxia (oxygen deprivation) and painful tissue damage affecting major organs. Hospitals, drug companies, and many researchers focus on the elimination of patient pain because physical pain and suffering are conceptually entangled. While pain can cause suffering, Eva shows that pain is not easily reducible to suffering. As Eva explained in our interview, "Before I got sick, my mom came to Dr. Flannery and Dr. Koan—Dr. Koan is my nephrologist—and she was saying how she

wanted to keep me [in the hospital], wanted me to have a kidney transplant and wanted me to have a bone marrow transplant. And they're
like, 'Well, she's not really at that state that she would need a kidney
transplant.' This was before they were thinking about it. And then
everything happened and I needed one anyway so. . . . But, the bone
marrow transplant, I was never really big on that. I don't know, it's like
. . . I wouldn't know what to do. I just think it's weird not to have pain
anymore. You know, not to have sickle cell anymore. I just . . . it's not
like . . . it's like I don't want it . . . not to have pain anymore, but it
would just be like . . . I've had it for like . . . twenty years, and straight
through for all . . . like . . . I don't know, constantly for like eight years,
so it would just seem really weird, if anything if just . . . you know, I
don't know how to explain it, it just seems weird, so . . ."

Pressing Eva, I asked, "Could it be because of identity, you know, like
it's part of your identity?"

Not convinced that identity is the proper way to describe what she
feels, Eva corrected me, "Yeah, it's like . . . I'm not saying I'm not anybody without the pain, but it's just like . . . to go on with not feeling
anything, which would be good, it would just feel weird not to have it
part of me anymore."

When I told Mr. Jefferson, Eva's social worker, that I had interviewed
an adolescent (I did not mention her by name) who identified with her
pain, his response was, "Secondary gain." The concept of secondary
gain in medicine was introduced by sociologist Talcott Parsons in the
1950s.[4] Secondary gain, which many health care professionals would
say includes identification with pain, is behavior used to hide a hidden
agenda, which could include seeking advantages or drawing attention to
oneself. From Mr. Jefferson's perspective, Eva derives utility from being
in pain, namely, attention from family members and practitioners.

Because 90 percent of sickle cell patient hospital admissions are for
painful episodes and because there are only surrogate measures for
determining if a patient is truly in pain (e.g., blood pressure), much of
the care for sickle cell patients involves issues of trust. Many practitioners doubt that their patients are in severe enough pain to require strong
opioids.[5] As a result, medical practitioners try to block what they consider unwarranted access to powerful narcotics, but to do so requires
constructing artificial paradigms of patient suffering. The paradigms
used by the sickle cell team mirror the psychiatric classifications that
position suffering as either psychogenic (hysteria, pseudosuffering),
somatogenic (of uncertain somatic origin), pathophysiological (biological

with certain origins), or sociogenic (a socially constructed disease with
a number of potential origins).[6] Using these paradigms, they then construct treatment protocols accordingly. But what if there are no clear
divisions between any of these paradigms of suffering? What if Eva
simply accepts her suffering as a facet of her existence, something
unclassifiable?

Secondary gain as a concept presumes that for sickle cell patients
there is no uncertainty with respect to pain. Patients are somehow supposed to know when a symptom indicates something dire or something
minor. Clearly this is not the case. Ninety percent of painful crises are
managed by patients at home, which means that patients access health
care when they "feel" a crisis is more severe than normal.[7] If a patient
accesses the emergency room and it is discovered that the crisis is not
urgent, she is given the message, similar to Eva, that she should be more
independent, more stoic in the face of a chronic illness. To turn refusal
to access health care into a rational choice, patient articulations of suffering are reduced to cost-benefit analyses. I asked Eva's mother, Flora,
why she encouraged Eva to manage her pain at home. "Did you ever
worry about her being labeled a 'frequent flier,' or . . ."

Flora responded, "No, I never thought about that because up until
she started going through [her crises] we never went. No, my concern
now, maybe it shouldn't be, but my fear after was like, 'Oh, my God!
What is my employer going to say? How is all this going to impact on
my insurance coverage?' I was afraid that I might lose my coverage
because of that. It was a concern. Or, then, you know, you would be
labeled as if you are using up everybody else's resources. You know those
things. And they still bother me, and I wish that I didn't have to use the
facility or the insurance coverage. But hopefully [laughs] the costs will
keep on decreasing."

Secondary gain is translated as health care overutilization, and by
articulating pain's utility, the health care system constructs a wasteful
object in need of reform. Eva is of course in need of reform, not the
system, because Eva's identification with her pain is ultimately wasteful.
In the long run it generally costs more to maintain a patient on chronic
transfusion therapy than to pay for a successful or unsuccessful bone
marrow transplant.

Secondary gain reinforces the idea that patients are emotional and
willful whereas practitioners are rational. It presumes that there are
rational desires, and identifying with one's pain or developing emotional
dependence on health care providers is irrational. In opposition, saving

lives, being a hero, and being beloved by one's patients and colleagues are never described as a practitioner's secondary gain.

Eva's identification with her suffering is not, I argue, reducible to quantifiable objects that need to be targeted administratively. Rather, Eva's identification helps her make sense of the medical uncertainties: uncertainty about lethal versus nonlethal pain, about what forms of intervention lead to what outcomes, about what she should and should not endure given her rights to health care and health care's claims to alleviate suffering. Articulating distinctions between real (rational) and imagined (irrational) suffering is a method for assigning blame. Real suffering can be quantified through blood cell counts and X-rays; imagined suffering results from poor patient choices and psychological problems. Through these distinctions, responsibility is assigned, and when the patient is held blameless, access to biomedical care is made available.

Linking Eva's identification with her pain to a secondary need for either attention or advantage represents a functionalist interpretation of the relationship between suffering and idioms of distress. Functionalism and structural-functionalism are approaches to studying culture that attribute behaviors, rituals, institutions, and ideas to enhanced well-being. Using these paradigms of social action, an ethnographer's job is to explain how a seemingly bizarre rite or practice enhances survival for the individual and/or the maintenance of the social system.[8] While functionalist explanations make sense at one level, we do things because they work, they are reductionistic—because we do things, they necessarily enhance our survival. There are in fact many cultural practices and beliefs that enhance our survival (the Protestant work ethic) or that are neither beneficial nor deleterious (singing in the shower), and then there are some that are detrimental (suttee, or a Hindu woman throwing herself on her husband's funeral pyre). Functionalist explanations, like secondary gain, reduce suffering to scientific classifications and moral judgments and, according to Nietzsche, contribute to a psychological state of nihilism: "The feeling of valuelessness was reached with the realization that the overall character of existence may not be interpreted by means of the concept of 'aim,' the concept of 'unity,' or the concept of 'truth.' Existence has no goal or end; any comprehensive unity in the plurality of events is lacking: the character of existence is not 'true,' is *false*."[9]

What I find particularly compelling in Eva's attempt to describe her relationship to pain is that she lacks, and culturally we lack, a language for expressing her form of suffering. Elaine Scarry, in *The Body in*

*Pain: The Making and Unmaking of the World,* describes the importance of finding a language to articulate pain. She describes the value of a *language of agency,* or verbal strategy, which allows people in pain to make their world, to name their suffering, and possibly to overcome their pain. Rather than describing language as solely a tool of self-empowerment, Scarry addresses the political potential of the language of agency:

> But we will also see that this verbal sign is so inherently unstable that when not carefully controlled (as it is in the contexts just cited) it can have different effects and can even be intentionally enlisted for the opposite purposes, invoked not to coax pain into visibility but to push it into further invisibility, invoked not to assist in the elimination of pain but to assist in its infliction, invoked not to extend culture (as happens in medicine, law, and art) but to dismantle that culture. . . . the two uses are not simply distinct but mutually exclusive; in fact we will see that one of the central tasks of civilization is to stabilize this most elementary sign.[10]

Although I agree with Scarry that a language of pain can be very political, I disagree with her characterization of this binary. In the case of sickle cell pain, language that makes some types of pain visible inadvertently, or advertently, foists other types of pain into invisibility. To cast one language of agency as benign and the other as sadistic is to open the floodgates for assigning the label of sadist to countless medical professionals who in randomized studies have been shown to diminish the pain of their African American patients. In the case of sickle cell pain, the language of agency embedded in treatment paradigms is framed by the language of goodness and rationality. Pain that does not respond to these treatment strategies is cast as psychopathological rather than real, making the sign, pain, an entirely unstable referent. This new language of agency, embedded in pain treatment paradigms, makes other languages, like Eva's identification with her pain, suspect and subject to ridicule or erasure. Research dollars and the allocation of resources are predicated on presumptions about suffering, but what if for Eva social isolation causes more suffering? What if for another patient poverty causes more suffering? What is at stake for the health care system when Eva identifies with an alternative view of suffering?

Two months after our initial interview, Eva received a kidney transplant. It turns out that her kidney problems were caused by sclerosis, or hardening of the kidneys. Her condition initially might have been caused by a sickle cell crisis. Or perhaps not. The medical causes of her suffering are less a concern to her than the existential questions and emotional turmoil. In an interview following her transplant, Eva revealed why secondary gain inadequately explained her identification with her suffering, which she herself realized had no comprehensive unity: "I think I'm happier now than I was throughout the initial turmoil. I'm more emotional than anything else. I just didn't know how to deal with it when I was younger because you have to blame somebody, and I blamed God for years. And I turned my back on him for a long time. So it's like, you're angry and you see what this is doing to your family because my mom, she still blames herself and she shouldn't blame herself. She didn't make the disease, you know? Because she's a nurse, and she knows what sickle cell is, and she knows that they were taking a chance, my dad and my mom, because they both knew that they had the trait. I don't blame them. I mean, she wonders if she should have had an abortion and stuff like that. And that made me even more angry toward God to even, like, let this happen in the first place. So, I had a lot of issues.

"I don't even remember what the turning point was, but I didn't hate him anymore. At first, I was depressed and angry, but then I got rid of the anger and there was still depression, and I still acknowledged him as being there and everything, but it was like, I was still sitting, I thought alone. And I think that the high school thing affected me a lot because you don't have that group of friends. I mean, I only had my church and my family and that was it. Which isn't bad or anything, but you still want what normal people, quote unquote have. So, um . . . I'm really not stressing out as much as I did before. I mean, if all of this happened when I was sixteen, it would be a different story and I would be a different person. But, since I've gone through all of this, and I've accepted all of the scars on my body and everything, it's just like . . . not even like I'm dealing with it, I'm just, going through life and happy down the line. I mean, I couldn't say that when I was younger because I was still angry and people would say, 'Well, you would have it worse somewhere else, you have to remember about that.' I used to be really selfish, like, 'Well, that's not helping me any.' I'm still going through this. Now it's, like, I acknowledge the pain and everything, but I can't let it consume me." Eva demonstrates that her physical suffering is only a small part of her overall suffering. To reduce her identification with her pain to secondary gain misses the fact that often with suffering there is no one and nothing to blame.

Regardless of the uncertainty of suffering, medical ethicists often try to locate a source of blame. Ethicist Ronald Green, for example, in "Parental Autonomy and the Obligation Not to Harm One's Child Genetically," argues against the completely value-neutral and nondirective approach to genetic counseling for a pregnant woman. He says,

"Whatever the outcome of these debates, emerging knowledge of genetics has recently raised a new possibility: that parents may be in a position to use genetic information in ways that not only have nothing to do with the prevention or cure of disease but also actively involve the infliction of harm or suffering on their child."[11] New medical discoveries, in this case genes linked to disability, have, for Green, changed what constitutes intentional infliction of suffering and ethical social action. Disagreeing with Green, disability rights ethicists reject the assumption that living with a disability constitutes suffering, and that, viewed over the course of a lifetime, suffering is the cost of being human.[12]

In a marvelous examination of what is described as "the disability paradox," Peter Ubel et al. show that people, whether sick, disabled, or recent winners of the lottery, report markedly similar levels of happiness.[13] The disability paradox has been described as the phenomenon in which people in poor health report levels of happiness that are much higher than a healthy person would predict.[14] We can attribute some of this paradox to scale recalibration, or the idea that people judge their quality of life relative to what, given their situation, represents optimal health. That means that if you have sickle cell disease, you may not expect to be in perfect health; therefore, when someone asks you to evaluate your level of happiness, you adjust the scale. Ubel et al. found, however, that scale recalibration did not fundamentally alter quality-of-life ratings. There were other confounders such as recall bias ("Aren't I happier now?") and conversational context (how quality-of-life questions are framed). Regardless, when the researchers studied the moods of patients throughout the day, moment by moment, the reported levels of happiness were almost indistinguishable from those of healthy people.

The disability paradox challenges the underlying logic of utilitarianism or the idea that people act rationally to maximize their happiness. According to this research, regardless of the outcome of any action, people believe that they have acted rationally to maximize their happiness. Anthropologists are well aware of how adaptable people are to their cultural and physical environments. Cultural relativism as an approach to studying various cultures presumes that people have the capacity to find meaning and value in practices as diverse as circumcision and monster truck rallies, and in environments as diverse as the Kalahari Desert and the Ituri Forest.[15] Similarly, people who are sick and/or in pain find ways to make sense of their physical state, and given the proper tools and a particular disposition, one can turn possible adversity into, in Eva's case, a hopeful future. This ability to adapt is at the heart of the disabilities rights movement, which challenges the idea that normative physical states determine well-being.[16] The disability paradox highlights the fact that objectifying suffering by locating a cause and a solution is a political act.[17]

Three years and three months after we first met, Eva and I reunited at her home the day after Independence Day. She was living with her parents in their quiet black middle-class neighborhood of single-family homes. Her two-story home was organized to accommodate four grown children and two parents. The living room was divided by couches, chairs, and desks into spaces that provide the user a modicum of privacy. If the goal of this arrangement was to increase family harmony, it worked. Eva and her siblings were extremely close, and her parents seemed in no hurry for them to leave. I was greeted by Eva's mother, Flora, who was sweating from housework. She was larger and darker than I imagined given Eva's lithe frame and light complexion. Flora is from Nigeria, and despite living in the United States for more than two decades, she has retained a fairly thick accent. Eva and I spoke alone for about an hour before Flora joined us.

Eva looked good. She was still thin and had a steroid-induced moon-shaped face, but she had a spring in her step. I had seen her at Camp Freedom, a weekend retreat for children and adolescents with sickle cell disease, the previous summer. She was a counselor, and although she told me she managed to get straight As again during the spring term, she had seemed tired that summer. She said that she was amazed that she had done so well given how sick she had been. This summer was different.

When we met, she had recently started dreading her hair, and she had a container of holding wax in her hand when I entered the living room. She had a boyfriend, Ray, who wore his hair in dreadlocks for spiritual reasons. Ray was a vegetarian and had a Web site devoted to black empowerment through knowledge. On the Web site he debunked what he believed were historical distortions of Africa and Christianity. Eva found Ray's approach to the body, health, black empowerment, and spirituality refreshing. Ray, who earned his living as an artist painting T-shirts at various tourist sites along the eastern seaboard, was the epitome of the new black bohemian. Eva's father, who received a degree from Princeton Theological Seminary, appreciated Ray's intellect but was challenged by his critiques of Christianity.

Ever since Eva was young, her father had been concerned about his children's success. At one point he took a job in New York, but when Eva's grades started to slip, he quit his job to stay home to help her.

He assumed responsibility for the domestic chores and child rearing while his wife continued to work as a nurse. It did not surprise Eva, therefore, that her father worried about her future financial stability. Her father's disapproval did not, however, dampen Eva's interest in Ray, who seemed to be opening Eva's world. Ray, who was in his thirties, also had sickle cell disease but was not as seriously affected by it as Eva.

I interviewed Eva in order to understand how school, family, and Ray fit into her perceptions about herself, her disease, her suffering, and her future. Smiling, Eva said, "I'm taking two philosophy courses, a religion course, business ethics, biomedical ethics, and intro to the Bible. Because my minors are philosophy and religion, I'm trying to get my minor done. Then I'll just have the fall semester and that's it."

Excited for her, I said enthusiastically, "Then you graduate!"

Eva laughed. "I'm gonna get a job. I need benefits, so that's what I'm doing now."

For the record I asked, "Your health is being taken care of by the state, right?"

Anxious to clarify, Eva replied, "Oh, the health care and everything? Yeah, but it's been three years, so I'm waiting on them to give me some type of paperwork or something because Mr. Jefferson said that they're supposed to, like, go over my case and see if I'm still clinically disabled. Since I've gotten the kidney transplant they will probably say that I'm not, but since I'm on apheresis . . ." Apheresis is chronic blood transfusion therapy that required Eva to visit the hospital every three weeks. The treatment differs from regular blood transfusion therapy in that the iron has been taken out of the blood prior to being transfused. Referring to the sickle cell team she works with at Children's East, Eva added, "They said that there might be a chance that I'll keep my benefits. They don't know, so . . ." After speaking quickly, Eva trailed off, not knowing what to add.

Wondering how a chronically ill young adult manages to pay for medications, I asked, "The antirejection medication is how much?"

"I don't even know. I think it's like $250 [per month], but I don't know if that's everything. I might be wrong, so . . ." Even Eva, who was very mature and in many ways very independent, was sheltered from the financial aspects of disease management.

Wanting Eva to clarify the law, I asked, "So they count you as not disabled three years after you get your transplant?"

More proud of how long she has survived the transplant than concerned about her changing status, she stated, "It's been three years this June. June 16 was the date."

Picking up on her pride, I asked, "What is it like after three years?"

"It's good . . . I mean, I've been going through my ups and downs and everything since January, when they first put in the port for the apheresis." Before January, Eva had received transfusions every four to five weeks for years, and they had been helping. Eva was very sensitive to increased levels of iron in her blood, and so for the first two days after her transfusions she would feel sick, but after that her energy would return. By the winter of 2003, she was no longer able to recover from the transfusions; as she described it, she felt as though the iron was causing tremendous pressure in her head. She said that in a meeting between her mother and Dr. Ross they discussed the fact that they were running out of options and decided to put in a permanent port, or what LaTasha called a "line." Because Eva had very few remaining accessible veins, she has had a port put in place so that every three or four weeks she can receive blood in which the iron is removed before it is transfused. Ports work well for cancer patients or patients with acute diseases that require extensive treatment, but they are delicate and can easily become blocked and infected. For chronic patients, ports are stopgaps.

Similar to LaTasha, Eva has had to have her port replaced. She explained, "The first one didn't work, so that was stressful. I had to have another surgery in February. This one has been working. I'm feeling much better, but um . . . time . . . time line memory is bad. I was in the hospital in February. I went into septic shock. There was something wrong with my kidney. I had an infection. I didn't want to go to the hospital, I thought I was just feeling, you know. . . . But it was like one in the morning when I was really sick. I felt cold and I felt feverish and everything, so my boyfriend came and got me and took me to the hospital. They said that I almost died and everything. But, I mean, I don't know because I was still conscious and talking. They said that my fever was like 105. So after that scare, everything started getting better. Dr. Ross said my bone marrow shut down, and that made the S count go down, so now I'm not having any more pain. I mean, it's been ten years basically that I've been in pain and then, maybe eight years since I've been in constant pain. Now that's all gone, and it's been like a real blessing and at the same time a weird adjustment because I haven't felt like this since I was thirteen. So it's been very interesting. Really good . . . really good."

Excited for her and curious about what happened, I inquired further, "So, your bone marrow stopped producing S hemoglobin?"

"Yeah, when I had the septic shock it shut down, and Dr. Ross said that the levels went down. So even after I got out of the hospital I felt better. I was really weak, but I didn't have any pain. Then I guess the transfusions are helping that, so. . . . And now they're also taking off the iron, so I'm feeling a lot better."

Eva now could describe the absence of pain: "I have so much energy compared to before, you know. Also, your mood is different of course. You're not in pain all the time. I don't have any words to describe it because it's completely different and it's . . . I don't even know. It's changed a lot. I've changed a lot. So I'm happy about that." While she was fearful about intervening to end her pain, the accidental side effects of a near-death experience were a welcome relief.

She also attributed her healthy new regimens to her improved health. "I started taking steps to strengthen myself like emotionally and spiritually back in December when I started fasting and things like that. I slowly started getting off food, so now I don't eat meat anymore. That's also helped my system, especially medications that I used to be on. Now, I'm taking more vitamins than actual medications prescribed by doctors."

Wondering how her physicians felt about her taking control over her treatment decisions, I asked, "Is that by choice, by your choice?"

"Yeah."

"But they would prefer you took more medicine. . . ."

"No, I mean . . . Well, the stuff that I am on, the immunosuppressants, I can't get off of that. I'm still taking penicillin, and stuff like that. But, I had migraines. Like, constant migraines all the time. The neurologist had me on two medications, and they weren't doing anything. I mean, the pain was constantly there, but it was just numbed. But, still, you know, nothing could stop it once a real attack came through, so a friend of mine suggested I should take ginkgo biloba, so I started doing that. And for the first time in years I actually had no headaches, and I could deal with the light and sounds. After that I was still on their medication, and I slowly started to get off of it. When I was going to go in for a refill and they said that I should come in and see the doctor, and I'm, like, why are you refilling this when I'm feeling so much better. I didn't want to be on medications anyway, so I stopped taking it, and I'm fine. So, I called him and left a message saying I'm not taking medications anymore."

"And what else did you take yourself off of?"

"Basically, that was it. I took myself off of the Tylenol. That was one of the things that I had for my headaches. First nephrology put me on that for my blood pressure. Then they said that I don't have to take that anymore, but then the neurologist kept me on it for my headaches. So just those two."

Trying to determine the relationship between suffering and the self, I asked, "When the pain disappeared, did it change your goals or your sense of how much future you have and what kind of future you have? Or did that really not change and you're still . . ."

"I'm still determined, but I guess it changed my outlook. I guess I'm more positive now than I was before. Like I still did what I had to do, and I wouldn't let anything stop me, but I was still in a depressed state, I think. I'm more positive, there's more I can do. I can do anything, so . . ." In Eva's case suffering did not change her basic ambitions but only limited the speed of her accomplishments.

Asking her to speak to the disability paradox, I commented, "It's interesting, though, because when you were in pain, you were getting straight As, you were going to school, you were planning your future . . ."

"Yeah, I'm still doing that. This last year was really crazy because of, you know, almost dying, the two surgeries, very stressful but I still came out with As. . . . I still look back at stuff like that, I'm like amazed and, you know, humbled by all of it because I don't even know how I got through all that stuff. And, trying to concentrate with the headaches and . . ."

"Yeah, how do you do it?"

"I . . . I can't even . . . tell you. . . ."

"You're smart, that helps."

"Yeah . . . I just did what I had to do. But no, I mean, with the headaches and everything, there wasn't much that I could do. We used to keep blankets on our windows to keep out the light, or . . . There wasn't anything that really I could take that helped with the headaches. So, I just had to deal with it. There wasn't anything really that I *could* do."

Eva's description of her powerlessness in the face of illness was interesting to me because it meant that she had to find ways to be agentive that did not involve fixing the problem. Therefore, I added, "It's interesting because somebody like me, who's never had to deal with a chronic illness, or life-or-death situations, or pain. I don't know how you do it. And for you, it's probably just your life. So, you know, how do you describe your life?"

"I mean, there's just a very big family structure, and there were people at church who helped me. I guess just my faith. Even though sometimes I just resign myself, 'Well, this is how it is, and this is how it's always going to be.' But, it changed, so . . ."

"It's interesting because in our first conversation, you were talking about a bone marrow transplant and you were saying that you didn't really think that that was for you. And you were saying that it's hard to explain, but you were saying that 'pain is so much a part of who I am.'"

"Yeah, I felt like that. I couldn't imagine this, how I am now. I couldn't imagine not being in pain or how that would feel because I couldn't remember how it felt to not be in pain. When they were talking about bone marrow transplants and not having sickle cell anymore, it just seemed like, it was just a weird concept of not having to deal with it. I didn't know how to . . . I don't know. . . . I didn't know how to react to that."

"Looking back, do you think that you would have gotten one, though, if you could have?"

"I think I was too old also, but at that time they were saying it was getting more dangerous because I was getting older. So the thought of those types of things that scare me or whatever, but . . . I probably would have. I probably would have. Probably more because my parents, or my mom, wanted me to do it than me wanting to do it."

Many medical decisions are based on submission to authority, whether a physician, parent, or normative social values. As we see in the case of Eva, her decision to have a bone marrow transplant would not have been her own but her parents'. She did not view a transplant as the key to ending her suffering.

## DISCOURSES OF SUFFERING AND DISEASE ADVOCACY

Suffering can be described as individual but inarticulable, and as articulable but culturally elaborated. The first form is individual suffering, which is unquantifiable and incomparable. Most sickle cell patients would claim that their disease causes them to suffer but in very different ways, just as poverty or experiences of tragedy cause incommensurate suffering. It is a reasonable question to ask whether people suffer before they have articulated the objects of their suffering, a question situated squarely in the linguistic debate over whether consciousness precedes language. I believe that they do, but because power shapes discourses of suffering, some suffering is poorly conceptualized, or even denied, while other forms of suffering are hypercognized and culturally authorized.

The second form of suffering is collective, by which I mean it is how people articulate their suffering through language and culture.[18] Philosopher Owsei Temkin organizes diseases into similar categories:

ontological and physiological. The ontological theory of disease is the idea that how patients experience disease is never related to the actual pathophysiology of the disease. In this case, disease symptomology is culturally determined. The physiological theory is the idea that individuals experience disease in unique ways. Ultimately, Temkin concludes that disease is neither a purely ontological nor a purely physiological event.[19] Similarly, suffering can be organized in relation to two conceptual categories, individual and collective, but suffering is an aggregate of personal experiences and culture.

Much of the anthropological work on suffering identifies how collective representations of suffering act to empower marginalized groups. Komatra Chuengsatiansup, in "Marginality, Suffering, and Community," writes: "The intersubjectivity of social suffering, by virtue of being rooted in a shared historical and structural predicament, constitutes a sphere of shared cognizance and shared practices which together forge a collective political consciousness of an imagined community of dissenters. Viewed from this angle, the social ceases to be a single structure of constraint or merely the source of unnecessary forms of human suffering. Rather, against the official politics of exclusion and indifference, society is better conceived as sets of multiple potential sources of collective empowerment and as multiple spaces of resistance."[20] While collective representations of sickle cell suffering—shared historical memory, disease/treatment paradigms, and political objectives—have been used to gain political advantage and increase access to resources and power, these discourses of suffering are clearly tied to their objectives.[21]

Philosopher Hannah Arendt contrasts compassion and pity in the same way I contrast individual and collective suffering. Arendt argues that compassion can only be for individuals: "It cannot reach out farther than what is suffered by one person and still remain what it is supposed to be, co-suffering." Pity depersonalizes and aggregates suffering into classes of people, and while the language of pity seems highly idealistic, it has a particular disingenuous quality. Arendt notes that "in contrast to the loquacity of pity," compassion has a "curious muteness." "Passion and compassion are not speechless, but their language consists in gestures and expressions of countenance rather than in words."[22] An important question, then, is, How does individual suffering get translated into cultural signifiers that then can be used for political purposes? And who controls the production of these discourses?

Setting a health care agenda where diseases that cause the greatest suffering receive the most NIH funding would be an impossible social policy. Suffering cannot be objectified, as we see in the case of Eva, yet our discourses of suffering cast some illnesses as more pernicious, evil if you will, than others. These discourses not only provide the idioms for weighing the relative weight of various forms of suffering but also provide a framework for how patients should perform their illness.

A compassionate approach to illness would, I believe, focus less on identifying legitimate suffering and more on helping patients who suffer remake their world, which is how Elaine Scarry describes the agentive aspects of language in the face of suffering. Individuals with severe illnesses and disabilities are capable of making their lives meaningful as long as they are given the tools to shape their futures, or lifescapes. Eva's strong supportive family fought to make sure she received an education so that her life did not revolve simply around managing her illness. But many sickle cell patients are not as fortunate. As an adult, Eva faced real structural barriers given her current health status. Eva had received her kidney transplant three years prior to our conversation, and the state now wanted to declassify her as disabled. If she did not find a job with health benefits right after college, her $250 per month prescription drug bill (already a stretch for a recent college graduate) would increase beyond what she could afford. How did Eva's status as a worthy recipient of state aid change? Eva was transitioning from being an adolescent who "suffers" from kidney failure to an adult who may be locked in an uninteresting and low-paying job in order to secure health insurance. Potential job loss was also a real concern given the severity of her illness.

The concepts of secondary gain, inappropriate dependence on health care services, and patient noncompliance are employed frequently at national sickle cell association meetings or in conversation with practitioners. By using these terms, the medical professionals I encountered unself-consciously acted as gatekeepers for the public trust even as they were trying to expand health care access for their patients. Their use of conservative terminology to classify difficult patients meant that their strategies for opening up access were not radical. There is, however, an advantage to being a reformer rather than a revolutionary. By not straying too far from the taken-for-granted, commonsense wisdom shared by the medical community, these reformers couch new understandings of the disease and patient care in safe, familiar tropes. These constructed discourses of sickle cell patient suffering are shared at national meetings where physicians learn to differentiate, for example, opioid *dependence* from opioid *addiction* or where they are taught to see pain as a separate disease rather than as a symptom.

Altering medical professionals' dispositions toward the disease and the patients is one method for standardizing and improving the quality of care nationwide. Ultimately, however, each practitioner develops and deploys a unique model of patient suffering in his or her home institution based on particular institutional needs and personal perspectives.[23] Hospital administrators need objects to target in order to improve the bottom line, and the sickle cell community takes control by defining these objects preemptively. Discourses of suffering are, importantly, strategic.

Consider the description of sickle cell disease used in a letter by the original cosponsors of the Sickle Cell Treatment Act of 2003. This act includes, among other things, federal matching funds for sickle cell–related services and the establishment of forty health centers. More than $100 million annually is at stake, which means politically the act cannot appear to be a new form of welfare or universal health coverage. The letter was signed by Senators Jim Talent, Chuck Schumer, and Richard Burr and Representative Danny Davis, but the description of suffering used to encourage other members of the Senate and Congress to cosponsor the bill comes directly from the national sickle cell association. The bullet points opening the letter dated April 10, 2003, include the following:

- Sickle Cell Disease is an inherited disease that is a major health problem in the United States, especially for African-Americans.
- More than 2.5 million Americans, mostly African-Americans, have the sickle cell trait.
- SCD occurs in approximately 1 in 300 newborn African-American infants.
- There is still NO CURE.

The letter continues:

Dear Colleague:
Please join us in helping the thousands of people who suffer from Sickle Cell Disease (SCD), a genetic disease affecting red blood cells. Approximately 70,000 Americans have SCD and approximately 1,800 American babies are born with the disease each year. The most feared complication for children with SCD is a stroke, which may affect infants as young as 18 months of age. While some patients can remain without symptoms for years, many others may not survive infancy or early childhood.

Many adults with SCD have severe physical problems, such as acute lung complications that can result in death. Adults with SCD can also develop chronic problems, including pulmonary disease, pulmonary hypertension, and kidney failure. The average life span for an adult with SCD is

45 years. Strokes in the adult SCD population commonly result in both lifelong mental and physical disabilities.

These first two paragraphs identify sickle cell patient suffering in order to sell the treatment act as an act of compassion. Compassion in this letter takes two forms, compassion for children and concern for loss of adult productivity. In the United States, children are icons of vulnerability and innocence, and as a society we believe it is our moral duty to protect them and to provide them with every opportunity to become productive citizens. Anthropologist Lesley Sharp describes how children are assigned such a high social value that we rarely question the extraordinary measures used to try to save them: "Within clinical contexts, children likewise are viewed overwhelmingly as extraordinarily precious human beings whose lives must be protected at all costs. Physicians speak regularly of going to 'heroic lengths' to save the lives of children who are severely physically damaged by a wide range of congenital complications or injuries."[24] Because we believe that the well-being of our youngest citizens represents the quality of our civilization, many states extend health care insurance to children of the working poor, but not to their parents.[25]

The plea for compassion for the adult population in the letter is more ambivalent, expressing concern both for the patient and for the American taxpayer. Missing in the letter is any mention of adult chronic pain so severe that it has been compared in the medical literature to bone cancer pain.[26] This pain at times requires extended stays in the hospital being administered OxyContin or morphine, or, even worse, the daily use of prescription narcotics.[27] To acknowledge this in the letter would threaten the narrative of suffering the community and the legislators are working hard to construct; instead, the letter continues, "Newborn screening, genetic counseling, and education of patients and family members are critical preventative measures that decrease morbidity and mortality, delay or prevent complications, decrease inpatient hospital stays, and lower overall care costs."

Since the rise of the modern medical system in the nineteenth century, powerful individuals have been encouraged to contribute to the health care of the poor in order to protect themselves. With the development of germ theory in the nineteenth century, European Americans realized that diseases refused to abide by the rules of segregation, and with this realization a new breed of the selfish, even racist, humanitarian emerged.[28] Today the fear is not the spreading of diseases by Negro cooks, nannies, chauffeurs, or butlers but the fear that diseases of poverty will deplete the financial resources of hardworking American citizens. Although sickle cell disease is not technically a disease of poverty, because the disease primarily affects blacks, and blacks are twice as likely as whites to be poor, to some extent sickle cell disease is a disease of poverty.

The letter finally urges potential cosponsors "to help those Americans living with SCD, and to fund research to find a cure for future generations." A cure eliminates treatment costs for disabilities, but directing funds toward the search for an elusive cure compromises comprehensive care, which many physicians argue holds the most promise. Through blood transfusion therapy, penicillin, hydroxyurea, and a greater understanding of the pathophysiology of the disease, life expectancy for sickle cell patients has increased. But these treatments require a commitment to people and not to the bottom line. In truth the disease pales in comparison to cardiovascular disease, which in 2001 killed 77,226 black people, at a rate 31 percent higher than that of whites.[29] Even hematologists who have devoted their lives to helping adults with sickle cell concede that the benefits of huge investments in sickle cell disease, particularly physician education, are uncertain given that sickle cell falls somewhere between an orphan disease and a major disease.[30]

Regardless of the disease's uncertain urgency, since 1970 the sickle cell disease community has been able to marshal support from the National Institutes of Health, the federal government (the sickle cell acts of 1972 and 2003), state governments (Title V block grants), insurance companies, and local institutions with phenomenal success. Hematologists have made tremendous progress in understanding and treating sickle cell disease on a virtual shoestring relative to the social investment in other diseases, including cystic fibrosis, which affects about half as many individuals: approximately 36,000, most of whom are European Americans. Their success is attributable to how the sickle cell community continues to work within the discursive regimes of biomedicine to increase patient access to health care.

Discourses of suffering inspire compassion in practitioners. Dr. Allen, a hematologist and the director of the sickle cell center at Children's Hospital West in California, who was mentioned earlier, said: "I separated the heme service starting 7/1/2001. . . . there is a separate heme [hematology] service so only SCA [sickle cell anemia][31] docs attend on SCA patients. . . . this means the residents get one approach to pain management, they get their teaching from docs who understand and care about SCA kids."[32] At Dr. Allen's institution, sickle cell patient access improved when he placed limits on who could treat his patients. Only practitioners well versed in a compassionate narrative about sickle cell patient suffering were allowed to work with his "SCA kids." His strategy has been to educate doctors by using what doctors consider objective measures of suffering, and with the additional support of funding, he has been able to turn disinterest in sickle cell patients into interest, even passion.

In an interview Dr. Allen said: "We have a neurologist now who was hired to do brain tumors, who was walking around the wards a year ago making comments about 'these damn sickle patients!' I've been referring all the stroke kids to [him] and we've sucked him in. Four months ago I had him see one of my stroke patients, but he was just devastated. [He] says, 'My God, Allen, this CAT scan looks terrible! You gotta do something about this disease.' Now he's part of the team. The psychosocial guys have always been plus/minus. We just haven't had the funding to bring them on board. One of our junior faculty members, one of our fellows who is in the clinic with me trained in molecular biology and gene therapy, we got her hooked on red cell disorders. She started growing sickle red cells from stem cells in the laboratory and now has developed her own research program in the area of gene therapy for sickle cell disease."

In order to operationalize a treatment protocol, Dr. Allen had to produce brain scans, which are considered objective measures of suffering. He did not, notably, encourage new approaches to identifying patient suffering through, for example, cultural competency training or increased numbers of hematology grand rounds. This approach worked very well for physicians, who privilege what they consider hard scientific proof.

Allen's counternarrative about suffering has improved sickle cell patient care in his home institution, but his approach privileges the validity of scans over practitioner-patient communication. For example, by using patient pathophysiology to define the limits of health care, the institution is freed from responsibility for alleviating sickle cell patient suffering caused by an aborted education or unemployment due to illness. I am not arguing that it is a hospital's or a physician's duty to provide holistic care. I only want to point out that Dr. Allen ultimately did what he knew would work within his institution. He did not revolutionize sickle cell care, but through his efforts he did provide patients better access to effective pain management and comprehensive care.

Dr. Taylor, who treats adult patients at Children's Hospital North, noted the same relationship between hard data and legitimacy. He began by mentioning how difficult his patient population is. "Marilyn Trask is such a great social worker, but she gets burned out too. She works so hard, and the people don't follow up and call back. And it's like, 'Ugh!'" As frustrated as he was by his patients, his knowledge of the brain damage caused by silent strokes helped Dr. Taylor maintain some compassion toward them. "And, it's actually interesting that a lot of people have so much brain damage in scanning and functional MRI scanning, that you have the have-nots, cannots, and will nots. And most of our patients are at least two of the three at some point. But, there's more going on than just being obstreperous, you know, and then add onto that poor coping skills. If you've got poor coping skills to start with and you get some central or frontal lobe damage, it's like I'm amazed we have as many functional patients as we do. . . . You can just tell when you have some clinical neurological damage."

Wanting Dr. Taylor to address the fact that the NIH does not consider it a priority to study subtle brain injury in sickle cell patients, I noted, "Marilyn Trask was saying that the NIH grant for 2003, that you have that piece—"

Taylor interrupted, "Yeah. [Our center director] has been working very hard with [our local university]. He's got some incredible preliminary data, but then the first thing we really need to do is to really document what's happening, how it's happening. Then the other question is, How do we help it, slow it down? Because it's such a damning thing for their long-term ability to care for themselves."

I added, "And your ability to care for them."

He responded, "Yeah, and that too."

I asked, "Would that translate into more funding for . . ."

Addressing how knowledge is legitimated in medicine and how funding always follows these methods of legitimation, Dr. Taylor replied, "It could. The more data you have and show, 'This is what's happening. Here is the data. This is the published, accepted, reviewed data. We need this because of this . . .' Instead of saying, 'We have yet another group of screwed-up people, give us more money.' What current funding climate we're going into, I don't know, but your best bet always is you can show a particular problem and have a reasonable solution that you can measure. That's one of our goals."

Not only does showing hard data such as imaging data provide the necessary proof for some that sickle cell patients suffer; it also fits well into the insurance reimbursement structure, which gives no reward to physicians for more effective listening. For example, physicians cannot bill an insurance company for conversing for twenty minutes with a sickle cell patient in order to properly interpret an array of complicated symptoms. But a physician can bill for a very expensive CAT scan or a chest X-ray. As patients grow older, longer consultations are essential because hematologists must determine if a patient's symptoms are caused by sickle cell disease, some other disease, or lifestyle. Health care for insurance companies is always tied to consumables, and a conversation leading to diagnosis cannot be broken down into objective codes. Dr. Taylor also revealed in his interview, "My first whole year here, I didn't get paid a penny from any of the patients that I saw because Medicaid apparently rejected my application because they had new forms but didn't tell anybody. And it's only because we have research grants that, you know, we're able to float this clinic. If we didn't have those, this place would be gone. There's just not enough resources [for us to put] the amount of time and energy we put into the poor patients who are truly needy."[33]

Dr. Taylor demonstrates how biomedicine creates idioms of distress and suffering for sickle cell patients. Biomedical imaging helps Taylor see his patients' suffering as real because he can measure it. With enough data, Taylor hopes to convince large funding sources, such as the NIH, to support a study into how the adult brain has been ravaged by the disease and what to do about it. But until there are enough statistically significant findings, Dr. Taylor accepts the current lack of interest into one of the things that makes working with his clients particularly difficult. Once it becomes common medical wisdom that the brains of sickle cell patients need to be studied and treatment protocols established to protect from long-term damage, Dr. Taylor will have the resources to turn his inarticulate "ughs" and his loathing for some of his patients into a treatment paradigm based on the new science of sickle cell disease and cognition. Notably, languages of agency around disease are helpful not only for patients but also for physicians, who often direct the anxiety that comes with medical uncertainty at their patients.

## PITY AND HEALTH CARE INEQUITIES

At the local level, the practitioner-patient dyad is extremely important for health care outcomes. Observing chronically ill children in a number of hospital-based clinics, it became clear that a practitioner had to imagine a patient's future before he or she could prescribe various physical or occupational therapy, preventative treatments, or, in the case of Eva's kidney problems, further testing. When Eva was thirteen, her physician would have had to care that she was getting sicker and that being sick was adversely affecting her schooling and therefore her future. Then he would have had to admit to himself that he needed help from a sickle cell specialist in order to reduce Eva's chances of long-term damage. Instead, he placed responsibility for Eva's deteriorating health on her shoulders. As Eva reported, "They would usually say drink, and they didn't really try to do any tests, or figure out why I was sick."

For the families I followed with sick or disabled children in the late 1990s, if the disease was not visible to the naked eye—a clubbed foot, spina bifida—their first encounter with a physician often ended in the physician reassuring them that if they just changed their lifestyle, the problem would go away. This happened quite tragically in the case of a four-year-old girl with a brain tumor. For nine months the girl's mother was told to change her daughter's diet and to be more sensitive to the girl's stress over the mother's impending divorce. These consumers of health care were treated, in essence, as nonrational beings. Although much of the medical anthropology literature stresses how dehumanizing biomedicine is because it ignores the mind-body connection, for blacks in search of a diagnosis for physical symptoms, Cartesian dualism has a certain appeal.

Physicians have various reasons for dismissing the physical complaints of their black patients more readily than those of other groups, including an inability to relate to or understand the patient, a lack of respect for the patient's intelligence, or the belief that blacks live in dysfunctional families and communities and therefore symptoms are the result of stress rather than real disease. The type of insurance the patient has also influences the physician's perspective and treatment approach. In the end, all these reasoned explanations fall, I believe, under one rubric, which is an inability to be empathetic to the suffering of black patients.

Deployed notions of suffering are a useful form of symbolic capital, but this ethnography does not presume that symbolic capital is a reproducible constant. The sign value of symbolic capital is not a product of nature but is cultivated with tremendous effort within fields of *doxa,* or within the realm of the self-evident. Intense imaginative labor goes into the construction of cultural signifiers, which then become means through which health care services are legitimated. For example, during their shift from child to adult status, adolescent sickle cell patients lose an essential form of social capital casting them as innocent and deserving. As adults they are asked to "pull their weight" and "contribute their fair share" in exchange for rights to health care. Now that sickle cell patients are living well into adulthood, the community is scrambling to construct the ideal adult sickle cell patient who is not childlike but is nevertheless innocent, and who is not always employable but is nevertheless a contributing and thus deserving member of society. This imaginative work is not done simply to change the minds of outsiders; many people within the community are actually working to change the way sickle cell patients relate to their illness, their schooling, their employment, and their health care.

But have these counterdiscourses found acceptance because they are a rational response to suffering, or because they are an aesthetic solution to a perceived injustice that embodies our beliefs about a life worth living, the role of medicine, and multiculturalism? I use the term *aesthetics* deliberately to situate my theoretical questions squarely in the Frankfurt school debates around revolutionary idealism and the limits of reason. The Frankfurt school (established in 1923) was composed of self-described critical theorists who struggled with Marx's historical materialism thesis in the wake of Nazism, Stalinism, fascism, and—the unanticipated problematic revolutionary subject—the proletariat. Theodor Adorno (1903–69), inspired by Friedrich Nietzsche, argued that all dogmas or authorized discourses that promote moral absolutes, rationality, and telos and that claim to promote progress and truth simply legitimate and consolidate institutionalized power. Both Adorno and Nietzsche found truth in aesthetics rather than in objectivity, science, and technology. For neo-Marxists interested in revolutionary change, dispensing with the idea of moral absolutes was particularly challenging, but each member of the Frankfurt school found his own way of critically engaging the question of the relationship between materialism on the one hand and individual existentialism on the other. Jürgen Habermas (b. 1929), for example, strongly condemned the rejection of reason by poststructuralists and postmodernists and proposed instead communicative action. For Habermas, during social interactions the conceptual strategies used by each individual are a purposive rationality that leads to consensus and progress.[34]

As an anthropologist, I know that culture is proof of the human capacity for creativity, and cultural diversity is proof that there exists an almost infinite array of ways for humans to act and to construct meaning in the world. Cultures are expressions of beliefs and ideologies, but while Adorno and Nietzsche would argue therefore that rationality is myth, I argue that rationality is relative or context dependent. Within context, reason can help guide us not to moral absolutes but toward determining whether something is consistent or inconsistent with our moral beliefs. This is simply a complicated way of saying that I want to have my cake and eat it too. I believe that ending racial health inequities is important, but I also believe that the discourses used to help ensure equal treatment are as steeped in problematic absolutes, telos, and questionable notions of origin and identity as the discourses they replace.

The decision to transform racial health disparities into an object of political concern and the discussions surrounding their elimination are, I believe, situated in the realm of a self-reflective aesthetics. Regardless of the fact that the discourse is not based in objective realism, if such a thing exists, I still believe that it can be fairly argued that health inequities are logically inconsistent with America's developing ethical system. Racial health disparities conflict with our democratic ideals in the sense that they disadvantage people who are supposed to have access to an equal playing field. In terms of power and empowerment, it seems reasonable to expect the discourses that encourage us to submit to the authority and violence of the state should be applied similarly in instances that oppress us as in instances that uplift us. Arguing that ending racial health disparities is a good thing is not based on objectivity; it is, however, reasonable given our cultural aesthetics (philosophy and ethics) to target this form of suffering.

That said, it is uncertain whether racial health disparities produce more suffering in the black community than does poverty, incarceration, or poor schools in the inner city. Racial health disparities have successfully been framed as anathema to our moral sensibilities, and thus transformed into a political object of concern. At the same time, other forms of suffering connected to poverty and inequality remain largely ignored or the discourse around them reworked to once again blame the poor for their laziness, moral and social dysfunction, and/or genetic inferiority.

Working within the discursive regimes of biomedicine, the sickle cell community strategically objectifies patient suffering to improve health care access for sickle cell patients. While this strategy opens up some forms of access, it also closes off other conversations about the relationship between health care and social justice. Instead of challenging the health care/capitalist nexus, these discourses of suffering simply say that given the current health care system, sickle cell patients are worthy recipients of care. In order to be transformative, these discourses would have to challenge the idea that suffering is even a necessary criterion for treatment.

The metaphoric disconnect between the hospital's ultraperformance broadloom carpet, signifying order, and the uneven tapestry of Eva's story of suffering speaks volumes about the unbridged gap between the uncertainty that defines the life of patients and the certainty and order demanded by the structure of the medical system. Greater medical efficiency is not the key to ending racial health care disparities because greater efficiency requires less rather than more attention to the complexities of patient suffering. Poverty, stress, racism, lack of a safety net, environmental pollution, and violence are not merely complicating factors; they may in fact be the primary contributors to suffering. It is essential for us to ask why we have chosen to tackle health disparities through medicine when racial health disparities are commensurate with educational and income disparities, and pale in comparison to incarceration disparities. The sickle cell community's attempt to reframe patients as victims rather than perpetrators of their own suffering is understandable given the discursive regimes of medicine. But placing patient suffering in another paradigmatic box is not revolutionizing health care.

# PART II

# Reforming the System

# CHAPTER 7

# Finding a Way Out of *Doxa*

*Anthropology of the Imagination*

To my frustration, after more than two hundred hours of observation and interviews in two different pediatric hospitals in California, the causes for health care disparities remained elusive. Race or racism played a part, but how much remained unclear. Medical uncertainty compounded by racialized discourses appeared to be a significant factor, but, again, trying to determine a pattern seemed impossible given that every case was unique and anecdotal. Over time I discovered that many of my presumptions about the intersection of race and health were simply wrong.

One assumption I had before entering the field, an assumption strongly supported by the literature, is that government-sponsored insurance for the poor is the primary impediment to quality care. The problem with this assumption was revealed early on in my research while observing a weekly spina bifida clinic at Children's Hospital West. Spina bifida is a neural tube birth defect causing minimal to severe paralysis and brain injury. On clinic days, neurologists, internists, orthopedists, occupational therapists, physical therapists, nurses, and nutritionists spent the morning traveling from room to room seeing outpatients ranging in age from birth to about twenty. The clinic occupied a wing of the hospital, and during its five hours of operation the hall would be bustling with children trying out state-of-the-art orthotics built by a former violinist turned outdoor sports enthusiast. Children who in the past would have been dependent on a wheelchair their entire lives were swathed in braces to maintain skeletal form and then sent down the hall to test out their new equipment. Teenage patients whose weight had hindered their ability to walk maneuvered their brightly colored aluminum wheelchairs through an obstacle course of little children and equipment. These same teenagers would often spend the morning being assessed by a physical therapist in hopes that they could literally "walk" for graduation. Moans could be heard from the cast room as children with contractures were being either put into or taken out of casts designed to reshape their feet. In addition to assessing each patient medically, this clinic was designed to maximize each child's mobility, which from the medical staff's point of view was a necessary step toward personal independence. This clinic, serving primarily lower-middle-class and poor Latinos, delivered state-of-the-art care to some of the most marginalized U.S. immigrants and citizens. At least 80 percent of the clinic clientele had public insurance.

During one clinic observation I was introduced to Sharon, a four-year-old-girl whose parents used a private HMO. Her parents, originally from India, were too proud to put Sharon on public insurance. The HMO refused to reimburse regular physical or occupational therapy, and every visit to every specialist had to be approved by a series of insurance gatekeepers. At four, Sharon had serious feet contractures, meaning her feet were shaped like those of a ballerina on pointe. To be able to walk using a walker or forearm crutches, she would require surgery and then casting to reshape her feet. During this visit I watched little girls and boys enthusiastically demonstrate their walking prowess to proud medical staff while Sharon sat and refused to even crawl. Because of her lack of mobility, she developed a furtive whine that her mother responded to on cue. From the perspective of the physical therapist, Sharon was physically and developmentally disadvantaged by her HMO. The lesson from this experience was that reduced access and poor outcomes are not necessarily reducible to poverty.

Another assumption about the cause of health care disparities is that physicians lack empathy and spend too little time listening to their minority patients. I questioned the role of physician empathy in disparities after observing an appointment in an outpatient unit. For several months I had been following Miles, a cute, chubby, dark-skinned five-year-old. On a number of occasions, I attended his physical therapy sessions and visited his home to interview his grandmother, Dorothy. Miles had a problem with circulation in his hip. At three years of age, Miles had begun limping, so Dorothy took him to the doctor, who immediately referred him to CHW. When I met the family, Miles was in his third year of treatment.

I was invited to observe Miles's appointment with his orthopedic surgeon, an appointment scheduled to dovetail with his physical therapy. In the examination room, the family and I sat in chairs pressed up against two walls while the surgeon and a resident inspected and talked about the X-rays just taken of Miles's hip. The two physicians spoke to each other for about ten minutes, then the family was told that Miles did not need more surgery. Before the women had time to ask questions, the surgeon and resident abruptly left the room. As an outside observer I was appalled that Miles's surgeon barely made eye contact with Miles, Dorothy, or his mother, Phyllis, and made no effort to explain his diagnosis or future treatment plans.

Surprisingly, in a follow-up conversation with Miles's grandmother about the appointment, she had nothing but praise for her grandson's doctor. From her perspective the only thing that mattered was Miles's recovery. During the encounter, while I was focusing on the dynamics between the patient's family and the practitioner, Dorothy was keenly interested in the surgeon's grilling of the resident. She even sensed that the surgeon, who was extremely even-tempered and unexpressive, was frustrated with the resident's diagnostic skills. Dorothy decentered herself, refusing to use her relationship with the surgeon as a litmus test for the quality of Miles's health care. Instead, because the surgeon demonstrated that the training at CHW was rigorous, the encounter elevated Dorothy's trust in her grandson's health care.

Medical anthropologists have long noted the importance of patient explanatory models and illness narratives for proper diagnosis and treatment.[1] Elaborating on Robin Horton's thesis on African forms of thought and Western science, Arthur Kleinman says,

> Vagueness, multiplicity of meanings, frequent changes, and lack of sharp boundaries between ideas and experiences are characteristic of lay explanatory models (Ems). The idioms, metaphors, and logics they employ are substantially different from those of scientific medicine. For example, rather than the single causal trains of scientific logic, popular Ems may involve symbolic connections like those of traditional Chinese medical thought: a logic of symbolic balance and resonant harmonies. Even the logical principles of "identity" and "contradiction," so fundamental to formal reasoning, may be contravened in popular Ems. Obviously, ethnicity, social class, and education influence choice of metaphor and idiom.[2]

Explanatory models are culturally elaborated idioms of distress. When a person becomes ill, he or she often uses these models to develop an illness narrative that places the causes for an illness in a complex web of personal, social, and biological meaning. Kleinman argues that because illness involves both mind and body, locating disease etiology and developing an effective treatment necessarily require that physicians identify how a patient understands his or her suffering. Is the pain physical, spiritual, or context dependent? How disruptive are the symptoms to the patient's life? Does the patient want to be cured of the disease or just want control over the symptoms?

Following this argument, biomedicine is often critiqued for reducing disease to pathophysiology when in fact the origin of disease may reside in social suffering: poverty, violence, inequality.[3] Even the simple act of identifying a sensation of a disease is a culturally mediated process requiring one to accept the biomedical objects and metaphors used to identify bodily systems. Carrying this thesis further, many medical anthropologists believe that if physicians fail to appreciate the connection between explanatory models and the body, their effectiveness as healers is compromised.[4] Based on my own research in North America, however, a clinical mandate for greater physician sensitivity toward alternative explanatory models may be a misplaced effort.[5]

Health care disparities are not, importantly, the result of the amount of time a physician spends interpreting a patient's illness narrative. For example, is illness always framed as narrative? Are physicians necessarily able to interpret any patient narrative? My informants could have chosen an alternative healing modality that relies on different explanatory models, but instead they chose to seek help from physicians who practice allopathic medicine. For these patients, to be accurately diagnosed and then successfully treated was an essential act of respect, and well-meaning but ineffective (sometimes condescending) empathy was considered an impediment to good care. In Dorothy's case, she did not want to be loved or pitied or validated by health care professionals. As long as the system worked, she was satisfied.

Along with a number of disconfirming observations about how race matters in the clinic, some of my observations confirmed that racial stereotyping among the professionals was significant. About one year into my research at CHW, for educational purposes a video I had taped of one of Miles's physical therapy sessions was shown to a roomful of white physical and occupational therapists. The ten-minute excerpt shown in a hospital seminar room was meant as an opportunity for professional therapists to discuss how to work with families. For purposes of anonymity, prior to the viewing the therapists were not given any details about the family or about the success of Miles's therapy. What they learned about the family in the process of viewing the video is that Miles's grandmother, who sits quietly in the corner, is overweight. Miles's mother, who is waiting for her dentures from Medicaid, appears to be a former drug addict; dressed in a red knee-length, short-sleeved dress, she is clearly anxious for the session to be over. In the tape, one also sees Miles eagerly working with his physical therapist on a number of exercises, while his grandmother looks on expressionless. Eventually, the therapist asks the grandmother to list the exercises they have been performing at home. The physical therapist responds in the affirmative to most of the exercises listed by the grandmother, but she warns that jumping on the bed is bad for Miles's pelvis. Unexpectedly, the viewing elicited assumptions about the grandmother's lack of knowledge and the mother's lack of interest in Miles's therapy.

Miles's white physical therapist, Mary, remained quiet during the one-hour discussion. Mary had tremendous respect for Miles's family, and when I asked her about the session a couple days after the event, she said that she was shocked and deeply hurt by the assumptions made by her colleagues. Mary had spent two years working in West Africa, and from my perspective Mary simply saw race differently.

Despite the inferences about family dysfunction made by the occupational and physical therapists who viewed the video, the family was very functional; the children were well taken care of, there was tremendous love between family members, and the grandmother was extremely disciplined about daily physical therapy. Miles had four siblings, and all, except one who was born prematurely, were performing well in school either academically or in extracurricular sports. The therapists seemed disrespectful of the family and seemed to discount the possibility that the family could have played a substantial role in Miles's tremendous progress. Most patients with Miles's disease develop severe difficulty walking, and some eventually require a wheelchair. With daily physical therapy the condition can be ameliorated, but in Miles's case, through the efforts of his grandmother and physical therapist, the condition actually reversed itself, and he was eventually considered cured. Given the family's socioeconomic demographic, however, most practitioners assumed that the grandmother was incapable of sustaining effective home therapy.

After four years of research during which I collected contradictory narratives about patient empowerment and disempowerment, I seemed to be no closer to understanding the origins of racial health care disparities. It was only after I was able to step outside the assumptions

framing all the disparities in health care literature that I began to recognize that my data had a form. I finally asked myself, "Why are we
trying to manage health care disparities through medicine?" or, more
bluntly, "Health care disparities, so what?"[6] The moral panic in the literature is that health care inequities are bad, perhaps evil, and therefore
if we want to consider our society just, we must end them. While I do
believe they are symptomatic of a number of other disturbing issues, the
moral panic is distracting us from basic health care distribution issues.
Crudely, one can think of our current medical system as one that rations
health care according to cost. Would a proposal to end health care disparities require shifting the burden from the poor to another group?
The elderly or the disabled, perhaps? Or should the medical system
allow unfettered access to an endless supply of resources? Before repair-
ing health care piecemeal, as proposed in *Unequal Treatment,* as a society we must determine how we position ourselves morally in this debate.
Occasional civil rights lawsuits or even the threat of civil rights lawsuits,
a form of intervention recommended in *Unequal Treatment,* are not
going to repair the system.[7] They are largely symbolic, and instead of
improving the system they will simply encourage the development of
more scientific discourses that obfuscate racial prejudice.

Understanding health care disparities, including black overrepresen-
tation in kidney disease, end-stage cancer, infant mortality, and cardiovascular disease, to name a few, requires stepping back and examining
black health overall. The Centers for Disease Control (CDC) reported
in 2001 that the life expectancy for white males born in 1999 was 74.6
years, whereas the life expectancy for black males born in 1999 was
67.8 years.[8] Studying mortality by age and race, in 1999 blacks under
the age of 55 had a 1.7 to 2.7 times greater chance of death. The average for those ages was 2.1, with the greatest difference in mortality
being for infants under one (2.7), and for adults between the ages of 45
and 54 (2.2). Put another way, blacks had about a 15 percent chance of
dying before 55, and whites had about an 8 percent chance. A 6.8-year
difference in life expectancy is hard to understand out of context; to
bring some meaning to this finding, one must examine the broader
social issues.

Life expectancy rates do not tell a story about quality of life. To assess
quality of life, I used statistics on education, wealth, and incarceration.
According to the U.S. Census Bureau, in 1999 the percentage of white
males between the ages of 25 and 29 who had obtained a bachelor's
degree or higher was 32.0 percent, and for black males the percentage

was 13.1 percent; thus white males were 2.4 times more likely to obtain a college degree.[9] With respect to wealth, white families had an average income of $51,224, and black families had an average income of $31,778, meaning white family income was, on average, 1.6 times greater. For people over 16 years old, unemployment in 2002 was 10.4 percent for blacks and 4.8 percent for whites.[10] In 2001, 22.7 percent of black families lived in poverty, as did 9.9 percent of white families.[11] Finally, the ratio of incarceration for blacks and whites, which is a troubling 8.2:1, puts the life expectancy disparities in a different light and makes the medical system seem worthy of significant praise. In 1996, nationwide 4.6 percent of black men were in prison; in Washington, D.C., the percentages ranged from 5.7 to 7.8 percent.[12] The proportion of black men who have ever served time is somewhere on the order of 20 percent.

Given the unequal social indicators for African American well-being outside of health, why should we expect medical access and health outcomes to be different? It is important to remember that class and race are deeply entangled in America, and the American medical system is, at least at one level, a capitalist enterprise. So, do we want hospitals to accept all patients regardless of ability to pay? Do we expect for-profit and nonprofit hospitals to go bankrupt in pursuit of a moral victory? Do we want physicians to treat patients even if that means they will receive no reimbursements for those services? Should we hold the medical system accountable for reversing the effects of poverty, environmental racism, and stress? In an effort to improve doctor-patient collaborations, do we want nationally mandated standards for how physicians should treat minority patients? These mandates would most certainly give physicians little room to find patient-specific solutions to suffering.

It may be illuminating to put these questions aside for a bit to address the issue of suffering. The American insurance system performs less like a canal efficiently moving goods, services, and people from place to place and more like a dike with numerous gaping holes. Public entities and nongovernmental organizations (NGOs) plug the holes, but at any time these organizations can, and do, take their fingers out of the dike. The point was driven home to me by several hematologists. Even within urban centers containing substantial populations of sickle cell patients, adult hospitals refuse to open sickle cell clinics because most sickle cell patients have public insurance. This means a sickle cell clinic may receive only about fifteen dollars per patient per year for routine checkups, which optimally are supposed to occur about four times a year.

Physicians treating sickle cell patients perform clinical tasks that are often not reimbursable, such as conducting long interviews about symptoms, treatments, and psychosocial issues. Dr. Taylor earned literally no income the first year he treated adult sickle cell patients at Children's Hospital North and very little the second year.[13] At Children's Hospital East the sickle cell clinic is funded almost entirely through grants, and if the Sickle Cell Anemia Control Act had not passed in 1972, the clinic would probably not exist. Since the act was passed, the National Heart, Lung, and Blood Institute has expended around $1 billion to support sickle cell disease research and treatment. Largely as a result of this funding, the life expectancy for sickle cell patients has risen since 1970.[14] In this case the rescue of a disease population by the government worked, an instance of success that points to a clear relationship between material resources and improved health outcomes.

Perhaps a solution to disparities in health care access should be modeled on the historic impetus leading to the control act of 1972. During and after the civil rights movement, the neglect of the black body became a metaphor for the neglect of the black community, and the Nixon administration decided that improving health care for African Americans was an important gesture of concern.[15] In order for the act to pass, the legislative and executive branches had to agree that "sickle cell anemia is a debilitating, inheritable disease," and that it is "a deadly and tragic burden."[16] Simply put, they had to agree that sickle cell patients suffer. While the benefits derived from the Nixon administration's support of the Sickle Cell Anemia Control Act are unquestioned, the fact that it was a symbolic gesture is extremely problematic. The Nixon administration did not simply increase national spending on health but diverted research and treatment funding from other diseases like heart disease, which continues to be the number one killer of black and white Americans.[17] Nixon ultimately scored political points for articulating an agenda that, ironically, did not add substantively to the overall health care budget. His symbolic efforts were able to appease particular constituencies, but this success introduces another concern: should expanding and equalizing health care access have to rely on the "politics of pity"?

Most theorizing about access presumes that suffering is a by-product of power and injustice.[18] Perhaps we can trace this perspective to Jean-Jacques Rousseau, who argued that social systems are constructed by agentive individuals and are therefore not natural or inevitable. As agents we can undo systems of inequality and injustice and end suffering.[19] Rousseau's conceptualization of the origins of suffering differed from that of Thomas Hobbes, who believed that through power and reason, rational systems can avert suffering caused by violence. As long as the system is ruled by reason, Hobbes believed the public need not condemn or eliminate suffering, but rather could accept suffering as an inevitable part of life. When issues of suffering are taken up in politics, the suffering of others is often glorified and compassion replaced with pity. Hannah Arendt describes pity as "the perversion of compassion."[20] At the same time that she condemns the politics of pity as at times cruel, she recognizes the ability of this sentiment to produce solidarity and social revolution.

Ultimately, the politics of pity is about perspective. The spectator identifies the persecutor and benefactor in order to locate truth and blame.[21] The spectator, therefore, situates him- or herself as the arbiter of the real. As a spectator, I find it very difficult to locate the real origins of racial health care disparities because medical institutions employ both scientific discourses, which determine who gets what treatment, and the politics of pity, which are symbolic gestures that, similar to the scientific discourses, conceal prejudice. Generally, Americans find intolerable the idea that the medical system would allow someone to suffer for the sake of the greater good. To a certain extent we can accept disparities in the justice system because the person is a criminal, or in the educational system because the person lacks merit, but in medicine the person is not at fault. We expect more from medicine because at a conceptual level a person who is sick is a victim; he or she suffers. Right?

Actually, I have found that the ways in which some institutions and physicians bridge the contradiction between health care rationing and the moral indignation about suffering is to blame patients for their suffering. Medical professionals will often shift focus away from the organic issues of disease and disability and toward family dysfunction, patient noncompliance, and psychosocial deficits. The director of CHE's sickle cell clinic, who happens to be black, said, "Without knowing the race of a patient, I can figure out the patient's race by the way doctors and nurses describe the patient and the patient's family, usually as dysfunctional."[22] It is important to note here that hematologists who specialize in sickle cell disease are particularly sensitive to racism regardless of their own race or ethnicity. They are a very sympathetic group, from my perspective, given that they focus on the less prestigious end of the hematology/oncology nexus. In retaliation for discrimination against their patients, hematologists deploy counterdiscourses about the legitimacy of sickle cell patient suffering. Because the medical system is discursively situated between discourses of rationality (neoliberal economics, medical science) and the politics of pity, the physicians I work with try to create a clinic space (literally) for sickle cell patients by embedding the politics of pity in the language of science. Physicians promote the idea that strong analgesics are not addictive when used to treat pain, and they use scanning technology to show that their patients suffer somatic injury. Not completely acts of selflessness, these efforts are often necessary for the physician to validate his or her own place in the institution.

Unfortunately, it is difficult to dress sickle cell disease in pink ribbons. Sickle cell is a congenital disease that in the United States affects about seventy thousand people, primarily black. Like the black population generally, more than one-third of patients are from lower-middle-class and poor families, and many are on public assistance. The number one symptom is pain, which requires strong analgesics, including opioids; one of the most effective is OxyContin. The adult population has lower rates of employment, and most do not have college degrees. From a cynic's perspective, they are a drug-dependent, welfare population, making it difficult to establish moral clarity when it comes to institutional debates about expanding sickle cell patient access.

The hematologists I have interviewed try hard to humanize their patient populations, and they do so by attempting to standardize care through the deployment of disease/treatment paradigms. The paradigms rely on particular conceptualizations of their patients and what constitutes a life worth living. Some have long-term views that focus on patient empowerment, education, employment, and reduced morbidity. Others emphasize short-term goals, including unfettered health care access for the prevention of secondary complications. The medical uncertainty surrounding pain and the long-term use of strong analgesics make it possible for physicians to take different positions with respect to patient suffering. In light of this moral ambiguity, how do I as a spectator take any position with respect to truth and blame?

Before careening into a Nietzschean "God is dead" thesis on suffering, an argument I find theoretically satisfying but socially unwise, let me return to the statistical analysis of the state of black America. Based on several key socioeconomic indicators, black Americans experience greater levels of suffering than white Americans. Infant mortality is almost three times greater in the black community, black men are anywhere from 9.6 to 49 times more likely to be incarcerated, and blacks are less educated, poorer, and have higher rates of unemployment.

Disparities in health outcomes are, in some respects, one of the least of the black community's problems. So, short of a renewal of America's collective consciousness about race and class, how do we think it is possible to mend the medical system without simply shifting the morbidity and mortality burden to another segment of the population? Why, in fact, does eliminating racial health disparities matter?

To date, the expansion of health care access to African Americans has relied, in large part, on the politics of pity. But, as with affirmative action, will reparations for black people's "unequal" suffering turn to resentment and retribution? Employing the politics of pity can be a strategy for expanding health care access, but is this an effective long-term strategy for shoring up the nonlucrative domains of our medical system? For the sickle cell community, the politics of pity worked in its favor, but at the expense of other health care issues. In addition, the politics of pity is often appropriated by pharmaceutical companies and insurance companies to redirect capital flows. Interestingly, the market politics of health care has at times been beneficial to the black community, further complicating the question of whether or not a national discourse is needed or if neoliberal economics and financial incentives can save the health care system from itself.

While there is much to criticize with respect to the politics of pity, in my examination, I situate myself as both observer and participant as I encourage a moral rethinking of the current system of rationing. After all, it is impossible to leave morality out of debates about health care. The ultimate question I want to address is, Is there another way to organize a medical system that does not rely on the politics of pity but does attend to moral discourses about justice?

Thus far, sympathy for health care disparities has generated reforms, usually at the local level, with mixed results. Employing translators in hospitals and clinics for non-English-speaking patients has been effective. Less clearly helpful have been cultural competency training programs, in which physicians are taught to be sensitive to cultural differences. Within the clinic, cultural competency discourses encourage the production of more and more euphemisms for patient and family dysfunction. Patients are no longer labeled irrational; now their cultures are identified as the source of their beliefs and behaviors. Blaming culture deflects attention from structural inadequacies and legitimates labeling and stereotyping.

Another proposed reform for ending disparities has been a push for ethnopharmacogenomics, or drugs designed for particular racial and ethnic groups. But the use of race and ethnicity as a proxy for DNA, from my perspective, is equal parts retrograde and offensive. The public is convinced that putting more resources toward medicine will produce a healthier populace and greater equities in health care when, in fact, two of the leading causes of premature death, obesity and smoking, could be reduced through political and social intervention.

The sickle cell community has to participate in the politics of pity at some level in order to be taken seriously by the medical establishment. There seem to be two effective responses to these pressures. Some medical professionals have responded by trying to take the politics of pity out of access protocols. Others have tried to fully immerse their patients in the politics of pity in order for them to use it to their advantage. Dr. Lennette Benjamin, an adult care hematologist at Montifiore Hospital in the Bronx, has removed the issue of patient worthiness from her pain treatment protocol, demonstrating that opening up unfettered access to health care can actually make patients less reliant on it. Benjamin's approach to adult care attends to health care justice while attempting to hold the politics of pity at bay.

Tall, light-skinned, with short, slicked-back hair, Dr. Benjamin has an ageless beauty. She is a well-known, respected leader in the sickle cell community, so prominent that I am unable to mask her identity through the use of a pseudonym. I first read about Dr. Benjamin's pain treatment protocol in 2000 while conducting a literature review. The article focused on how Montifiore's sickle cell pain protocol saves the hospital millions of dollars annually in inpatient expenses. The protocol requires that a patient entering the treatment facility be assessed right away and that pain medications be administered no later than twenty minutes after the patient's arrival. Every twenty minutes the patient's pain is reassessed to determine if the treatment is effective, and pain medication is adjusted accordingly. Most patients are discharged within three or four hours after arrival.

Dr. Benjamin designed her protocol after hearing a colleague at the Rockefeller Institution describe how pain should be considered a separate disease. Pain is often considered a symptom of organic damage, but in the case of sickle cell pain, Dr. Benjamin treats the pain as if it is unrelated to underlying physical assault. She argues that pain causes secondary complications, and that one should not confuse the secondary complications with the primary cause of the pain. By treating sickle cell pain effectively and quickly, Dr. Benjamin has virtually eliminated

malingering, drug addiction, and patient dysfunction and has reduced
the morbidity and mortality that come with undertreating sickle cell
pain.

Dr. Benjamin's new patients who have recently transitioned from
pediatric to adult care are often confused when they first enter her day
hospital for treatment for a painful episode. Sitting in a conference room
in her sickle cell center in the Bronx, Dr. Benjamin provided important
insights into her treatment hermeneutic: "We start seeing patients as
early as sixteen. That's very interesting because they come with different
ideas about what's supposed to happen. Most of them come expecting
that they're going to be admitted no matter what. Even if we relieve their
pain they say, 'Oh no.' They [feel they] have to go in because we didn't
do anything. We just treated their pain, 'And it's gonna come back!'
(imitating an upset patient). But, over time, they learn that they don't
have to come in. That it's okay."

I was skeptical at first. Dr. Allen at Children's West designed his own
pain treatment protocol based in part on Dr. Benjamin's research, but
Dr. Benjamin's approach is in many respects more radical. Dr. Allen
still relies on practitioner empathy to secure patient access to effective
pain treatment. Dr. Benjamin removes staff subjectivity almost entirely
from the health care access calculus. Speaking about her adult clients,
she said, "Self-advocacy means that they've got to understand this medication. They've got to understand their treatment. They've got to
understand the potential pitfalls. If they happen to go to somebody
who starts reintroducing some of these things, they have to say, wait a
minute."

"These things" Dr. Benjamin refers to are what she considers dependence on physicians who often withhold or dispense pain medications as
a method of controlling patient behavior. While I do not believe that
patient autonomy is necessarily empowering, knowledge is a crucial
piece of what I would call her implicit patient health care contract,
which basically states, "If you can learn to articulate your pain medication needs, then I will provide you with unfettered access to effective
pain treatments."

Listening to Dr. Benjamin at the association meetings and at an NIH
conference, I have always been interested in her feelings toward her
patients. Buried in treatment protocols are assumptions about patient
agency and temperament. In an attempt to explore these connections, I
asked Dr. Benjamin how physicians feel about their patients: "A lot of
people still seem really angry at their patients for having pain. And very

dismissive. . . . It's a frustration because, you know, they aren't really *angry* with the patients. They don't realize they're kind of angry with themselves. Because it's not something that we've been really trained to deal with." Dr. Benjamin traced physician frustration to a lack of knowledge about the relationship between pain and analgesics. Similar to Dr. Allen, she noted that physicians need to be trained to empathize with sickle cell patients in pain, and the most effective method for doing this is through science education. "Because of the nature of the medication that we're treating them with. You've got these opioids. So, if you're using a sort of morphine equivalent for treating severe pain or even moderate to severe pain, there are a certain amount of people just by virtue of what you're using that are going to respond well to it. But it does not mean that you have a plan that enables you to deal with that person continually. So, what happens a lot of times is people plod along. They have pretty good success and then, all of a sudden, things start happening." Dr. Benjamin found that when treatments lose their effectiveness, physicians unfamiliar with the science of pain blame the patient. "The dose gets escalated, they need more and more prescriptions and then these people say, 'Wait a minute. I'm not doing that anymore. I'm not participating in this because you have a problem.' Part of the time it's because we have not assessed people. When you do that, you pick up on little things and you can intervene appropriately."

Dr. Benjamin placed responsibility for effective pain management on the shoulders of her colleagues, many of whom continue to subscribe to older, inflexible models of pain relief: "Another thing that people don't understand is even with these opioids and switching from one to another, they take these tables literally. So they think that if you're on this [dosage] with this drug and they switch you over to whatever, the corresponding dose would be $x$ on another drug. If you didn't respond, you know, that's your fault. So, they don't understand that different people handle [medications differently]."

Dr. Benjamin, who comes across as very cerebral and preoccupied with research, does not seem to have the patient hand-holding skills that many pediatric practitioners exhibit. But does hand-holding necessarily lead to good patient outcomes? In an attempt to understand this relationship, I asked, "How do people die here?"

She responded, "Of the people who die here with deaths related to their disease, a lot of times there is at least a pulmonary component. The other issue is, where did they die? You know, who died at home? Why did they die? If they didn't have autopsies, you don't necessarily know. There's an occasional suicide, an occasional murder, and other kinds of things. But I would say that the recurring element is some kind of pulmonary something."

Recognizing that the data are incomplete, I nevertheless pushed her to extrapolate about a possible relationship: "And do your patients die later, since you have this protocol?"

Dr. Benjamin answered, "Well, yeah. And these people, when you compare them to the others, there was one death in this protocol group. There were three in the in-service patients who were followed at the same time, and six of the private patients who were followed. Remember that there were only thirteen private patients, so that was six out of thirteen."

Looking aghast, I said, "That's a lot."

She agreed and said, "That's a lot. Those are people that were followed privately over several years. Also, there is a difference in their use of illicit drugs. The one person who died within the protocol had very severe pulmonary hypertension. When I say protocol patients versus service versus private, he was a private patient, but he was then referred for participation in this protocol. So, he still is a person who, over the years, had been banished by the private physicians." Adult patients are similarly punted from care like pediatric patients. "He had really severe pulmonary hypertension that, until he had his pain under control, was not even recognized as being part of his problem. This is what happens a lot of times with the people that visit frequently, that whatever their associated [conditions] are, they are often missed because there is such a focus on they're always coming in for pain."

Continuing, Dr. Benjamin reflected on the quality of the data: "So clearly there is potentially some bias. One thing that we know is that the people [in the protocol group] are [rarely] being admitted into the hospital [because] they did not have acute chest [syndrome]. Because that's not a thing that you treat at home, so there was a decrease in all that. We're still trying to go through the data and looking at all of the kinds of things that they had before. I know one of the people from the study, he had many episodes of acute chest and he was severely iron overloaded. And on the protocol, we not only got his pain under control so that he wasn't in, but we eventually got his iron burden down to speed, but it took about four years."

Trying to understand the reason patients choose private practice over Dr. Benjamin's center, I asked, "If they have private insurance, they have jobs, right, or not necessarily?"

"Not necessarily. Sometimes there are some people who are followed by private physicians who still have Medicaid. But a lot of them do have jobs, and they either have Blue Cross/Blue Shield [or] they have some kind of insurance."

Dr. Benjamin demonstrated that physicians do not need to wear their patient empathy on their sleeves in order to be effective practitioners. In fact, it seemed that her emotional distance from her patients made her more able to accept the sort of demands for pain medication that drove Dr. Taylor at CHN to reread Wittgenstein. Trying to understand what passions Dr. Benjamin has embedded in her treatment hermeneutic, I asked her, "And why did you choose hematology?"

"When I was an intern, I got these great hematology cases, so I was always running down to hematology and doing this stuff. My very first week as an intern, I had this great case, and they made me present it at grand rounds. The first week! So, I presented it and it went well. So I got off on a good foot with that. Then I started getting these cases, so I was always running to heme and going over things with the fellows and the head of hematology.

"Then I went to a meeting on sickle cell disease that was held at the Sheraton Hotel in New York. There were people from all over, and I was so upset by what I saw occurring there, and it seemed to me that the field was almost divided in black and white with one exception; the white people were doing all of the science, and the black people were clinical people. I could just see that [black] people were frustrated that they were kind of left out, or shut out. Then some of the ideas that some of the black people that were attending had were, frankly, disturbing as well. It was like one said, 'Well, these cells get in the body and they explode.' I looked at that and I said, 'I'm going to change this.' I said, 'I'm going to go and get very well trained. I'm gonna come back and I'm gonna to do something to change this.' I felt this obligation or responsibility to do something in sickle cell disease to change this because I was very happy doing my little [lab research] stuff. But when I finished that and got ready to get a job in the area, I said, 'Okay, this is it. I've got to go work in this area.' So I ended up at Rockefeller." I should not have been surprised that beneath the calm exterior characteristic of a bench scientist lay an impassioned humanist inspired by the notion that she could change the field.

She continued, "I went to Howard Med School. We had like Roland Scott and people like that. Dr. Scott was preeminent in the field. So, I remember one thing that he said when we were having one of those

NIH-sponsored sort of think tanks. And we were talking about thera-pies, and so he stood up, and he said, 'I want to know, when are we going to do something about the pain?' People are kind of controlling the field because they don't really understand, but they know that it's really important. They would rather work on pathophysiological things that are related to the disease. Never mind that to me this is like a defin-ing feature of the disease. There is still a reluctance to really tackle it. It's something that people take for granted. I've had people who are very, very prominent in the field tell me that they don't assess pain, 'I don't assess it, I just treat them.'"

Wondering how one can translate Benjamin's passion to other physi-cians, I asked, "You have an energy that other physicians don't neces-sarily have with respect to their patients. So how do you translate this?"

Dr. Benjamin replied, "Since we haven't had any money allocated for anything we do, we just do educational things at the meetings. So, I think that we've done a pretty good job. I think that a lot of people don't realize where they have gotten this information." Most medical profes-sionals talk about the need to educate patients. Benjamin focuses on the need to educate practitioners.

"Your panels are always packed," I added.

"Yeah, but it's stuff that once people get it, they take it for granted. When I first started going to [the meetings] they had the medical stuff over here, and then they had the psychosocial stuff over here. But, you can't deal with pain like that." Benjamin would like to see her pain pro-tocol adopted as the national and international standard. "It's become a real passion. I'm hoping that over time we will be able to share what we've done here and kind of change the face of how pain is managed in sickle cell disease in this country and in other parts of the world. And, you know, I have done some stuff in Africa and Trinidad and Tobago and in some other places."

Benjamin's protocol demonstrates that evidence-based standards of care can improve health care access and health outcomes for sickle cell patients. Her approach to treatment also demonstrates that overatten-tiveness to patient psychology or dysfunction is often a fallback position when there are gaps in the scientific knowledge. Whether a patient is addicted to powerful analgesics or has pseudoaddiction, tolerance, or dependence on pain medications, Benjamin believes that physicians have a role as scientists to understand why and then to hone therapies to address the issue. Benjamin sees her role as a problem solver rather than as a gatekeeper protecting the institution from overuse.

It would seem that Dr. Benjamin's evidence-based approach simply needs to be replicated by other hospitals. I argue, however, that single-payer universal health insurance, which reduces rationing health care by cost, and evidence-based medicine get us only part of the way toward reducing racial disparities in health care. In addition to the science of drug titration, there are qualitative aspects to Benjamin's treatment hermeneutic that, if absent, could nullify the effectiveness of her program. Importantly, Benjamin's approach cannot be divorced from either her respect for her patients or the efforts by her team to socialize her patients to her treatment hermeneutic. Benjamin's treatment success is very real, as demonstrated by the millions of dollars saved in averted treatment costs and the longevity of her patients. Even so, in the hands of another physician, her protocol could be misapplied. For example, physicians read patients differently, and therefore pain assessments will vary even when physicians think they are following Dr. Benjamin's protocol. Pain assessment is an area where racial assumptions can impact physician choice.

Dr. Benjamin's protocol also does not work without the cooperation of the patient. Socializing patients to Dr. Benjamin's disease/treatment paradigm is crucial to the success of her program. I am not arguing that all medical knowledge is socially constructed, but in order for treatment protocols to work for chronically ill patients, the patient must participate in all the exigencies. Dr. Benjamin considers the science of sickle cell disease as well as the education of practitioners and patients of equal importance. Her protocol requires that patients learn to clearly articulate their symptoms, but many institutions lack the infrastructure for patient education. Because the protocol is built on trust, patient education must also be ongoing because changes in response to pain medication may indicate changes in overall health status. Without a strong commitment to patient education, Dr. Benjamin's protocol has the potential to reproduce staff resentment toward patients. Patients who are unable to work with a team to determine why they require higher dosages of pain medication are in danger of being labeled drug seeking.

Patient socialization, therefore, is very important to improving treatment success. In pediatrics, the movement toward adolescent transitioning is an acknowledgment that the culture of medicine is real and that patients must be acculturated to medicine's language, rituals, and performative demands in order to receive the best care. The next chapter focuses on adolescent transitioning and what health care access issues are solved and what problems are reproduced as a result of this approach to improving health outcomes.

# CHAPTER 8

# Adolescent Transitioning

*Acculturating Patients to the Culture*
*of Medicine*

In a sylvan corner of a rural northeastern town, doctors, nurses, and various hospital staff members prepared for the arrival of campers to Camp Freedom. About 120 young campers and 30 adolescent junior counselors with sickle cell disease traveled from the inner city to rehearse adult independence. For five days children between the ages of seven and fourteen were freed from having to explain sickle cell disease to their peers—freed from explaining what a sickle cell crisis feels like, why daily folic acid is important, or why swimming can be one of the most painful summer activities. About 24 counselors were lead or senior counselors. They were pulled from the ranks of hospital staff and included a hospital chef, a janitor, and a computer consultant. These sympathetic souls, predominantly African American, had bonded with members of the sickle cell clinic. The junior counselors, in contrast, were adolescent sickle cell patients. During the five days at Camp Freedom many of the junior counselors would succumb to painful crises or adolescent flights of fancy, from flirtations to emotional breakdowns expressed in the idiom of a painful crisis.

Campers lived in cabins organized by age and each day they would rotate between several activities. They fished, played tennis, made art, rode paddleboats, played golf, cooked, and swam. During their down time they often practiced for the culminating event, the talent show. On the last night of camp each cabin put on a performance, which usually involved dancing, singing, and testimonials of overcoming illness or the temptations of inner-city America. The two summers I stayed at the camp I was truly impressed and thoroughly entertained by the campers.

From the perspective of the campers and many of the counselors, Camp Freedom was a satisfying retreat that they looked forward to year after year. For five days the presumptions about health, disability, and race were suspended, and sickle cell patients felt empowered to let go of some of the performances that gave them a sense of control over their lives in the city. From the perspective of the medical professionals running the camp, it was an optimum time to reshape how patients understood and responded to their disease.

When I arrived in the infirmary, Dr. Ross and Ms. Barns, a nurse, were organizing charts in order to operationalize the medication regimens of 150 patients. This is a rather daunting task because if it is not done correctly, the repercussions are potentially lethal. As the women transferred tablets of folic acid, hydroxyurea, and a rainbow of various medications from large jars into 150 little plastic cups, Dr. Ross brought up the story of Emma.

> *Dr. Ross:* Dr. Achebe told me yesterday that Emma died last month.
>
> *Ms. Barns:* Emma?
>
> *Dr. Ross:* You know, the girl you transferred to us for punching an orderly.
>
> *Ms. Barns:* Oh, yeah, Emma. I remember. I came into her room once, and she was drinking out of a baby bottle with one hand, and with her other hand she was sticking her breast with a needle. It was the strangest sight.[1]

Emma was sixteen when she was kicked out of Ms. Barns's hospital for punching an orderly and transferred to Children's Hospital East, where Dr. Ross works. Dr. Ross told us that Emma used to store old food trays under her bed, but despite these difficult behaviors, Dr. Ross grew fond of Emma, whose neuroses she compared to her own. By the time Emma was transferred to adult care at seventeen, she and Dr. Ross had forged a common bond.

Over the course of the four days at camp, the story of Emma emerged in three more conversations without my prompting. Emma, it turns out, was not crazy, but she was a difficult patient. Ms. Packer, a nurse who had cared for Emma on the adolescent unit at Children's Hospital East, revealed that Emma tried to intimidate staff members with loud street talk. The girl, it seems, performed her age and race for the hospital staff and was rewarded with their contempt. At seventeen Emma became pregnant and was by mandate transferred to adult care, where, although by all accounts she was relatively healthy, she died in her early twenties.

Describing Emma's death, Dr. Achebe, the director of CHE's clinic, said: "In the last four months we've lost two kids in their twenties at one of our adult hospitals. Kids that we graduated in the last three or four years, who were doing great. The stories are absolutely identical. The child was in the hospital, came in with pain. The doctor called and said, 'Oh, he was doing great. All he was getting was pain medication and IV. The nurse went in an hour and half after seeing him and he was dead in bed.' What kind of a mystery is that? That has never happened at Children's Hospital East. . . .

"They put you there and the more morphine you give me, the quieter I get. I don't complain I'm sleepy. Nurses don't want to disturb me. They probably didn't even check to see that I'm breathing so shallowly. I'm going unconscious. I don't bother them because I'm asleep. I vomit, choke in my sleep, and nobody notices. . . . This is how kids die. That's why I try to scare young people. I say, 'I want you to avoid depending on us so much that what you get back from us is our dislike for you, and our thinking that our job is done when you stop complaining.'"[2]

It must be noted that in addition to withholding pain medications, overmedicating is also a significant problem for sickle cell patients. Dr. Benjamin's day hospital protocol requires monitoring IV pain medication dosing and effectiveness every twenty minutes. This level of attention is not something that many nurses can manage on busy wards. Physicians can institutionalize these protocols, but it is much easier to demand careful monitoring in a pediatric hospital, where the staff-to-patient ratio is higher than in an adult hospital.

The eerie story of death told by Dr. Achebe motivates the clinic to transition adolescents or to educate adolescents to advocate for themselves. Unfortunately, the available adult services around CHE are so grim that he has begun refusing to discharge his adolescent patients. As his patient-to-staff ratio continues to grow, however, Achebe is under increasing pressure to let his older patients go. Achebe's only hope is that his clinic's transitioning program is preparing patients for adult care.

In the last thirty years, medical advances have increased life expectancy for sickle cell patients to about fifty years. By providing chronically ill patients an extra thirty years of life, the medical community is now faced with having to make those years meaningful. Clearly, thirty years of added pain and suffering is a scenario the community wants to avoid. In the 1990s, the sickle cell community responded to the shift in patient demographics by developing more adult services. Adult sickle cell centers, once extremely rare, are now being supported in many states through Title V block grants. Local associations are also being funded by states to help deal with the social repercussions of disability in adulthood. These community-based health organizations help adults deal with impediments to employment and education, economic hardship, and emotional and personal difficulties. With this expansion of services, adult doctors were noticing that their recently transferred patients were ill equipped for the demands placed on them in adult care.

Adolescent transitioning is a thoughtful attempt to improve patient-practitioner collaborations and health care access by looking beyond standard causation narratives that blame either the patient or the professional. Most professionals in the sickle cell community believe that for patients to have the autonomy they need to lead fairly typical American adult lives, they must reduce their dependence on the medical system. To accomplish this goal, adolescent patients are transitioned, a process through which teenagers are given greater and greater responsibility for their own care. Blum et al. describe transitioning as "the purposeful, planned movement of adolescents and young adults with chronic physical and medical conditions from a child-centered to an adult-oriented health care system."[3]

Through peer counseling, group meetings, and individual education, patients are taught the specifics of their disease and appropriate treatments. In addition, parents are encouraged to start giving their children more responsibility for taking medications and for communicating with professionals. Most argue that this process should begin around age thirteen until patients are discharged into adult care between the ages of eighteen and twenty-five. This model, of course, fits nicely with American conceptualizations of appropriate developmental goals for adolescents, including emotional, financial, and social independence.

Late adolescent sickle cell patients represent an extremely vulnerable population akin to canaries in mine shafts. They have just gained the right to vote but are typically a disenfranchised subsection of the electorate. They struggle with a disease that often interferes with their schooling and employment, thereby increasing their economic vulnerability. The majority also have public insurance, which means that in the strange hierarchy of our even stranger health care system, they are perceived as recipients of handouts and therefore less worthy of care.

In *The Miner's Canary: Enlisting Race, Resisting Power, Transforming Democracy,* Lani Guinier and Gerald Torres argue that individuals should use crises such as Emma's or Max's as a diagnostic tool for determining the presence of structures of inequality.[4] Just as a canary that dies warns a coal miner that the air in a mine shaft is poisonous, Max's ultimate discharge should have led to an investigation of the hospital's culture, not to the labeling of Max as a sociopath. One would never pathologize a canary that dies in a mine shaft; similarly, Max's experiences should have inspired a reflexive examination of institutional practices.

Organized by the two clinic social workers, transitioning at CHE is conceptualized as a program to increase patient maturity and medical sophistication. In an interview, Mr. Jefferson, the lead social worker, said, "A lot of disability is caused by families saying, 'This child is not going to live to be twenty anyway, why should I make him go to school?' Then the child becomes twenty, untrained, uneducated, parents now fully disgusted."[5]

From the point of view of the clinic, families reinforce habits that prevent patients from developing the skills necessary to assume adult roles. Anthropologist Helen Gremillion observed the same sort of blaming in a treatment center for adolescents with anorexia. Gremillion notes how women were often blamed for overmothering or for being too enmeshed in their daughters' lives.[6] Part of therapy involved extricating mothers from their daughters' lives, which meant that therapy, in effect, justified limiting parental access to medical treatment information. Anorexia, or in the case of sickle cell disease "disability," is often attributed to learned helplessness.

In the same interview Mr. Jefferson said: "The biggest thing that we teach here or preach to a lot of our families is consistency. If a child is showing that they can do certain things and then other times they can't, watch and learn. Unfortunately, sometimes some of the families, just to make it day to day is a struggle for them. So it's easier to send him to the hospital. It's harder for somebody to get up three, four nights out of the week to keep the child out of the hospital. Hot socks and towels every four hours, Tylenol with codeine every three hours, that requires getting up and doing this. It may also require taking off some days from work. So they say, 'What the hell, send him to the hospital, let them handle it. That way I get some sleep, and I can go to work the next day!' So if we have active participants at home who are willing to teach self-reliance, the child usually develops into a child who functions on a higher level."

Jefferson, like Dr. Achebe, stresses that patients should learn not to depend on the hospital or on doctors to relieve most pain, including frequent, severe pain. Accessing health care often is, for Jefferson, an indication of a child's diminished capacity to function at an age-appropriate level. Jefferson continued, "A mother who knows that her child has the ability to work through pain, 'No, you can go to school today. Take your Tylenol with codeine the night before, take your Motrin in the morning, and you are going to go to school today! You are not going to stay at home.' The child then has the ability to after a while say, 'I'm not gonna be able to get away with it, so I might just have to go ahead and suck it up!' These are the kids who go to college, these are the kids who do well, these are the kids who say, 'I'm in pain every day, but I can't let it stop me. I know I have a bad disease, I know this disease is probably one day gonna kill me, but I'm not gonna stop now.' Versus somebody who sits around, 'Oh me, oh my, I have no hope for tomorrow, no hope for the future. I must go to the hospital, get some morphine.' These are unfortunate situations. We do have kids acting like that."[7]

Fostering patient self-reliance, or teaching patients to comply with institutional treatment protocols, is for Jefferson tantamount to helping a child develop adult competencies. Maturity in the context of medicine is presented as a correspondence between the way the medical community understands and treats the disease and the way the patient understands and treats the disease. Patients who comply are viewed as rational because their treatment risk calculus corresponds to the risk calculus of the medical community. For example, Achebe and Jefferson's ideal patient accepts chronic pain as inevitable and self-manageable. Depending on physicians to treat every ache and pain, they argue, sets a patient up for other risks, including a loss of respect that can lead to poor medical treatment. What patient transitioning ideally does, in other words, is teach patients both to advocate for themselves in adult care and about the culture of medicine.

Flipping the notion of cultural competency on its head by arguing that patients need to learn about the culture of medicine as opposed to physicians needing to learn about the culture of their patients is a needed intervention. The problem with many transitioning programs, however, is that they are not framed as programs to teach patients about the culture of medicine. Instead, their focus is medical compliance. As a result, compliance information is rarely counterbalanced with information about medical uncertainty, practitioner personality issues, and institutional politics. Most transitioning programs simply reproduce the power differentials between patients and practitioners, which discourage patients from forming collaborative relationships with their doctors.

Another problem with transitioning discourses is that risk is often viewed very narrowly. In Mr. Jefferson's narrative of the parent who sends her child to the hospital so that she can get a good night's sleep and go to work the next day, he ignores the risks associated with compliance, which include loss of employment if a parent misses too many days of work or is too tired to function at work, or the risks associated with leaving a sick child at home alone. Compliance generally requires that patients conceptualize risk in the same way that physicians and institutions do, and Jefferson socializes his clients accordingly. But, as in the case of Emma, to conform to an adult hospital's conceptualization of risk puts sickle cell patients in a vulnerable position because obedience to institutional protocols, designed to reduce staff work load, can end in death.

At this point it is helpful to switch from using cultural competence in the medical sense, referring to the institutional mandates to sensitize medical professionals to cultural difference.[8] Given the focus on adolescent transitioning, it can be helpful to instead consider cultural competence in the developmental sense. Howard Gardner defines cultural competence as a set of skills that must be mastered in order for people to assume culturally determined roles.[9] Maturity, productivity, and intelligence are generally associated with cultural competence given that in order to be employed or to start a family one must have a complement of these attributes. Compliance, on the other hand, is obedience to a set of skills and roles demanded by cultural institutions. Within medicine, a patient's compliance to treatment regimens and institutional structures is considered a positive indication of maturity and intelligence. Indeed, notions of compliance and cultural competence are generally indistinguishable within the culture of medicine. Transitioning programs are billed as a method for helping adolescent sickle cell patients develop adult patient cultural competence, but most programs teach submission to medical authority, which has little to do with cultural competence in the developmental sense.

G. Stanley Hall wrote the first textbook on adolescence, in which he characterized it as a period of "storm and stress."[10] In the United States, adolescence sometimes begins with a rite of passage: elementary school graduation, a bat mitzvah or bar mitzvah, or a Quinceañera. Children are given more responsibilities and privileges, such as dating, later bedtimes, and more freedom to make independent choices. Douglas Kimmel and Irving Weiner, in *Adolescence: A Developmental Transition,* note that the time frames for the transition from childhood to adulthood differ cross-culturally. Kimmel and Weiner observe, "Currently in the United States, the period of adolescence is usually defined by what it is not; that is, when one is too old to be a child, but too young to be an adult, then one is an adolescent."[11] Referring to the confusion surrounding how to define adolescence, Kimmel and Weiner note that biological age tends to mark the beginning of adolescence whereas social age marks the end of adolescence. Adolescence opens with puberty and ends when one is legally eligible to marry, drink, vote, and drive. After the legal age of majority, punishments for crimes become more severe, and health care access diminishes.

The shift from minor to adult status accompanies changes in social expectations of appropriate behavior. There are of course exceptions, as one can enter the age of majority and still be viewed as an adolescent or child in social settings. College students, because they usually are not financially independent and often are not married, have mixed status. Similarly, a legal minor might assume adult responsibilities and roles, and in rare instances a judge may grant a minor some adult rights. It is unclear, in other words, if adolescence is a universal developmental stage or a culturally defined and socially determined transition. It also remains unclear whether internal or external factors have a greater influence on development during the teenage years, or what features of adolescence besides physical maturation are universal.

If there is no clear definition of adolescence, why do we employ the term? The idea of adolescence developed in the United States during the industrial revolution as a way to conceptually frame a shifting demographic. Before the nineteenth century, children remained in subordinate roles to their parents until a son inherited land. A man often would not marry until acquiring his inheritance. The industrial revolution and diminished landholdings changed the relationship between private property and adult status and allowed propertyless individuals to make a living in growing urban centers.

With new skills needed for emerging trades, education became vital. Education kept youth at home until they were qualified to practice a trade.[12] The changes in educational attainment that began during the industrial revolution were dramatic. According to Kimmel and Weiner, "In 1890, one out of every eighteen young people between 14 and 17 was in school; by 1920 it was one out of three; and by 1950 it was four out of five."[13]

Whatever adolescence is, it is clearly connected to material culture. Technological advances have meant that people have to spend more time in school in order to be employable. This has meant that a larger and larger percentage of people delay assuming what Americans would consider traditional adult roles: marriage, parenthood, employment. For people of a particular economic and educational class, graduate education further extends the transition to adulthood. At the other extreme, for poorer people with less education, adolescence seems to be contracting, a phenomenon revealed by the push to try minors as adults in our criminal justice system and, on a much smaller scale, by the phenomenon of punting adolescent sickle cell patients.

Rather than viewing black adolescent sickle cell patient behavior as age-appropriate, health professionals view disruptive behavior as dangerous, and a threat. The punishment for transgressing authority is loss of access to health care. The fact that access to material resources is connected to how a patient's behavior is coded means that being designated an adolescent is also a right.

American beliefs about childhood and adulthood are reflected in the organization of health care services. Children's hospitals are structured differently than adult hospitals, with perhaps the main distinction from the patient's perspective being staff availability. Adult hospitals tend to have larger patient-to-staff ratios and fewer psychosocial, educational, and family-friendly services than pediatric facilities. Adult physicians who treat sickle cell patients resent that their newly transferred patients still require a tremendous amount of hand-holding and that they are not coming into adult care prepared to accept greater responsibility for their health care. This clinical perspective is consistent with a general American perception that adulthood is the end result of a successful transition from dependence to independence and self-sufficiency.[14]

But are these transitioning programs really trying to foster cultural competence or patient compliance? Are these models teaching patients to be obedient to an adult health care system with problematic resource distribution and institutionalized biases? Or are they teaching patients skills in how to demand and receive services necessary to maintain optimal health? In the case of transitioning, is cultural competence compliance or noncompliance? Additionally, given the fact that adolescence is complicated by chronic illness, should chronically ill patients be expected to participate as adult citizens in the same way that typical healthy adults are? Put differently, should society hold them morally responsible for the same levels of productivity and self-sufficiency as a typical adult? This question is implicit in the discourses about adolescent transitioning. The debate is split between pediatric and adult practitioners who have unique perspectives based on the structural and moral presuppositions that inform their practice and institution.

## TRANSITIONING AND DISPARITIES

Adult sickle cell patients are expected to have high levels of self-efficacy, a psychological measure of a patient's ability to independently manage his or her own health and health care. The patient's knowledge of his or her pain treatment and compliance with institutional culture are read positively as independence and self-efficacy. The fact that self-efficacy and compliance with institutional culture are read as a good thing speaks to what is at stake politically, economically, and socially in adolescent transitioning. Objectified notions of what constitutes a good or bad outcome, or what constitutes a culturally competent adult sickle cell patient, are only partially concerned with patient needs. Primarily, notions of cultural competence are tied to proper acquiescence to structures, including health care delivery and resource distribution.

I have observed in pediatric care that physicians generally only want their compliant adolescent patients to practice independence. If an adolescent refuses to comply with medical treatment, the team blames the parent for not taking responsibility for her child. In my observations at CHW and CHE, the majority of weekly pediatric clinic meetings were spent dealing with adolescent issues, and in almost every meeting I observed, the parents were denounced for being either overinvolved or underinvolved in their child's treatment. Different conceptualizations of adolescent autonomy were employed at different times to promote specific institutional and clinical agendas. Regardless of the conceptual inconsistencies around transitioning discourses, the community feels as though acculturating adolescents to the culture of medicine is necessary to improve health care access.

Currently, many institutions consider sickle cell patients too difficult and simply refuse to treat adult patients. For more than three decades Dr. Achebe has tried to encourage several hospitals to establish adult sickle cell centers where physicians are professionally invested in knowing the latest treatment protocols and where, importantly, the staff cares about the patients. Unfortunately, even the university medical center next door to CHE continues to transfer to other hospitals all adult sickle cell patients who seek treatment. For adult hospitals in the area that do accept Dr. Achebe's patients, sickle cell patients add little to no symbolic or financial value to the hospital, and so the hospitals accept one or two premature sickle cell deaths a year.

Missing from these adult institutions are support services for sickle cell patients who must deal with the effect of health on job and family. Given the structural deficits, including lack of a viable adult sickle cell program, lack of workplace support for adults with serious health problems (or for parents who have children with serious health problems), and lack of any symbolic capital associated with treating sickle cell patients, how, in fact, is transitioning going to help adolescent patients? If we imagine cultural competence as the skills necessary to assume adult roles, cultural competence may, in the adult hospitals, be non-compliance. Parents who send their children to the hospital so they can go to work are competently managing risks. They are ensuring future income and reducing their child's risk of morbidity or mortality. Adult sickle cell patients use some of the same calculus as parents with children who have sickle cell because to do otherwise reduces the burden on the health care system but increases the burden on the family.

Adult medicine is built around the belief that given America's equality of opportunity, adults must take responsibility for their own destinies. Citing a counterexample, health care policy scholar M. Gregg Bloche credits Prussian leader Otto von Bismarck with "forging a compact to ensure that citizens called on to risk everything [in war] had their needs met in return."[15] Bloche notes that after sending troops to Paris in 1870, Bismarck created the first social insurance system, which included medical coverage for all German citizens. While rarely the explicit focus of health care debates, the association between risks made by citizens for the state and the state's responsibility to protect their welfare is at the heart of the issue of whether health care should be a right or a privilege. For African Americans who are perceived as lesser contributors to the public good, these conceptual entanglements affect their health care access.

Culturally, pediatric institutions are charged with a different set of ethical mandates than adult care. Pediatric care is rooted in Americans' near-obsessive desire to protect the lives of innocent children while simultaneously denying adults what some consider basic human rights like food, shelter, and health care. The clearest example of this is the government's continued expansion of health coverage for minors, including now fetuses, but not pregnant women.[16] This is not the case in adult medicine, where patients must assume responsibility for their own suffering. Perhaps the most succinct way to describe the differences would be to say that in adult care patient suffering does not produce a moral panic.

While Emma's behavior in pediatric care, sucking on a bottle and sticking herself with a needle, indicates an adolescent enacting several different developmental stages, the medical system deemed her mature by transferring her to adult care after she became pregnant. Emma's pregnancy was symbolically read as an act of noncompliance. The punishment for her sexual transgression was removal from the one institution that was equipped to help her through a difficult time. She was thrust into adult care, where dependence was not allowed. With that transfer, whatever physical, social, or psychological suffering she endured as a result of illness, family neglect, or the added burden of taking care of a baby alone went from an issue of societal responsibility to one of individual responsibility.

The tension between pediatric professionals and adult professionals over responsibility for socializing patients into adult care is akin to a tribal war. When I asked a child specialist the difference between pediatric and adult care, she responded: "On a pediatric level, our docs will tell you they're not going to get rich doing hematology, especially in an academic center. Docs who want to care for patients and really want to do things that are meaningful, they gravitate toward pediatrics."

This is far from an atypical response. At a structural level these differences are perceived to manifest in terms of treatment. Several CHE practitioners told me the story of an eighteen-year-old girl who was so "snowed" by all the pain medications prescribed by a rural doctor who sees both children and adults that it was, in the words of Mr. Jefferson, "a malpractice suit just waiting to be administered." The rural doctor had prescribed OxyContin, morphine, and Tylenol with codeine simultaneously. The CHE team decided the best course of action for weaning this girl off the heavy narcotics was to give her an epidural. Proud of the way his sickle cell team handled the opiate withdrawal, in the middle of the story the social worker said, "If they [meaning the patient and her mother] would have walked into an adult hospital . . . she would have told them what she was on and they would have had her going into a straitjacket, detoxing her cold turkey." Adult hospitals are perceived as less patient- and family-centered, less responsive to suffering, less flexible, more focused on "managing dollars rather than managing care," a phrase often repeated by Jefferson. From the adult providers' perspective, the pediatric institutions are to blame.

At an NIH quality of life workshop in Maryland, Dr. Lennette Benjamin challenged the common wisdom shared by pediatric practitioners.

This foremost pain specialist agreed that the services are fewer because there are more pediatric specialists, but she argued that patient dependency is being fostered in pediatric care. "These patients want adult doctors to interact in the same way as their pediatricians. These are expectations. . . . We tend to think pediatricians have covered it, but adult doctors, we have to cover things that were not done in pediatric care." When I pulled Benjamin aside to ask her to elaborate, she said that pediatricians tend to hold on to their favorite, or model, patients in order to maintain their patient rolls. Punting, she believes, is part of a market calculus.

Returning to the story of the overmedicated eighteen-year-old, one gets the sense that while professional pride is wonderful, it is not always accurate. The sickle cell team was shocked by how poorly managed this patient was by the rural doctor and equally appalled by her parents. The child had been in a wheelchair for six months because of the overdosing, and the parents had won guardianship over her based on the testimony of the rural doctor. The team felt a desire to help this child liberate herself from her parents and resented what they considered the parents' overinvolvement in their daughter's care. This reaction fits well into the American mandate for adult self-reliance but does not make sense given the team's response to other cases. In particular, the team was overwhelmed by adolescents who did not comply with treatment. One case discussed during a team meeting, for example, was of a fifteen-year-old whose parents had given him responsibility for taking his daily dose of hydroxyurea. The adolescent was lying about taking his medicine and was refusing other treatments. One team member proposed investigating the parents for neglect, a proposal that contradicted the philosophy of transitioning.[17]

At a breakfast workshop on transitioning that met during a national conference in Beverly Hills, California, attendees introduced themselves by describing why transitioning mattered to them. These brief introductions demonstrate how differently medical professionals view the adolescents they work with. Some viewed them as victims of the medical system; others viewed them as drug seekers who take advantage of the system. An African American nurse who worked with children said, "We find that there are problems with children going from pediatrics to the other section. We just don't know what to do because I think that they are spoiled rotten in pediatrics, and by the time they are adults and have to go over, they're not quite happy with it. So we find that again they stop coming into visits [at the adult center]. . . . They still come to us if they're in trouble."

A white woman who worked for a sickle cell association in California said, "We're currently in the process of putting together a transition program." She hoped the workshop would give her some ideas about how to design their program.

A black woman who described herself as someone who works for a pediatric hematology/oncology program in the Midwest commented, "We do not have a structured program for transitioning, and there are problems with transitioning. Basically we may recommend our patients to adult hematology, but they will not go there. They will utilize the emergency room. In [pediatrics] we have the entire team approach. We have the nurse, we have the doctor, we have a child psychologist, we have a social worker. With adult hematologists, there's basically only the doc. So I'm hoping to get some ideas about developing a structured program for adolescents."

A white woman from a state department of health who works for the department's newborn screening program said, "I've been interested in transitioning since we had Health Resources and Services Administration (HRSA) grants for service. [We] didn't seem to get anywhere both getting the adults interested and also getting the kids' mind-set different, to be more independent. But the problem that comes to the fore for us is that of the repeat offenders, the abusers of Medicaid, a number of them are adult people with sickle cell disease. Our Medicaid has said, 'Well, what can we do about these people who go from ER to ER to ER to admission to admission to admission and cost the state millions of dollars every year? How do we help those people, and how do we help other younger people from not . . . getting in that situation? I'm hoping to get some ideas, hoping to get some strategies, and maybe we'll be able to work up some programs."

A black woman who works for the sickle cell initiative in her city said, "We have a partnership with the pediatric hematology clinic, and there is no structured transition program, and one of our problems is the adult hematologists don't want to take sickle cell patients. So, I'm hoping to get some ideas that when I approach them again, that maybe I could kind of sway them to change their minds."

A black nurse commented, "We have a structured program for transitioning, but the fact of the matter is that when a pediatric child is seventeen, eighteen, nineteen, they begin to act up. Then the pediatric hematologist threatens to send them prematurely to the adult hospital. So, it's like a punishment type of thing. And even with the structure, you're not able to measure the kind of success that you have. . . . I'm looking to pick up something that we can include in our program that might help us to have a greater success."

A black male psychologist said, "I had a transitioning group for two years, and hopefully I plan to start another one. I'm here . . . to find out what everyone else is doing so that I could bring it back to the clinic. . . . I find that a lot of time you'll have staff say, 'Yeah, we want them to go.' But the child will show up for his appointment, or that child will call in for a prescription, and they'll write it. They are just as difficult to train to say, 'Let them go,' as the kids are themselves. Also, I'm interested in working with the parents too because parents have a hard time letting go and letting the child be a little bit more independent. So it's kind of a child's transition, the parents' transition, and the medical staff stepping back."

Finally, a white adult hematologist reiterated the importance of transitioning and then noted that his center was recently denied funding from the Robert Wood Johnson Foundation to develop a comprehensive transitioning program. He believed, however, that the foundation was interested, but that following the stock market crash it had to cut back on a "particular category of grants." I interpreted "particular category" as meaning psychosocial research and patient support.

These introductions revealed a number of issues that have hindered the development of comprehensive transitioning programs: (1) lack of institutional support in adult hospitals to establish comprehensive adult sickle cell programs; (2) inadequate services in existing adult programs, which encourages adult patients to skip appointments, to avoid routine care, and to manipulate the system in order to relieve their suffering (resistance strategies that are dangerous medically and that feed prejudices about how sickle cell patients are a burden on the health care system); (3) patient punting when children start asserting their independence; and (4) lack of funding for research regarding what services truly help patients transition.

Even for the dedicated professionals at Children's East who believe strongly in the philosophy behind transitioning, the pragmatic issues of care often encumber the actual practice of transitioning. In an interview Eva could barely articulate how or if she was being transitioned to adult care. During our first recorded interview in 2001, I asked her about her status at CHE, "So what's your status in terms of, like, being a patient at CHE? Are you going to be transitioned, or . . ."

With uncertainty Eva responded, "I'm going to have to be soon, I'll be twenty-one this year, so, I don't know how they're going to do it. I mean, they've talked to me about it because they think that the best might be going to St. Peter's [pseudonym] because they have a better sickle cell program or something." Eva received care at CHE, where the staff pride themselves on their efforts to transition adolescents. "No one's ever said anything specifically or when or what time. So, I don't know. Plus, all this was talked about before my kidneys failed completely, so now it's like I might be here longer, I'm not sure. Because, I mean, there are people who I've met in dialysis who are twenty-one now who are turning twenty-two and are still here, so I don't know what the cutoff is. Maybe twenty-two, twenty-three. Jefferson says that there are, like, still like adults coming back here." The American Medical Association leaves it up to physicians and institutions to set their own standards. I discovered patients discharged from pediatric care as young as fourteen years of age and as old as twenty-six. I was told that there were some patients who were even older than that.

I asked, "How do you feel about going to another hospital?"

Eva expressed concern: "I have mixed feelings because this is, like, more home or whatever. But, I know this has to be done. Then it's like you're wondering, how are all the doctors over there? Because, you know, adult hospitals are different than kids' hospitals. I mean, it's automatic. They're going to treat you as an adult, and things are going to be more, I don't know, step by step, and curt. And that's it, just this is the plan and that's it, and you're going to walk away and that's how they might treat you. My friend went over to St. Peter's and he hated it."

In the interview I conducted three years later, in 2004, when Eva was still receiving care at CHE, I asked her if she was going to be transitioned to adult care. With more confidence she said, "That's the next step. Because this is supposedly some type of new port [she recently had a port inserted in her chest]. . . . And it's, you know, the guinea pig thing all over again. So, everyone is trying to figure out how to do, I guess, do what they have to do to be on the apheresis. And the nurses there are all being taught . . . I guess it's different from the other ones. I don't know why. Um . . . so . . . I don't know, I mean, I think about going and transferring. . . . I don't know. At first, sometimes I say, 'Okay, it's time to go,' and other times I'll be like, 'No, I've been here so long, it's like kind of home.'"

I wanted to know if Eva felt in control of the decision to transfer her. "Are they waiting for you to say 'I'm ready to be transferred'? Are they introducing you to different doctors?" Given that nobody had really informed her about transitioning, the answer was fairly obvious.

Eva said she had not met an adult physician and did not know if she could initiate her own transfer. Eva is a very compliant patient, so it is not surprising that the practitioners at CHE are not anxious to see her go. In addition, there are no other institutions that provide the kind of care her doctors believe she needs or deserves.

In their current form, are adolescent transitioning programs the best approach to improving health care access for sickle cell patients? In an article published in the *Journal of Health Care for the Poor and Underserved*, Joseph Telfair et al. describe what physicians perceive to be the problem with their patients. Physicians expressed concern about "(1) families and youth being overly dependent on pediatric providers, (2) pediatric providers fostering dependency, and (3) a lack of communication between pediatric and adult providers."[18] A diverse group of 227 providers from different specialties who serve very different populations participated in Telfair's study. Of those, 67 percent said that they "did something to demonstrate transition" such as "(1) ceasing to see patients with their parents, (2) encouraging patients to accept more responsibility, (3) providing literature, (4) making the patient more financially responsible, and (5) having family conferences to discuss transition."[19] In the article, a provider's race, gender, and specialty seemed to make a difference in terms of expectations and transitioning strategy. For example, 81 percent of minority providers expected their patients to be knowledgeable about their illness versus 51 percent of European Americans. With respect to strategy, hematologists employed method 5 (family conferences) whereas providers treating both adults and adolescents employed method 3 (providing literature). The authors note that strategy differences by specialty are statistically significant ($p < .05$).

The authors conclude that most sickle cell patients are not transitioned in a comprehensive manner. The closing discussion notes what a comprehensive transitioning program should include:

> The goals of the program for support in the form of case management must clearly describe relevant activities. These activities include adolescent, young adult, and family asset and risk assessment; coordination (liaison) with providers and specialists; coordination with other institutions (e.g., schools and mental health, vocational rehabilitation, and community resources); and negotiation of health care and related systems. Listening; demonstrating respect for opinions, concerns, and cultural values of the young person, family, and community; providing advice specific to problem solving; and including family and significant others in decision making are all important in providing support to the adolescent in transition.[20]

Telfair, who has been writing about the importance of adolescent transitioning since 1994, is considered a top expert on transitioning and is called upon by the NIH and the sickle cell community to share his expertise at national meetings and invitation-only research workshops. Regardless of his professional recognition, providers still do the bare minimum when it comes to transitioning sickle cell patients. In a telephone interview in 2003, Telfair described several reasons for this lack of commitment to transitioning, which mirror the complaints listed at the workshop.

First, institutional infrastructures generally do not support transitioning, which means successful programs must be run by tireless individuals with missionary zeal. The majority of the physicians who would like to institute a transitioning program are simply overwhelmed managing the physical aspects of the disease. As Telfair explained in the interview: "I found early on that people who do the community-based work—those who are out in community-based organizations like cancer societies and cystic fibrosis foundations and sickle cell foundations—do a lot of the groundwork. Do a lot of the problem solving day to day, dealing with sort of the dirt-level stuff. Providers, in terms of doctors, nurses, those sort of folks are more along the lines of providing physical care. They try, I think, to a good degree, particularly pediatric ones, to understand what they call psychosocial work. But, through no fault of their own, I've come to understand that they have some [difficulties] between caring for the physical side of it, at the same time trying to understand that there are all these other factors in the kids' and families' life that really interfere with their ability to follow through with the care."[21]

Second, research scientists have a qualitatively different approach to patient care than clinicians, but clinicians are the ones who receive grant funding. As Telfair noted, "Within the NIH system, the bench researchers and the proposed bills that are sort of one step away from bench research, pretty much dominate the research question, which is really why you will have people saying, 'Well, yeah, we think that quality of life is important,' but at the same time, they don't quite understand it. They do stuff that has nothing to do with quality of life, but as sort of a good research question. So, to me there is sort of this dissonance going on within the body of which you work where you have the constant battle between, you know, trying to come up with a good research question for a clinical trial, as opposed to putting the patient and the family first and trying to resolve and work with them to have a good quality of life versus, you know, paying attention to their body parts."

Third, in pediatrics there is what he described as a catch-22: "On the one hand, doctors and nurses, physician assistants, physiologists, other folks, teach adolescents to do pain tolerance and to know what their medication is and things like that. But, on the other hand, when they're in there being treated for pain, they don't necessarily think that the patient can say, 'Oh, I need more,' or 'Oh, that's not enough,' or 'Oh, that's the wrong medication.' You know what I mean? So, on the one hand, they're saying, 'We want you to be yourself . . . to really be independent and really kind of control how you get it.' But on the other hand, 'We are still in control and we know what's best.'"

Telfair noted that the responsibility for transitioning falls to both the physician and the patient, but while providers easily point fingers at patients for lack of cultural competence, they rarely reflect on their own deficits. One of the reasons for this anxious paternalism is the misperception that everything in a patient's life revolves around medicine. Telfair noted that providers need to recognize that most patients spend less than 20 percent of their time dealing with health care issues, and as a result, patients make decisions about their treatment based upon far more than the statistical significance of a drug study.

Telfair described transitioning as a cultural shift: "If you look at transition, which is a cultural shift, which means you have to think differently about the adolescent. Not starting when they're sixteen, but starting when they're eleven or twelve or thirteen and begin to work with them and to understand how the systems work and move forward in a lot of the arenas, you know. Working on their relationships with their families, with their friends. Talking to them about human sexuality, you know, education as opposed to vocation. And, it's a process, long term, instead of a short kind of deal. But, it's a cultural, it's a social cultural shift."

Telfair's strategy for legitimating his research has been to turn a very complicated set of factors that he believes contribute to successful transitioning into single quantifiable codes. Telfair led the breakfast workshop at the National Sickle Cell Association meeting in Beverly Hills in 2003. His presentation was suffused with updates about how funding bodies and the scientific community had been receiving his work. He explained, "The behavioral science people are finally willing to look at the sort of grants that do not get traditional-type funding, which is what I do. I've tried three times to get individual studies, and no one said that it's a bad grant. They never tell me that. What they tell me is that essentially this is not the kind of thing we fund."

Following Telfair's assessment of his funding issues, the male hematologist at the meeting who himself had been turned down for a grant to fund adolescent transitioning opined that Telfair's lack of support was probably due to his lack of data, meaning statistically significant data. Telfair, who regularly must defend his work to scientists, reacted with equanimity, explaining, "See, now we have data. See, I think we had very little or no data. We knew what we were doing, there's no question about it, but they said that questions always come up. . . . Even though you've done a pilot study."

Despite being somewhat marginalized, Telfair remains optimistic that eventually his comprehensive model will be adopted by all pediatric sickle cell centers. He has reason to be hopeful. He has managed to produce statistically significant results for his transitioning research. Working within the discursive regimes of biomedicine, he has brought legitimacy to his research and his results. Yet, I wonder if hospital administrators and funders interpret his findings in the way that he hopes they will. Telfair's ideal transitioning program requires that providers be sensitive to patient development; he presumes that providers will treat their patients with respect; he believes that providers should empower their patients by allowing them to make their own treatment decisions within reason; he believes that transitioning programs should be holistic and should include education about topics that many in the health care field would consider outside their domain. In sum, Telfair would like practitioners to have a particular disposition toward their adolescent patients that is as unquantifiable as compassion.

Reading Telfair's articles, which include lists of things patients and providers do or should do, all associated with P values, one gets the sense that transitioning can be operationalized in the same way that protocols for drug treatments are operationalized. I discovered, however, what I consider a misapplication of his work during a conversation with an administrator at CHE who was unaffiliated with the sickle cell clinic. She was designing a transitioning diagnostic through focus group workshops with practitioners. She anticipated that the outcome of these meetings would be a checklist that providers could use during an encounter with a patient, perhaps on the eve of his or her transition. The physician would be required to ask the patient questions such as "Do you have a car?" and "How will you get to appointments?" Talking with her, I imagined that after the checklist is filled out by the physician and signed by the patient, the pediatric hospital is released from any sense of responsibility. With the signing of the checklist, perhaps in triplicate, the patient is officially transitioned. The checklist approach is clearly not what Telfair has in mind, yet Telfair's presentation of data, coded to produce statistically significant results, seems to reproduce the very bureaucratic forms of care he hopes to change: the rational accounting that produces a health care system that is less attentive to patient suffering than it is to the bottom line.

So while there are many things to celebrate about transitioning as idealized by Telfair, in practice transitioning remains a protocol for teaching compliance to authority. The potential strength of transitioning is that in addition to teaching patients about their disease and treatment, patients can be let in on the secrets of the culture of medicine. They can be introduced to medical uncertainty, professional hierarchies, hidden agendas, and institutional politics.

Another weakness of transitioning is the foundational presumption that adolescence is a time when sickle cell patients should become more independent. This expectation is challenged by the steady decline in health that begins at birth for these patients. Most bone marrow transplant protocols reject sickle cell patients over the age of sixteen because of the likelihood of irreversible damage to at least one major organ. Instead of taking into account this "natural history" of the disease and the life trajectory of the patient, transitioning models and adult health care services are being built on cultural presumptions about adolescent development interlaced with institutional needs for patient compliance. Transitioning programs work in concert with a political economy that punishes adults with certain types of dependencies. By focusing on improving patient compliance to institutional culture, transitioning programs teach patients that dependence on systems and people is pathological, but they do not teach patients to challenge the structural pathologies in adult medicine. Confusing the lack of dependence on the health care system with compliance is not, I believe, an act of purposeful omission or institutional collusion on the part of the clinic team. Instead, the team, somewhat unreflexively, socializes their patients to obey discourses within the medical system, hoping that patient conformity will produce better health care outcomes.

In at least one other cultural institution adolescents are asked to demonstrate compliance in order to be deemed competent. In judicial bypass hearings, a minor seeking a waiver to have an abortion without notifying her parents must demonstrate her maturity to a judge. While the vast majority of girls attending these hearings have been allowed to seek abortions, generally the girls who do not show compliance to mainstream goals are considered less mature.[22] Similar to the experiences of sickle cell patients, obedience to cultural notions of adolescent development are rewarded institutionally. Punishment for nonconformity in both health care and law is an institutional push into adulthood. In the case of the law, pregnant adolescents who are unable to demonstrate maturity are sometimes thrust into parenthood by being denied access to an abortion. In the case of the hospital, teens who become pregnant as well as teens as young as fourteen who are noncompliant are punted into adult care. In adult care, more often than not, patient demands for more pain medication or different types of treatment are thwarted simply because of reduced access to care.

Trying to determine why medicine and the law treat black adolescents more harshly than their white peers, it is necessary to examine the slippage between cultural competence and compliance.[23] Black adolescents are generally read as less culturally competent, which in the culture of medicine is translated to mean they are less compliant. They are, in sum, hopeless with respect to developing the skills necessary to assume appropriate adult roles and to become self-sufficient. They are punished by being stripped of their child status and forced to assume more responsibility, the result of the contradictory logics at the intersection of adolescence and institutional pragmatics.

Chronically ill adolescents who are noncompliant often have tremendous cultural competence with respect to the health care system. By all accounts, patients who have been transferred continue to buck the system in order to receive the care they need. In 2001, Dr. Achebe told me about a recently transitioned adolescent who in three months went to three different hospitals for pain treatment. At each hospital she gave a different case history. In one she said that she was a Jehovah's Witness so that the physician would not ask her if she received regular blood transfusions, which she did. Most physicians believe that a person who regularly receives blood transfusions cannot have pain because the percentage of sickled hemoglobin in his or her blood is lowered by these treatments, but many hematologists who specialize in sickle cell disease, including Dr. Davis, dismiss this as folk knowledge.

Finally, the most potentially devastating aspect of emphasizing patient independence and equating autonomy with cultural competence is that reliance on a family member or a strong advocate can mean the difference between life and death. In an interview with Eva's mother,

Flora, it became clear that even after Eva reached the age of twenty-four, without Flora's involvement in her care, Eva would not be alive.

Trying to put myself in Flora's shoes, I asked, "So, when I hear your stories, I feel like if I had been Eva's mom, Eva probably wouldn't have been alive because I wouldn't have caught some of the crucial things that you caught."

Flora, who considers her knowledge hard won, responded, "Well, maybe if you were her mom, you would have. When she was thirteen, before she collapsed, she was seeing a doctor here. [In the doctor's voice] 'She can go back to school on Monday, just rest for a few days and then come back, just send her back to school.'"

"He didn't know anything?" I offered.

"No . . . they didn't even check her blood level to see what it was, okay? Friday, I came home from work, she still wasn't looking well. By then, she was sharing a room with one of the other children. I told the other child, 'Can you sleep in my room today because I want to sleep in her room with her.' This is Friday night. They liked to watch *TGIF,* she didn't even want to watch *TGIF.* She went to bed. I slept on the bed with her. For the first time she was unconscious and probably because I was there, I found out because I was calling her and she wouldn't respond. So, as a mother, regardless of what the medical books say, you feel drawn to what is happening to your child, and maybe in that case get some help. So when I saw that she was unresponsive I called two rooms down I called my husband, 'Call 911,' that was our first trip to the emergency room."

I asked if that was the first time they were sent to CHE. Flora responded, "No, it was when we went to Regional because with 911 the ambulance just takes you to the nearest hospital, so we went to Regional Medical Center. They couldn't find a vein on her. They couldn't do anything because they told me, 'Oh, you go ahead and sit in the waiting room, we'll get you.' Finally, she came out with oxygen, she was unconscious during transport, but she came out enough to tell them, 'Go get my mom.' They came out and got me and I saw the IV on her and I said, 'Give her some fluid before the transfusion.' Then they checked her hemoglobin. Her hemoglobin was 2, which means there was no oxygen. There was not enough oxygen-carrying capacity to renourish the brain, and probably that's when all the kidney problems happened too, because there was not enough hemoglobin to carry the oxygen to nourish her vital organs. So, but then, they wanted to transport her to RHA. There was no ICU bed at RHA, I mean they were trapped. That's how we ended up at CHE."

Flora also conveyed a more recent story of an event that occurred after Eva was well past the age of majority. "Even as an adult, there would be moments when you cannot speak for yourself, when she was very ill. In February when she was admitted she was already an adult. I went in there and they were giving her dopamine, they were giving her epinephrine. I know that those two have a synergistic effect because they were giving it to her all day and she did not respond blood pressure-wise. So they were adding epinephrine. The effect is instantaneous, so her blood pressure rose from the bottom to off the roof and it's not something that you give and walk away. You have to be there, you have to watch it. I know they have monitors at the desk also, but I am here constantly, bit by bit I'm seeing the changes and you have to get in touch with the resident first."

Concerned about Eva's treatment with these synergistic drugs, she asked, " 'I'm sorry. . . . I'm a nurse and there are things that you have to do and then get the order later. How long do you want the blood pressure to stay so high before you finally get your official order to either turn it off or turn it down?' They get upset. I know there is a protocol. I know that everybody is legally bound, but it would be worse if because you haven't gotten an order, you cannot say that the blood pressure is beyond the range of normalcy. And they would check her blood sugar, for example, when they started she was MPO [nothing by mouth], nothing to drink because of what they had to do. But she drank and drank and drank, and with all the instabilities her blood sugar went off the roof. I said 'If you just give it time, she will come back down.' Of course, they won't listen. They had to give her insulin and then she bottomed out! [claps hands, laughs] So stuff like that is like . . ."

Flora continued, "I'm not a doctor, but I'm in the situation where I can make judgments all the time. In anesthetics we do all these things on a daily basis and we don't need an official to tell you what to do. And that's where it's a little bit different for me. We make decisions all the time even before the residents could respond. We are able to say to the resident, 'No, this is wrong,' or 'This is not good enough,' or 'Do this.' Or you go above the resident and call the attending. That's how it's practiced in my country. But when I come and see certain things being done, [uses deep voice] 'Oh, we'll have to wait for a resident to come.' What happens to those who don't know anything at all? Or to children who don't have parents who could be there some of the time? What health care are we presenting to people? Yes, comparatively to other parts of the world, it is the best. But, even in that best, there are scary moments."

Recalling another incident, Flora described when she almost lost Eva: "I remember when she was in the emergency room. She had been downgraded from critical to normal. So, she was no longer being monitored for air and blood flow. It's ten P.M. I have to work the next day. I say, 'Eva it's okay, they are getting your room ready. I'm leaving. This is where your glasses are. Do you hear me?' No response. 'Eva?' Probably she was seizing at that time, or she had become unconscious. I called for help. Everybody comes and they all stand. How could there be such a rapid change like that? I had to say to them, 'She's not breathing.' I had to grab the ambu bag and started bagging her. Suction, they couldn't even hook up the suction. With one hand, on the other hand I'm doing the suction trying to put it together. When it was all over, the nurse said to me, 'Who are you, anyway?' I said, 'I'm the child's parent, that's why that counts.' [I'm] somebody who is intimately going to stand up by this child's safety."

It is important to critique presumptions about independence and self-sufficiency, since they are ripe with elisions and obfuscations. Sociologist Karl Marx believed an integral part of the development of an enlightened social system was the recognition that we are all dependent on one another for survival. One need not be a Marxist, however, to conclude that having a job, being married, owning a home, and having children also makes one dependent on employers, individuals, and lending institutions. Just as there is no unconditioned free will (freedom), no one is ever freed from dependence. Bill Gates is as dependent on Microsoft consumers as the consumers are on the products produced by his company. Adult sickle cell patients must depend on health care in order to reduce their risk of morbidity or mortality.

The institutional need to bracket a period during which patients are supposed to transition from dependence to independence ignores patients' risks. Emma, Max, John, LaTasha, and Eva are rational actors who find ways to adapt given the limits of the system.[24] Sometimes they require parental involvement; other times they resist those in authority based upon a reasoned assessment of risks. Performing compliance or noncompliance is not a demonstration of greater or lesser cultural competence. Rather, patients know the consequences of their performances and act accordingly. Ultimately, a transitioning program designed to reduce disparities in health care would be attentive to the wisdom of noncompliance and patient dependence.

# CHAPTER 9

# Thought Experiment

*What Does It Mean to Save a Life?*

The quality of health care is based in large part on the imagination and on the culture of hope.[1] But although in the United States hope is generally associated with good things, the culture of hope in medicine can be monolithic and hegemonic. As a result, discourses of hope in medicine have the capacity to drown out other perspectives about what constitutes health and well-being. For example, anthropologist Lesley Sharp describes the ways in which the social imperative to save innocent lives has led to risky medical experimentation: "Transplantation in the United States is driven by a strong professional ethos that insists on saving and extending human lives, sometimes, it seems, at all costs (and here 'costs' may be financial, social, and emotional). Currently, an especially pronounced focus for concern is the ailing child. This is particularly challenging when the need for a heart or a set of lungs arises."[2] Reviewing the histories of the first transplant surgeons, Sharp notes how radically experimental their surgeries were. Most of the early transplant patients died on the table; those who survived spent the remainder of their lives in intensive care, most likely in pain. It is difficult to label these experimental surgeries nefarious because at the time the physicians, institutions, and families were hopeful. But these procedures point to the power of medical authority to shape our sense of what constitutes good and appropriate care even if the care is neither. Clearly these early transplants were less about saving or improving the quality of these children's lives and more about creating a successful transplant protocol. We need to consider that hope can blind us to, at the risk of sounding overly dramatic, medicine's cruelty.

In the case of chronic illness, what if medical treatments were sold not as good or bad but as a series of trade-offs? Patients are told that they can pick from a smorgasbord of forms of suffering, and the physician complies with the wishes of his or her patients. When physicians collaborate to help a patient reach his or her life goals, whatever they may be, a doctor has ceased using medicine to control a patient and has begun using medicine as a tool for patient empowerment. I argue that treatment decisions should be based not on socially ratified discourses of suffering but on sensitivity to a patient's lifescape or a hopeful narrative about how medical intervention in the present will help shape a self-defined future. A physician helps frame a patient's lifescape by facilitating access to biotechnologies that he or she believes are worthwhile and that can potentially generate a patient's desired goals. A lifescape should help a physician decide what it means to save a particular life. The biotechnical embrace helps physicians and patients determine how to do it.[3]

To explore in more depth the role of the imagination in deciding what it means to save a life and how to do it, I asked thirty-seven physicians, nurses, psychologists, sociologists, social workers, researchers, patients, and family members to respond to a hypothetical ethical dilemma. Recognizing that what Dr. Benjamin has accomplished in an adult care setting might not be so easily achieved in the pediatric realm, I became interested in what types of epistemologies and structures stand in the way of unfettered access to health care for adolescent patients. Tracking the origins of these age-based structures led me to sites of power and authority, which in this case brought me back to issues of law, risk, medical authority, and social responsibility. The questions I posed dealt with the issue of when a chronically ill adolescent should have the right to consent to a risky medical procedure. My goal was to address the perceived appropriateness of adolescents weighing in on present-day treatment risks given an uncertain future of suffering and possible early death.

There seems to be tremendous confusion about what sickle cell adolescent patients need protection from: their parents, unethical medical experimentation, irrationality, or themselves. Because of this confusion, the legal age of majority seems to be inconsistently used as a factor in decisions about whether to delegate authority to parents, physicians, or patients. The patient empowerment trope, family-centered care, which was born, I believe, out of a desire to reduce health care costs and physician/institution responsibility, has not replaced medical paternalism. This thought experiment revealed that the sickle cell community is struggling to create an approach to adolescent suffering that they consider rational, if perhaps a bit paternalistic. Adolescent transitioning is one method, but I wanted to know how the discourse about adolescent autonomy or self-efficacy is reframed in light of the culture of hope. In this case, I was interested in how the long-term consequences of current treatment decisions are factored into beliefs about adolescent autonomy, and whether the biotechnical embrace of an experimental therapy alters people's risk calculus. Again, is adolescent transitioning about empowering adolescents with agency, or about acculturating young patients to the risk calculus of the medical community?

At the National Sickle Cell Association meeting in Los Angeles in April 2004, I posed three questions to members of the sickle cell community in order to understand how members conceptualize risk and the ethics of adolescent consent. Over the course of three days I interviewed thirty-five patients, community advocates, researchers, and medical professionals.[4] Eleven interviewees were doctors, seven were researchers, five were patients, six were nurses, four were psychosocial staff, and two were community-based activists.[5]

To make sense of the data, I had to divide the respondents into two groups. The first subgroup of thirty included professionals and advocates who do not have sickle cell disease and do not have immediate family members with sickle cell disease. The second subgroup of seven included patients and one family member (I include Eva and Flora). Of the thirty respondents in the first subgroup, ten were born and raised outside of the United States.[6]

The following three scenarios were presented to my respondents:

Dilemma 1: Jasmine is fifteen years old. Her physician has told her that she is an excellent candidate for a bone marrow transplant. *She wants the transplant, but her parents refuse to give their consent.* For her the risk seems small. Two friends received transplants and are now doing well. Her parents believe the risk is too high. *Should Jasmine be allowed to get a transplant without her parents' permission and why?*

Dilemma 2: Simon is fifteen years old. His physician has told him that he is an excellent candidate for a bone marrow transplant. *Simon's parents want Simon to have the transplant, but Simon does not want to have the transplant. Should Simon be required to undergo the transplant and why?*

Dilemma 3: Jasmine is now twenty-eight. She was not allowed to have the bone marrow transplant, and she was not offered another opportunity to have a transplant. *At twenty-eight, Jasmine is severely ill and spends six months of every year in the hospital. Given her present condition, should Jasmine have been allowed to have the transplant at fifteen and why?*

I chose these dilemmas because respondents have to juggle beliefs about patient autonomy with a medical risk calculus that varies with age. For example, in one study the survival rate and the disease-free survival rate for a bone marrow transplant for patients fourteen years and younger were 93 percent and 82 percent, respectively.[7] The ideal age for transplantation is eight years or younger, when the survival rate is around 99 percent and the success rate is around 90 percent. As a patient ages, the survival rate declines; by the age of sixteen many patients have end-organ damage, like Eva's renal failure, such that they are ineligible for a transplant.

For parents, the decision about whether or not to transplant becomes in a sense irreversible. Put differently, a patient's destiny is determined before he or she has a right to consent to a myloablative transplant. Parents often do not consent because a myloablative transplant is excruciating as the child's bone marrow is destroyed with toxic dosages of chemotherapy drugs. When the patient is on the verge of death, he or she receives donated marrow, often from a relative. The most painful part of the procedure lasts about three months, but it usually takes at least one year before the child is deemed healthy enough to return to normal activities. If the patient is lucky, his or her new marrow will not produce a sometimes acute, sometimes chronic, but always painful rejection response called graft-versus-host disease (GVHD).

There is an alternative treatment. After the age of sixteen, the child may still be eligible for a nonmyloablative transplant, which involves a less toxic dosage of marrow-destroying drugs and does not completely destroy the bone marrow. This type of transplant is still being tested, however, and the outcomes thus far have been poor.

Because of the uncertainties about how severe a child's sickle cell disease will be over his or her lifetime, and uncertainties about the morbidity and mortality resulting from transplantation, parents often ask themselves whether the treatment risks are worth it. In one study, only 49 percent of parents said that given the current rates of disease-free survival, the risk was acceptable.[8] In practice, parents express an even greater reluctance to put their children at risk for dying or GVHD. So the question becomes, Should children as young as ten be able to independently consent to a transplant? Overwhelmingly, the responses to the three scenarios in the thought experiment were informed by beliefs about what constitutes a rational desire to preserve the body, a rational sense of autonomous agency, a rational quality-of-life calculus, and a rational need to protect the interests of both the state and the institution.

The responses of the medical professionals ($n$ = 30) differed from those of the patients/family ($n$ = 7). The differences were substantial and suggestive of how patients and medical professionals perceive suffering from very different vantages. With respect to the first question, 30 percent of nurses ($n$ = 7), patient advocates ($n$ = 8), physicians ($n$ = 11), and researchers ($n$ = 4) said that Jasmine should be allowed to freely consent to a transplant regardless of her age. Including the seven sickle cell patients and Flora, that figure increases to 40.5 percent. All who answered yes to this question stipulated that Jasmine should be given authority only if it is determined that she is fully knowledgeable about the procedure and its risks.

Although I chose to divide the respondents into two camps, beliefs about patient autonomy did not divide neatly between patients/family and medical professionals. Within the medical profession, occupation matters with respect to perceptions about patients. Fifty-seven percent of the nurses said that Jasmine should be allowed to consent, whereas only 10 percent of physicians said they would bypass parental authority. This disparity makes sense given that nurses, who generally get to know their chronic patients well, often assume the role of patient advocate. The physicians interviewed, on the other hand, view bone marrow transplantation as a risky elective procedure, not a treatment panacea, and therefore not a procedure worth fighting for. Dr. Allen, the director of the CHW sickle cell clinic, typified the physician response: "I think that the promise of gene therapy is on the horizon as well. And so, if the parent asks me, 'Dr. Allen, can you keep my child on chronic transfusions until gene therapy is a possibility within twenty years?' the answer is yes. So, then the question becomes, not to transplant or not, but you're weighing one treatment which is . . . granted you're taking a chance that the gene therapy won't come through, but, you know, I've seen some of the data, including data from my own faculty, that suggest that this is going to happen. She says in five years, I think fifteen, so I'll give you twenty. So, your patient is thirty years old. Many transplanters are cowboys. I had a patient with chronic graft-versus-host disease [an immune rejection disease caused by a transplant] that went to do a transplant in a nearby state. [The doctor] said, 'Sure, I can do a transplant for his disease. What is that, by the way?' Honestly. . . . This is conveyed to me by the mother. I mean, they're transplanting end-stage brain tumors for God's sake. I think that's unethical."

Five percent of the medical professionals ($n = 2$) said that outside authorities (science and the law) should determine whether Jasmine is allowed to have the transplant. These respondents, both males, did not believe that parental autonomy should take primacy over patient autonomy. Instead, they argued, a parent's objections should be considered simply one of several relevant factors. The physician from Nigeria said, "I come from a background that says, 'It takes a village to raise a child.'" For him the community must be involved in decisions of this magnitude. The research geneticist from Ghana argued that people, whether the age of majority or younger, must earn the right to make decisions by demonstrating their knowledge. He made a positivist argument that through science one discovers truth, and therefore, in the end, Jasmine's decision must be based on an evidence-based risk calculus. The majority of all the medical professionals, 70 percent, said that Jasmine should not be allowed to make the decision without parental approval. Most thought that the procedure requires such extraordinary commitment, including up to a year of isolation and semi-isolation, that it would simply be impossible for a fifteen-year-old to go through the procedure without the full support of either a parent or a guardian.

Overwhelmingly, respondents believed that Simon should not be forced to undergo a transplant. Seventy-three percent of medical professionals thought that Simon must be willing to assume the risk, endure the pain, and commit to the follow-up regimens; otherwise it is unlikely that the treatment will succeed. The respondents who would refuse Jasmine's request but honor Simon's believed that patient commitment and will were so necessary to treatment outcomes that their different approaches to patient rights were not contradictory. The 17 percent of medical professionals who argued against Simon's independence contended that Simon's answer demonstrated his fear and lack of knowledge. Given what they perceived as immaturity, they believed that Simon should be required to undergo the transplant. Three medical professionals, or 10 percent, argued that an outside authority should decide for the family. These respondents included the two from West Africa, as well as a female physician from India who believed strongly that parents should have authority over their children until the age of eighteen. This belief is modified by her insistence that if a transplant is strongly indicated, then it is not an "ethical question." She explained, "I feel that this decision is very medical rather than ethical. So I'm biased. I feel that this depends on the medical situation of the patient." Because she puts parental autonomy on par with medical expertise she believes that the decision should be made by an outside authority.

The respondents were almost equally divided when it came to whether prognosis should play a role in Jasmine's right to freely consent to treatment as a minor. If Jasmine's terminal status at twenty-eight had been predicted, 53 percent of medical professionals believed she should have had the right to consent to medical treatment as a minor. In other words, 23 percent of the people I interviewed changed their answer from no to yes—that Jasmine should be given the right to consent. The respondents who did not change their minds argued that the choices about whether to perform a transplant are not clear even knowing the long-term odds of survival. In addition to never really knowing the exact disease trajectory of any one patient, there is the issue of whether or not to wait for the next available cutting-edge therapy or treatment. Others felt that there is no way to accurately address any of my three scenarios because each case is unique. Parental issues, disease severity, treatment options, and patient maturity produce a different constellation of variables around which medical professionals work.

When first embarking on this thought experiment, my presumption was that the maturity of the minor would feature as prominently as it does in the case of abortion. In certain states, minors who seek an abortion without parental consent must submit to a judicial bypass hearing, at which time a judge determines whether a teen is mature enough to make this decision. If the teen is deemed immature, the judge can still allow the abortion based on a belief that an abortion is in the best interest of the minor. In the case of bone marrow transplants for sickle cell disease, I assumed patient maturity would be a prominent issue because maturity is often used as a surrogate for rationality, particularly in adolescent transitioning discourse. There is definitional slippage between maturity and rationality because acculturation and cultural competence are generally conflated even though one can be culturally competent in the developmental sense of maintaining a job and household, but not necessarily be acculturated, which would mean accepting the cultural beliefs of the surrounding community. The most relevant example in this case is the refusal of Jehovah's Witnesses to allow their children to receive blood transfusions.

In the case of this thought experiment, not only was maturity rarely mentioned, but all presumed that Jasmine and Simon understood the procedures and the risks. Within the first subgroup, only five respondents stated that they believed Jasmine and Simon lacked the maturity to make their own decision; of those five, only three stated that Simon should be forced to undergo the transplant. The majority of those who would deny Jasmine the transplant stated either that it is not a legal fight worth having or that transplants are such difficult procedures that they require full parental support. The physicians interviewed who have had to obtain court orders to give children what they consider lifesaving blood transfusions over the objections of parents and guardians placed transplants on a different order. Rather than being lifesaving, successful bone marrow transplants are life-enhancing. Therefore, for many medical professionals it does not make sense to take temporary custody away from parents for a risky transplant.[9]

Those who supported Jasmine's choice often cited one or two transplant success stories as proof that transplants have a very low risk-benefit ratio. The only physician, a white woman from the South, to assert that Jasmine's parents were acting irrationally, and therefore that the child needed court protection, relayed the story of a girl she treated for leukemia. This patient, who had had a traumatic childhood, initially rejected a bone marrow transplant even though she had a sibling donor match. Her brother convinced her to have the treatment, and now "She's a junior in college and she's making straight As." A black registered nurse from the South who had also witnessed a few successful transplants and no failures believed that Jasmine's parents needed to be educated. A white registered nurse from the Northeast said that based upon her experiences, she believes that chronically ill sickle cell patients from a very young age understand what they need in order to control their quality of life. She cited the example of one of her five-year-old patients who in an emergency room demanded a topical numbing cream before being stuck with a needle. This was a procedure he had learned from his nurses at his sickle cell clinic. In the emergency room this child was initially rebuffed by the house staff. The child persisted, however, and ultimately received the cream. Based on this anecdote, the nurse argued vehemently that Jasmine should have the right to consent to a transplant.

The best way to understand these varied responses is to recognize them as different approaches to saving a life. For example, respondents who referred to the dilemmas as "medical" rather than "ethical" considered the preservation of the physical body paramount. Medical for them meant evidence-based, which quantifies risk in a way that eclipses the experiences of individuals. For those who collapse saving a life with saving a body, there is a firm distinction between rational and irrational choice. The second group of respondents defines saving a life as increased

patient agency to determine one's own future. These respondents want
patients to have the autonomy to paint their own lifescape regardless of
the risks. Finally, the third group of respondents includes those who
define saving a life as an act that enhances both the life and the survival
of the patient but not at the expense of the community. These respondents recognize that the law is arbitrary, but for them the law frees medical professionals and institutions from taking risks that may destroy the
legitimacy and authority of the profession.

Dr. Kassim, a physician from India, noted, "Well, you know, parents
are given complete control over the destiny of their children, and that is
the ethical framework in which all of civilization, not only Western civilization is based, so . . ." He added, "Any line that you draw in the sand
is a line drawn in the sand. The wind can blow it away, you know"
[laughs]. Physicians who rejected Jasmine's right to consent as a minor
are not unaware of the arbitrariness of the law; rather, for them the law
provides a solution for social impasses. For Dr. Kassim there are so
many uncertainties with respect to bone marrow transplantation that
he would be unwilling to fight for either Jasmine or Simon. For him, the
law protects all parties: the patient, parents, physician, and institution.
Dr. Kassim appreciates the enormous amount of medical uncertainty
surrounding sickle cell disease. For him the law provides clear structural
and legal demarcations that help him navigate in foggy terrain. His
approach to saving a life became apparent in his final remarks on why
he believes a bad prognosis should not change the legal rights of chronically ill minors. He said, "Hindsight is twenty-twenty is the only reason
I can tell you why."

I added, "But they are trying to find new ways of developing prog-
nostic tools . . ."

Grinning, Dr. Kassim responded, "Sure, but that is still really in
development you know. Okay, so . . . I gave a talk on unrelated donor
transplant to the ethics institute at the University of Minnesota. Jeff
Kahn and all those people and Art Caplan had been there before.[10] I
talked to them for an hour and I said, 'Answer my question, is it ethical
to do unrelated donor transplant for sickle cell disease?' They said, 'Ah,
nice talk.' You know . . ."

I laughed, "They avoided the question!"

"They said, 'Can we write a paper?'" Gesturing wildly, Dr. Kassim
said, "'What do you mean? You're ethicists. You're supposed to tell me
what to do!' They said, 'No. Ethicists can allow you to phrase the question. We can't give you the answer.' So, that would be why I have this

little bias, and I'm sorry that I haven't answered any of your questions the way you wanted me to! [laughs]." Anthropologist, ethicist—what's the difference? I did not bother to correct him. In exchange for his time I was happy to be the butt of his joke.

Pediatric hematologists made up the majority of those who preferred clear legal and structural boundaries. Putting a patient's life at risk is not something most physicians want to do without clearly demarcating spheres of authority. For a physician to use the law to limit a minor's agency is not unimaginative or self-serving; the physicians I spoke with are unnerved by the idea that their actions could lead to a patient's disability or death. Dr. Allen from CHW said during his interview, "I lost a patient to sickle cell disease in our center. I think that was four years ago, five years ago, and that was from a screwup."

"Too much morphine?" I asked.

"No," Dr. Allen responded. "The kid with a fever who wasn't given antibiotics when they should have. And now I know that the internist . . . you know . . . Pediatrics, you know, we're a little bit insulated from that, but . . . So . . . And I . . ." What Dr. Allen was trying not to say is that the physician who improperly treated his sickle cell patient was an internist and not part of his team. Abruptly changing the subject, Dr. Allen said, "You know, hydroxyurea has made a huge difference in their overall survival. According to Steinberg's paper last summer, there is a 40 percent decrease in death."

I asked him if he has observed similar decreases. "Oh, yeah," he said with pleasure. "I see kids that were admitted all the time and they're not coming in at all anymore." Dr. Allen's risk calculus changed when he considered what type of care Jasmine would receive. For Dr. Allen, patients should not be seen by internists who know little about sickle cell disease. In situations like these, he argues, it is better to push treatments like hydroxyurea and bone marrow transplantation that keep patients out of hospitals. He elaborated, "If the choices were to have a transplant or go off to Indiana, where there isn't a sickle cell patient in the state, then. . . ."

In summary, the health care professionals viewed underage consent as a question of rational choice, patient autonomy, or individual versus institutional checks and balances. With the exception of physicians, who generally want to balance saving a patient's life with preserving the legitimacy of their profession and institution, health care professionals see parental autonomy as one of a number of decision-making factors. Only three health care professionals considered parental autonomy alone a decisive factor. Twenty-three considered parental authority part of a system of checks and balances. Four believed that in the case of these dilemmas, the legal age of consent should be extended to minors.

## THE PATIENTS

For the patients and Eva's mother, Flora, patient or parental autonomy was the only relevant category. Medical professionals, from their point of view, should never be given the right to override the authority of parents and patients. They believed the job of medical professionals is to present enough detailed information to allow families to make decisions. Institutional concerns, from the perspective of families and patients, are obstacles to be negotiated. Patients know from experience that medicine is more art than science, and that treatment decisions are simply a series of trade-offs. These patients had been on the receiving end of treatment errors and misdiagnoses, forever destroying the mystique of medicine.

Doris, a Jamaican woman in her fifties, relayed several personal stories that revealed why she no longer considered medical advice authoritative. Doris is a petite woman who punctuates her stories with an infectious giggle. After the birth of her now adult child, Doris developed sickling in her lungs, or acute chest syndrome, and has since had significant problems with asthma, pneumonia, and bronchitis. For Doris, chronic pain and lung damage remain her most significant health problems, but in spite of these challenges, she remains active. Currently she counsels sickle cell patients on nutrition, academic success, and how to tolerate pain and get on with life. In the telling of her health history, Doris described her last doctor visits before finally being diagnosed with sickle cell disease at the age of twenty-five: "I was in California and I went swimming. I got on the plane [the next day], and I had this excruciating pain on the whole left side of my body. I thought I was having a heart attack because I could turn this way, but I couldn't turn that way. When I got back to New York, I couldn't even sleep in a bed. I had to sleep upright in a chair because laying down was so painful. So, I went to the hospital again, and I'm like, 'I don't know why I'm having all this pain, but I went swimming.' The doctor didn't even take a stethoscope to check to see if my heart was beating. He told me I sprained my neck. So, I said to him, 'If I sprained my neck, why is it I can turn to one side?' I said, 'This is totally ridiculous. You're prescribing something for me and you have no clue why I'm feeling all this pain?' So I went to this other clinic. I just kept going from place to place just to try to find out what was my problem. I went to this doctor. The doctor there *did* say that he could see that I was having sickling of the cells. He said, 'Oh, you don't look like someone who has sickle cell disease.' So my next question to him was, 'What is a person supposed to look like if they have sickle cell disease?' He just didn't answer, but they were ready to have surgery on me. I said, 'Nobody is cutting me until I know what is my problem.' So I said, 'You know what, I'll just go deal with my pain.' And that's why I was so glad when that friend told me about this place. She said, 'Just go there and find out, and they will tell you whether it's the trait.' And, that's when I went, and that's the first time I found out that I had the C hemoglobin."

When considering a doctor's risk-benefit assessment in bone marrow transplantation, Doris said, "There are times when they really don't know. Because in my case, from my experience, the doctor had said, 'This is going to happen if you do this!' and it never happened." Doris's experiences with poor physician prognoses and questionable treatment advice informed her belief that Jasmine and Simon should have the right to decide whether or not to have a transplant. With a smile on her face Doris stated, "If the child is willing to take the risk and is willing to go for it, then I really think that in that case, yeah." She later acknowledged that doctors and hospitals might be sued if they performed the procedure without parental consent, but ethically she believes strongly that a chronically ill adolescent should be allowed to shape his or her own fate. She did not, however, believe that prognosis should determine whether or not minors have the right to consent. Again, from her perspective doctors are often wrong.

Until Doris left for New York at the age of eighteen, her great-grandfather in Jamaica treated her frequent pain crises. When she was in pain, her great-grandfather would rub her with essential oils. Having read a tremendous amount of literature on nutrition and the importance of maintaining a particular body pH, Doris believes that her diet in Jamaica was the best thing for her sickle cell disease. Doris has chosen to return to the health regimens of her youth and now rejects standard treatments. She explained, "If a person really wants to do it [have a transplant], let them at least try. My thing is, like, hydroxyurea, I personally make a choice. I don't want it. I'm going to try something else." I asked Doris if she had been offered transfusion therapy. Doris replied, "Yeah, I didn't want it because to me that would be like adding more stuff to my system than my system probably can deal with. That's the way I look at it. I said, 'Let me try another route, and then I will see how that works.'"

Jan, another patient who participated in the thought experiment, also refuses standard therapies. She sought refuge from health care in religion after deciding that the chronic blood transfusions prescribed to treat her sickle cell disease were wrong. "After I had my second child and they wanted to give me blood. I was so sick of taking blood transfusions. My sister who lived in the Los Angeles area at the time said, 'Why are you crying?' And I said, 'Because I've got this bag of blood hanging here and I'm so sick of taking blood I don't know what to do.' She said, 'Talk to a Jehovah's Witness. They do not take blood.' The next year, I got into a Bible study and everything."

Jan was an exuberant light-skinned women in her fifties whose vitality hid her precarious health. In addition to having frequent pain episodes, she had had two artificial hip replacements, had had thirteen operations, was almost completely blind in one eye, and had double vision in the other. Despite her aches, pains, and physical limitations, she was pursuing a degree in counseling. When she finished her degree, her goal was to begin educating physicians about sickle cell patients.

At the beginning of the interview Jan argued that parents should have autonomy when it comes to medical consent. "Jasmine shouldn't be able to get a transplant without her parents' consent because Jasmine is still up under the age limit to where she is considered her parents' responsibility. The risks that are involved, I don't think that Jasmine fully understands them all, so she does need that adult backing. Her parents are going to be the ones who are going to have to suffer with her with the decision that she makes, so, no, she should not leave them out of this."

Responding to whether Simon should be forced to undergo a bone marrow transplant, Jan said, "No, I would not force Simon to undergo that. See, then I'm messing with his spiritual side, and that's going to make it more difficult for Simon to even heal through this process because you forced him to do something that he didn't want to do." Her response, I believe, surprised her, and as a result Jan moved away from her original assertion about parental authority and became emphatic that patient autonomy was essential. "Don't treat the person as though they are not involved, okay. That is their life, all right, so don't sit back and make decisions on a child who is able to think, all right. They are able to think and function and say, 'I've read something about this. I know some things about this. If I don't have all the information and

everything, then help me there so that I *do* make the right decision.'
That's what I'm saying."

Finally, Jan tried to make sense of the questions and her answer by
revealing a story that speaks to issues of how ethical knowledge is
produced. "At the age of six, when they found out I had sickle cell disease, when they gave me that first bag of blood, my body and mind
said, 'No, this is not the way to go.' It's like you said, you're a child, so
you have to. I put my trust in my parents, okay. They were my leaders.
They were my directors. Because God knew they were ignorant to the
fact of what was going on, I did not get punished for their doings. He
doesn't do that to us. He doesn't punish us for what other people are
doing. He punishes us for what *we* do. So, I think that she [Jasmine]
should have been able to make her decision as long as, like I said, she
was knowledgeable."

Jan turned the discussion into a question of one's soul. She referred to
the Bible, in which the age of consent, according to her reading, is
twelve: "It's still the individual's choice, according to the Bible. We are
out from under our parents' thumbs, so to say, after we get to the age of
twelve because by then they should have taught us right from wrong.
And if we don't have all the knowledge necessary, and we still need our
parents' backing. . . . In teaching our children, we should have taught
them the respect to, 'Mom, Dad, I'm going to make this decision;' or
'Mom, Dad, I'm going to listen to what you say, but know that the final
say-so is mine.' That's the way I trained my children, 'Whatever you
want to do in this world, that's up to you. If you do something that's
wrong, you're the one that's going to answer, not me. But before you got
to be twelve years old, I had to answer for everything you did.'"

Saving a life in Jan's case means allowing someone the agency to save
his or her soul even if it means physical death. For Jan, suffering, the
consequence for disobeying God, was far more frightening than facing
one's mortality. About her family she said, "I'm the only Jehovah's
Witness *in* my family. My older sister before she passed wanted to know
more about it. Unfortunately, she passed away as we were getting close
and everything."

Similar to Doris, Jan recounted instances where physicians gave her
bad prognoses and unnecessary treatments. As a result, physician and
institutional demands and concerns did not inform her ethics calculus.
She believed herself to be, in many instances, more rational than her
physicians. Her evidence for what was or was not rational came from
her own experiences, coupled with her interpretation of the Bible.

Similar to Doris, Jan relied on alternative therapies to quell disease symptoms. For both, evidence-based medicine caused pain and suffering, both physical and psychic. From the perspective of Doris and Jan, statistical probabilities have nothing to do with their day-to-day experiences with sickle cell disease and sense of wellness, which is why they believe that saving a life means supporting a patient's autonomy. Even though they recognize that legally Jasmine's and Simon's parents have a right to determine their children's future, ethically they believe that as soon as patients are able to understand the repercussions of their choices, they should be granted agency. Medical professionals who privilege saving bodies over saving souls consider Doris and Jan nonrational actors, and patients like Jan and Doris are often described in their charts as problematic and noncompliant.

Ella, another interlocutor, was at the sickle cell association meetings to learn as much as possible about blood transfusion therapy. Petite and beautiful, Ella had a surprisingly solemn disposition. She was married, had three children, and was in her late twenties. Female sickle cell patients often have a difficult time with pregnancies and the physical demands of child rearing, but Ella had an extensive support network that helped her juggle family and chronic illness. She had flown from Colorado to acquire enough scientific information to challenge her hematologist.

Ella said, "It's a conflict between whether I stay on transfusions or not. I feel like the transfusion program is being protected for political reasons, and they need as many patients on it as possible." I asked her what she thought was motivating doctors to put people on transfusion therapy, to which she replied, "Grants . . . dollars."

She told me that she did not think she needed transfusions. "I've been told that I don't need to be transfused. I've had the option of staying off, but my doctor is like, 'Well, I don't know . . .' I have private insurance, and my copays are high even though I have private insurance. And so, that's why I really don't appreciate the way people make me feel. I mean, they make me feel like my money is not as green as other patients' that they see, oncology patients. They make me feel like if they're doing their job they're doing me a favor, and anything I want I don't deserve. So, maybe I said too much."

Ella's conspiracy theories are the only way she makes sense of her experiences with medical care because her physicians do not communicate well or take her requests for information seriously. Because in her city there is only one place that handles long-term care for sickle cell patients, Ella confesses that she has come to the meeting to find a new physician.

"I am very dissatisfied. I feel that it's unethical because at what cost do you put someone's life . . . because I've had residual issues from having blood. When I was younger I didn't have blood transfusions that much. It was like every six months. The same person donated, so I knew where my blood was coming from."

She compared her prior experiences, which she believes were handled well, to her more recent care. "And [now] these are exchange transfusions. There are six units of blood every four weeks from six different people. I have concerns about hormones if six different individuals are donating blood. How many of them are men? How many of them are women of childbearing age? And so, how many are actually replacing the hormones that you lose in your blood when they take it out? What's replaced? I have issues about those things, and when I bring them up, they make me feel like I ask too much. I get brick-walled, 'No, no . . . no . . . of course you don't know. We know a lot about that.' Right now, I've been very well advised as to what to say, what not to say, and the only thing that is keeping me patient is the whole thing is so political. It's just really ugly and really, really nasty. You know? We've had an individual retire, and she had been there for almost thirty years, and she's been replaced with individuals that have no care in the world about patients with sickle cell."

Unlike Jan and Doris, Ella is just beginning to reject medical authority. She considers her hematologists entrepreneurs first, compassionate physicians second. Ella wants to empower herself with enough scientific information to reject medical paternalism.

In response to the ethical dilemma, Ella began by firmly positioning herself in the parental autonomy camp, saying, "I mean, the parent is the parent until that child is eighteen." It is important to note that Ella was interviewed along with Martha, another sickle cell patient, who argued that a fifteen-year-old should have the right to consent to treatments. Martha said, "I'm just thinking of the average fifteen-year-old these days, they're pretty intelligent, they are pretty informed kids, at least, maybe the fifteen-year-olds that I encounter. The parents, they mean well, and in no way, shape, or form are they being bad parents to say no. But maybe a part of that 'no' is 'Well, I don't want to lose Jasmine.'"

Martha, in her late thirties, has severe pulmonary hypertension; as a result, her sentences are broken up by loud, deliberate inhalations from a nasal cannula, a thin, hollow tube connected to a tank and positioned under her nose to deliver concentrated oxygen to her damaged lungs.

Martha, who has a seven-year-old daughter, described her health as follows: "At twenty-seven I had my first hip replacement. I was supposed
to have it replaced [again] two years ago, but because of the pulmonary
hypertension it's very difficult and dangerous to put me under anesthesia because of the stress on my heart. So, I'm just living from day to day
in a lot of very severe pain because my left hip is totally gone. I've had
an infarct in both hips really bad and infarcts in my lungs."

Martha, who had thus far been much more severely affected by her
disease than Ella, concluded that nobody should stop Jasmine from creating a better life for herself. Ella never explicitly acknowledged that
Martha is a living reminder of Jasmine; nevertheless, Ella did modify
her position slightly after listening to Martha. Ella added that if an adolescent can prove that he or she is mature and knowledgeable about the
procedure and risks, then perhaps authority can be granted to the
minor. In neither case did either Martha or Ella mention physician input
or institutional risk assessment. In fact, Ella emphasized that if a minor
is granted rights, a judge should mediate not because the judge would
make the most rational decision but in order to make it clear to the parents that this was the child's decision. The judge's ruling, Ella concluded,
would hopefully diminish future parental guilt.

Martha, who is originally from Belize, has had positive experiences
with her physicians. Initially she was followed by Dr. Davis, but recently
she switched to Dr. Jackson because he works in a hospital that allows
her daughter to visit. I found it extremely interesting that Martha had
had positive experiences with Dr. Davis. Dr. Davis, an adult physician
who was described earlier, believes strongly in patient agency and in
encouraging patients to choose whatever treatment fits their definition
of a life well lived. Only one of his patients is on chronic transfusion
therapy. Over the years, Dr. Davis has observed that his adult patients
reject chronic transfusion therapy. Between the numerous trips to the
hospital and the daily eight-hour Desferal treatments, adult patients
simply do not want to abide by the transfusion regimens. Others believe
that Dr. Davis subtly discourages his patients from transfusion therapy
simply because he believes it reduces patient quality of life. One could
ask, therefore, if Martha would have been healthier had she had been on
chronic transfusion therapy. There is no way to answer that question,
but if we examine narratives of chronic patients, patients like Martha
seem to value treatment decision agency much more than they value the
possible health outcomes that may have resulted from medical paternalism, as we see in the case of Ella.

Tamika, a sickle cell patient in her thirties, best summed up the differences between health care worker and patient perspectives. Responding to Simon's dilemma, Tamika said: "There might be a reason why this child does not want to have the transplant. He might be scared, he might be nervous. That's a kind of hard question actually because the parents want him to have it and he doesn't want to have it. I think that if that child has sickle cell, and that's the way that child feels, then the child shouldn't have to have it. Because I'm like this . . . I have the disease myself and everybody says, 'Oh, you know, there might be a cure for sickle cell,' and stuff like that. I was born with this disease, I'm gonna leave here with that disease, and the reason why I feel like that is because this is something that God gave me. Also, when they say that they find cures and stuff like that, I always hear that there is a side effect. I have enough problems, I don't need anymore. Honestly."

Eventually she added, "If Simon died, it was Simon's time to go [Tamika and I laugh]. It was Simon's time to go." Summarizing her response, I said, "Just accept it." With a smile on her face but without equivocation, Tamika said, "Right. Because I've been in the hospital, and I've been overdosed and stuff like that. And they would have to pump my stomach and bring me back. I could have died, but it wasn't my time to go. So, if Simon died, it was Simon's time to go, I believe."

This pragmatic fatalism was something that the health care professionals did not address. Perhaps they felt uncomfortable expressing the real fact that sometimes people die as a result of treatment. Whether their silence was the result of oversight or decorum, what can or does get said by whom is important.

Analyzing my data, perhaps there were no real surprises. It makes sense that physicians who have a professional stake in the success of their sickle cell centers, institutions, and reputations consider the needs of not just the patient but also the community and institution. It makes sense that nurses appreciate the importance of patient agency given that they witness individual patient suffering and treatment uncertainties at a personal level. Pediatric nurses who treat sickle cell patients often watch their patients grow from babies into adults. Over the years they get to know the families and the intimate lives of their patients. It also makes sense that patients and family members focus on their own autonomy. Finally, it makes sense that physicians who are both clinicians and research scientists prioritize evidence-based approaches. The data demonstrate that perceptions about what factors should be used to determine whether a minor should be allowed to consent to a transplant are informed by one's professional or personal position.[11] There is clearly an element of structural-functionalism shaping sentiments around minor consent. To reduce it to structure and function alone, however, is to miss the relationship between philosophical understandings about the origins of suffering (theodicy) and accountability.

The three categorical responses to the dilemma can be reframed in terms of philosophical approaches to knowledge. I use the term *rational choice* to describe respondents who focus on saving bodies and who privilege evidence-based approaches. Their strong belief that empirical knowledge is truth makes them committed modernists. For them, patients need to be alive in order to make choices and to empower themselves. Therefore, to allow a teen to make the decision to take unnecessary risks makes no sense. In a number of legal cases, a judge made a decision to override an adolescent's wishes. In "Acknowledging the Hypocrisy: Granting Minors the Right to Choose Their Medical Treatment," Christine Hanisco describes a number of recent cases in which adolescents tried to refuse medical treatment:

> In Massachusetts, a sixteen-year-old boy ran away from home to avoid chemotherapy treatment despite his parents' consent. In California, a fifteen-year-old girl fled her home after being physically forced to succumb to chemotherapy, despite both her parents' and her lack of consent. Another fifteen-year-old who, with parental consent, chose to discontinue his medication and decline a third liver transplant, was forcibly removed by police from his home and hospitalized. Another fifteen year old, suffering from end-stage cystic fibrosis, was placed on a ventilator despite his repeated wishes against life-prolonging measures, such as intubation and mechanical ventilation.[12]

Implied in these rulings is the notion that the choice to refuse medical care is irrational, and that only adults are mature enough to (senselessly) end their own lives. In all these cases, the adolescent believed that medical intervention inflicted more suffering than if the disease had been allowed to progress naturally. In fact, the fifteen-year-old girl, a Hmong refugee who rejected the treatment for spiritual and cultural reasons, described the chemotherapy she was forced to endure as "torture."[13] What the rational choice respondents seem to forget is that quality of life is quantifiable only if one ignores personal variables.

"Patient agency" best describes the second category of responses. These are the individualists, often patients and patient advocates, who believe that adolescents who understand the risks should have complete control over their treatment decisions. There is legal precedent for this approach to the question of adolescent consent. In *Union Pacific Railway Company v. Botsford* (1891), the U.S. Supreme Court ruled that individuals had a right to refuse medical treatment.[14] Recent right-to-die cases, including *Cruzan vs. Director, Missouri Department of Health,* uphold the *Botsford* ruling, but these rights are granted to adults and parents of minors. What patient agency advocates often overlook is that patients are never fully autonomous. Patients rely on physicians, people, and/or institutions they trust in order to develop opinions about treatments. Their agentive choice, in other words, is very much situated in a particular social matrix that includes the valorization of a particular set of scientific facts embedded in a particular set of social and material relations. Adolescents who request bone marrow transplants are not independent thinkers. Instead, they have been given a culturally inscribed set of choices that are neither subversive nor revolutionary.

"Structural pragmatism" describes the third category of responses. Respondents in this category try to balance the needs of the patient, guardian(s), institution, scientific community, and sickle cell community. These individuals are hesitant to give minors the right to consent not because they think fifteen-year-olds are immature but because it presents a legal quagmire. If something were to go wrong, the institution could be threatened, the physician could lose professional standing, and the sponsors of bone marrow transplants (e.g., the NIH) could be forced to abandon experimental studies.

The courts consider six things when trying to determine who should have authority to consent to medical care:

1.  the patient's expressed preferences, if any;
2.  the patient's religious convictions, if any;
3.  the impact on the patient's family;
4.  the probability of adverse side effects from the treatment;
5.  the prognosis without treatment; and
6.  the present and future incompetence of the patient in making that decision.[15]

In this way, the pragmatists mirror, in many respects, the legal approach to underage consent. This very diplomatic approach is rarely if ever socially transformative, and in many ways, following this approach places individuals in the position of subjugating their own interests to protect the interests of powerful institutions.

There is a presumption, even among the respondents, that courts intervene only in exceptional cases, when a child's death is imminent. In fact, in a number of cases a parent has lost temporary custody of a child for refusing nonemergency treatment. In California, a parent lost custody for refusing to have his child monitored for the possible recurrence of cancer. In Iowa, a father lost custody for refusing to allow his child's tonsils and adenoids to be removed. In New York, a mother lost custody of her child for refusing to allow risky surgery to partially correct a facial deformity. In another case in New York, a mother lost custody for refusing medical and dental care for an umbilical hernia, fractured teeth, and cavities. Finally, in Texas, a mother was charged with neglect for choosing spiritual healing over medical treatment for her son's arthritic knee.[16] These parents all claimed to reject medical treatment for religious reasons, which may have simply been a defense strategy. But for someone who does not consider religious beliefs significantly different from secular beliefs, one can read their defense as a statement about values. Every year thousands of people die as a result of medical care, and so rejecting nonemergency treatment is not necessarily an irrational choice. With respect to the facial surgery, one wonders if the court is protecting the child, or if the court is enforcing normative values regarding appearance.

In some exceptional cases, a judge has accepted the religious convictions of a minor. In Illinois, a girl identified as E.G., who suffered from leukemia, and her mother, both Jehovah's Witnesses, refused a blood transfusion. E.G. was deemed a mature minor and therefore was allowed to refuse the transfusion. Ultimately, the Illinois Supreme Court ruled that since the U.S. Supreme Court had not recognized that either adults or minors have a constitutional right to refuse lifesaving medical treatment, the court based its decision on case law and Illinois statutes to conclude that a minor, with judicial approval, could refuse medical treatment. The court stated that in the absence of a statute, a trial judge should determine "whether a minor is mature enough to make health care choices on her own." However, the court stated that the right must be balanced against four state interests: "(1) the preservation of life; (2) protecting the interests of third parties; (3) prevention of suicide; and (4) maintaining the ethical integrity of the medical profession." Since E.G. was no longer a minor, the court did not remand the case to the trial court.[17]

The different perspectives about Jasmine's and Simon's right to consent are not based on whether or not a teenager is mature. People frame the solution to the dilemma differently based on where they locate truth and power: science, the individual, or institutions. The fact that people within the sickle cell community have varied approaches to making sense of abstract risk-benefit analyses means that there will never be a single approach to treatment ethics. What remains uncertain is the question of whether chronically ill minors will ever be given the right to determine their health care futures against the wishes of their parents or guardians. New treatments and therapies that must be performed before a patient reaches the age of majority present a new ethical challenge for the sickle cell community, but what would it take to transform the current status quo? Lowering the age of consent? Creating better prognosis tools? At the NIH, I heard a physician discuss another possible solution that her center is trying, which is to encourage parents to arrange transplants for their children before the age of ten to avoid the hassles of adolescent consent and compliance.

## A FAMILY DEFINES RISK

To illustrate the data here ethnographically, I return to the story of Eva and her parent's difficult decision to fight for a kidney transplant, a real-life equivalent of my hypothetical scenario. In the summer of 2004, I asked Eva's mother, Flora, hypothetically if Eva had been fifteen years old, still a minor, and had demanded a transplant against Flora's wishes, would she have allowed her daughter to make her own decision? Flora began answering by citing the rights of judges to overrule parents' wishes if the survival of the child is at stake. She mentioned the example of a Jehovah's Witness refusing a blood transfusion for a deathly ill child. Then she noted how difficult it was for her to answer the question because, unlike the hypothetical parent who refused, Flora was very much in favor of a bone marrow transplant. In fact, ever since Eva's condition deteriorated when she was around twelve years old, Flora repeatedly showed a willingness to experiment with risky procedures to improve the quality of Eva's life. While responding to my hypothetical dilemma, Flora could not sustain the voice of the impartial observer and began to explain her rationalization for what some of Eva's doctors believed was an unnecessary transplant: "I didn't have any data to support my inkling. But it seemed as if since she was not progressing, what was the next step for her? Now if I was ignorant, or . . . not ignorant . . . well, if I was not knowledgeable enough and she wanted it, and the medical people felt that it was necessary for her to have it, I think they would have gone ahead and given it to her."

Following Flora's lead, I switched from the hypothetical to Eva's life. "Let's say she died as a result of it? Would that make you angry given that your wishes were overruled?"

A bit flustered, Flora responded, "It's difficult to answer that because I am not in that situation, and . . ."

Realizing I might have gone too far, I pulled back and asked, "I guess the question would be . . . when you assume a risk, do you just assume it and just whatever happens happens, or do you . . ."

Flora's answer made me realize that she was not offended by my question but wanted to draw as best she could from her real-life experiences. Once she could recall a similar story, she began, "It's whatever happens happens because even when she was in the intensive care unit at one point, I called the doctors and told them, 'I want her to have a DNR.' She was bleeding everywhere. She was unconscious. I said, 'If she cannot maintain her own life, if she cannot breathe on her own, I do not want any extra measures to keep her alive.' At that point, my husband came in from work, saw her, he started crying. I said, 'This is what we are discussing, what do you want us to do at this point?' If you have to give up, you give up. And I told the doctors, 'This is my child. You do not love her more than I do. And if she has to die, then she will die, and it will be okay with us.' Even before then in '95, when she was critically ill and we had to go to Nigeria, I said to her, you can die anywhere, you can be here in America and die. You can be anywhere else and die. You don't need to be afraid of death. Eventually we all will die.

"One of my children, the youngest one, said, 'Oh, you don't love her if that's what you think!' I don't want her to die, but everything we do is risky. We step out even from our bedroom, we are taking a big risk. Driving a car, we're taking a risk. We don't think about that. And when your time is up, your time is up, no matter what you do. I don't want her to be vented and dependent on extraneous measures to keep the blood circulating if she's no longer there."

"This was after she was eighteen?" I asked.

"Yes."

"And you could do that, they allowed you to do that?"

"Yes, because she wasn't there to make the decision for herself," Flora said as she turned her palms up to the ceiling in a gesture of resignation.

Turning to Eva, I asked, "Is that something that you would decide as well?"

Without hesitation, Eva agreed with her mother, "To not be on machines or something? Yeah . . . yeah. . . . I don't see the point. If you're not there, it's just a body."

Returning to physician authority versus family autonomy, Flora clarified her feelings: "So, would I be angry that they went against my advice? I mean, they've gone against my advice before on other things that almost cost her her life, but it's part of life."

Flora immediately recognized that posing transplantation consent as a dilemma distinct from everyday practices in medicine is naive. The focus in medical ethics on the extraordinary hides more mundane truths, which in this case would be that overriding parental authority, similar to physician-assisted death (suicide), is something that happens on a daily basis, and any substantive discussion of medical ethics must consider the complexity of choice in practice. What Flora reveals is that for her chronically ill child, uncertainty exists even in the procedures deemed routine and safe.

Continuing with the thought experiment questions, I asked, "What if Eva hypothetically didn't want a transplant at fifteen, but you really wanted the transplant?"

Flora replied, "Well, does she understand enough to make that decision? We would have had a conference." Switching almost seamlessly from the hypothetical to the real, Flora continued, "[Eva] said, 'I want whatever is gonna make me well.' That's all she kept on saying. She couldn't even talk. She couldn't even sit straight. That's how worse off she was. And they were trying to veer the conversation from me to her. Which I understand, but, what is it if you're not there to think straight? What can you say? Mostly if you're always on the official narcotic, you cannot think straight to put two sentences together. That's why we have who we have [meaning family]. Together we can all make one good sentence.

"In the final analysis, it didn't come down to her asking for [a kidney transplant], it was us pushing for it. When things go wrong, they always think that maybe we didn't make the right decision. [Every time] she develops all these complications, I'm like, 'Oh, my God, was it the right decision to transplant?' I mean, I questioned myself that she has to be on all these medications all her life. That doesn't mean that we did not make the right decision, but everything has its consequence. There are no free rides. We have to deal with each decision that we make all the time."

I asked Flora if Eva's health outcomes were more predictable or uncertain. I used the example of Eva emerging from a near-fatal septic infection pain free. Flora disagreed with Eva that the pain went away as a result of the infection and the suppression of sickle cell production in her marrow and argued instead that the apheresis was responsible.

There seemed to be tremendous uncertainty about even the origins of the pain relief.

Eva defended her explanation: "The only reason why I say that is because even when I was in that hospital, I was tired, yes, but the pain wasn't there. And, it was very weird to get used to it, because I didn't know . . . I didn't know where it was coming from. I just didn't have any more pain." Instead of disputing Eva's assessment, Flora redirected the conversation to how little the physicians know about the causes and effects of illness. "And the only thing I know is that with the sepsis the bacteria had to colonize the kidney, which should have made the kidney function worse. When they did the kidney function test, the creatinine was even lower with the sepsis." That meant that the kidneys, according to the tests, were functioning more efficiently.

On the heels of this description of medical uncertainty, Flora recounted another story of how physicians often do not know why Eva's body responds as it has to illnesses and treatments: "When she went to the hospital with the shingles, one of the renowned doctors came over and snobbishly implied that a transplant is not always the answer, 'Transplant doesn't always mean that you are free of problems.' Something like that because she developed these shingles from immuno-suppression. I think he was probably one of those who didn't think she should have had the transplant. I mean, he made that statement, I just heard it, and that was all there was to it. I refused to take it any other way."

The doctor used Eva's shingles as proof that his earlier assessment of risk was right and as an indication of his superior medical knowledge. Flora, who has had to make many life-or-death decisions for her daughter, objects to his exploitation of an unanticipated outcome to assert his professional authority. Flora must live with the fact that her decision may have shortened her daughter's life, so not only is it callous to push responsibility for Eva's continued suffering onto Flora, but the physician clearly does not understand the lifescape that Flora is trying to create for Eva.

I tried to elicit Eva's feelings about dialysis. "But the other choice is you would have gone to dialysis three days a week."

Flora responded, "Yeah, that was for years and years and years."

I asked Eva, "Is that a choice you would have made?"

"I didn't like it. I was only on it for six months. From . . ."

Flora finished Eva's sentence, "From . . . yeah, six months because you started it in January and it ended in June, yeah, six months."

I asked, "You couldn't go to school or anything like that?"

"I was very tired . . ."

Flora was reminded of people who lived their lives while on dialysis. She commented, "I know those would do it and still go to work. There was that boy who was going to school. But, anyway, we're talking about a lot of issues here, not just sickle cell or . . ."

To contextualize Flora's story, I said, "For him maybe it was just the kidneys. . . ."

Eva confirmed my guess, "It was just his kidneys."

Flora repeated, "Just the kidneys, yeah. . . ."

The fact that the normally quiet Flora kept interrupting questions I directed at Eva indicated to me that Flora remained on the defensive about her decision to force a transplant.

From the perspective of the family there was no clear division between pediatric and adult care. Eva, who was almost twenty-four years old during this interview, relied on her mother to advocate for her and help her make choices. To label this dependence immaturity is to ignore the complexity of the decision-making process. Eva enjoyed relative health and productivity most of the year, but without parental support she would not have people around her who could help her out when her cognitive status was compromised by severe illness.

In transition discourse, the transition from adolescence to adulthood is presented as a sharp line. Chronically ill patients are to assume the role of self-advocate after turning eighteen, and those who do not do so are presumed in the health care setting to lack maturity. This is an arguable presumption particularly in the case of Eva, who exhibited numerous adult competencies in the areas of her life unrelated to health management. She was successfully working toward a career, and despite numerous brushes with death and disability, she was only a couple years behind her peers. Speaking with the director of another sickle cell clinic at a late-night fried chicken dinner at sickle cell camp, Dr. Duncan said that the teens he treats whose parents are the least involved, the worst advocates for their children, are often the most self-sufficient by the time they reach eighteen. Patients like Eva, whose parents proved to be powerful advocates, often continue to rely on their parents for health care decision making. Dr. Duncan's point seems at one level obvious, but what is not so obvious is which patients have better outcomes. The valorization of independence in the American health care setting may in fact be much more beneficial to the hospital than to the patient.

It is important to note that Eva was never pressured to transition. I believe it was because she was extremely compliant to medical authority and continued to perform well outside of the health care setting, making her the model patient. The decision not to transition Eva was not simply a self-serving act; the Children's Health East team also worried that in the hands of a weak adult sickle cell program, a complicated patient like Eva might not survive. Eva exemplifies why for chronically ill patients the structural distinctions between pediatric and adult care are problematic. Dependence and autonomy are not mutually exclusive and should not be treated as such. Giving a fifteen-year-old who suffers daily from excruciating pain the power to consent to a risky procedure regardless of her financial and emotional dependence on her parents is not necessarily a confused policy. Similarly, opening up a space in adult medicine for family and parental involvement in the care of chronically ill adults who are not developmentally disabled should not be viewed negatively.

## A PHYSICIAN DEFINES RISK

To better understand how physicians interpret risk, I asked Dr. Davis, the adult hematologist from California, how he would determine acceptable risk.

> *Carolyn:* They don't give bone marrow transplants to people over sixteen, right? Because there's too much organ damage already.
>
> *Dr. Davis:* The chance of you having an organ damaged, that would double or triple your mortality from the transplant, you see. Because you get lung disease. It's subtle. I don't care who you are, you can't get through a transplant. Normal people. If you had to have a transplant for breast cancer or something like that, and you have pulmonary fibrosis, even though you weren't symptomatic, you see, because of the weird pulmonary infections that you get, when you have no pulmonary reserve to carry you through, because you're already operating at maximum deficiency. So, any kind of pulmonary insult and you're gone.
>
> *Carolyn:* Do you think bone marrow transplants are going to be the wave of the future?
>
> *Dr. Davis:* What mortality and morbidity . . . morbidity being serious complications . . . what level and risk are you willing to take? You take a three-year-old, and you tell the family, "We can do a bone marrow, or a stem cell transplant on this kid, cure him of sickle cell disease, but he is going to have an XYZ chance of death or serious disease following it."

*Carolyn:* Yeah, but it has only been the most drastic cases where the parents have been like "okay, trans—"

*Dr. Davis:* Well, remember the mortality was 30 percent.

*Carolyn:* It's not that high.

*Dr. Davis:* It's not that high anymore. If they get it down to around 5 percent mortality, 10 percent serious morbidity . . .especially in under five year olds, who can tolerate transplants better than us older folks—older being anybody over six. If you're talking about those kind of risks, that's getting pretty damn low. See, even if I don't know my kid is going to have severe sickle cell disease, and if you look at what could happen to this child by age twenty or twenty-five, stroke or this that and the other, marrow transplant starts to look damned attractive. Thirty percent, 20 percent mortality is not all that attractive. When you get down in the 5 percent, you can sell it better.

*Carolyn:* It's still high.

*Dr. Davis:* Uh . . . see, but you tell me what you would do with your second kid because the first one died.

*Carolyn:* Yeah, if my child before had died, I would have a different perspective.

*Dr. Davis:* You see? Each family is going to have a totally different perspective. If you had a family who had a kid who wasn't even diagnosed until age seventeen, right, there's no point in even talking to you about a marrow transplant because your experience is going to be, "Well, sickle cell disease ain't all that bad." But, if your first kid died at age two from sepsis, your willingness to accept risk is going to be entirely different.

*Carolyn:* Right. Very interesting.

*Dr. Davis:* You want hard-and-fast rules; this is the most fluid subject in the world. Many physicians would argue that bone marrow transplantations, which bring a possible fourteen years of life free of disease, but possible suffering from the side effects of antirejection drugs and/or graft-versus-host disease, is better than eighteen years of life on chronic blood transfusion therapy. Some physicians believe that a 8 percent chance of death from the treatment surrounding a bone marrow transplant is worth the risk even when the patients who benefit most from the treatment are under the age of fourteen.

This thought experiment demonstrated that medical providers would like to support adolescent patient autonomy to improve future outcomes, but they recognize that medical uncertainty limits their ability to transform existing beliefs about adolescent immaturity and patient autonomy. The most radical and potentially transformative meditations on these dilemmas came from patients who acknowledge that following any medical advice does not protect one from morbidity or mortality. Death was an outcome they had come to accept; what they wanted was the power to choose their own risks.

Is it possible, I wonder, to release physicians and institutions from an overwhelming sense that they need to protect patients and society from irrationality? Is it possible to disentangle the politics of pity from health care such that sick and/or disabled people are not pitied but are encouraged to determine their own health futures using whatever resources are available? Some will choose unemployment and dependence on hospitals to relieve their physical suffering, but so what? Why do we judge this behavior as dysfunctional and the patient as a burden on the system?

The proliferation of discourses about patient dysfunction used to deny patients access to health care ultimately generates more waste. Dr. Benjamin described to me a phenomenon known as pseudoaddiction, a behavior that appears to be addiction but is actually the result of undertreating a painful crisis. The patient returns frequently for pain relief because the pain was never sufficiently treated, and he or she subsequently is identified as an addict or malingerer.

The state of health care for blacks in the United States produces symptoms of pseudoaddiction. Underfunded schools, environmental racism, lack of well-paying jobs and affordable housing in the inner city, and, finally, the attempt to control black people's access to health care by dismissing patient suffering as manipulative lead *not* to greater autonomy for blacks but to more dependence. Trying to protect educational, social, and health care resources from "undeserving blacks" only deepens the need. This thought experiment demonstrated that socializing health care providers, patients, and families to accept a new health care paradigm that limits medicine's moral duty to relieve suffering but expands medicine's duty to provide efficient and effective health care will not be easy.

# CHAPTER 10

# Rethinking Suffering

*Community-Based Health Care,*
*Alternative Medicine, and Faith*

When medicine was becoming professionalized in the nineteenth century, African American nurses and physicians made very explicit connections between medical access, social justice, and black redemption. At the time, disparities with respect to health care access were marked by Jim Crow. Hospitals, medical schools, and doctors' offices were typically segregated, and resource-poor black institutions provided diminished quality of care. Blacks would have to confront these racial barriers or continue to suffer the effects of unequal treatment. Since the 1960s, civil rights legislation, which protects blacks from institutional racism, and affirmative action, which created a stronger black middle class, mask the fact that race still matters. Racial health disparities are the canary in the coal mine, demonstrating at the level of physical health that something is amiss. The disparities between black and white life expectancy before and after Jim Crow remain strikingly similar, but because we perceive that racial inequalities are no longer institutionalized, discourses connecting health care access to social justice have been marginalized. Now discourses of equal treatment have been sublimated into scientific questions of evidence.

The evidence-based movement in medicine has pushed questions of social justice further to the periphery. Evidence-based medicine is built on the presumption that the choice of what diseases and drugs to study, the study design, the analysis of the data, the dissemination of the results, and FDA approval are somehow beyond politics. The medical community believes that through statistically significant P values it can organize a rational health care system in which all are treated equally. But social justice is difficult to code, has very messy variables, and would be difficult to prove statistically. Regulations in the form of FDA oversight and peer-reviewed scientific studies are thought to hold corruption, racism, and classism at bay. But BiDil, the first "ethnic" drug to treat cardiovascular disease, tells a different story. The drug has been offered as proof that the market can be responsive to, and ultimately benefit from, eliminating health care disparities. The scandal with BiDil is not that it is ineffective, but that it is a combination of two cheaper generic drugs, which begs the question of how BiDil received a patent in the first place. The novelty of the drug is the reassertion that race equals biology. In fact, nobody knows how effective BiDil is for other races, and giving the drug to anyone who does not self-identify as black constitutes off-label prescribing. The scientific community's eagerness to blame health care disparities on genetics rather than to look more deeply at social causes is one reason why a growing number of blacks are skeptical of medical science. While some hold firm to the belief that investing more money in treatments like BiDil is the best approach to reducing health inequities, many do not see themselves or their communities fully represented in the narrow categories used to construct clean scientific variables.

The gap between the promises of biomedicine and the benefits of biomedicine for the black community is significant. Blacks most sensitive to this disparity often turn to alternative medicine, where patients with tempered enthusiasm determine for themselves what constitutes treatment efficacy. Creating their own measures of evidence, blacks are designing regimens that they believe benefit them physically and spiritually.

For years I have witnessed the popularity of alternative health care among blacks. In 1994, while I was conducting research on African American Muslims, a number of conferences were dedicated in whole or in part to alternative medicine and alternative health regimens. When I asked a woman why so many Muslims subscribed to alternative medicine, she said bluntly, "A lot of people are dying of cancer and heart disease in our community."[1] At a sickle cell association meeting in Los Angeles in 2003, patients gave public testimonies describing how they treat their pain and quell the symptoms of their disease using a number of alternative therapies. The physicians in the audience not only did not interrupt or challenge these testimonies; one physician echoed that he, too, uses magnets to treat his pain.

The use of alternative medicine has been and remains a significant part of the African American experience. Historically, churches and mosques have been significant places of healing, and not simply spiritual or psychological healing. They have been places where very particular health regimens have been promoted as a necessary path to redemption.[2] This chapter explores why alternative approaches to healing offer promises to sickle cell patients that biomedicine does not. In particular, I will focus on the community-based sickle cell associations, a holistic health care center, and a church. These institutions, I argue, help patients make sense of their suffering in ways that biomedicine does not. These alternative discourses reinsert politics and social justice into health and health care by locating power and identifying a possible relationship between power and physical distress. As a result, they allow patients to feel agentive, as subjects rather than medical objects, and at the same time they embrace uncertainty rather than attempt to conquer it.

## COMMUNITY-BASED HEALTH

The behemoth housing the sickle cell association offices was once the headquarters of an insurance company that refused to insure blacks. The fact that this nineteenth-century, neoclassical replica of a wing of the U.S. Capitol complex is now home to a number of institutional entities that primarily help black and ethnic minorities speaks to how structures can literally be reembodied and ultimately transformed. Oddly situated beside a housing project, dilapidated row houses, and an aboveground rail system, this tribute to ancient Greece and Rome is treated less like a historical landmark than an accident of urban geopolitics. Situated about three miles from Children's Hospital East and the intellectual and financial heart of the city, this building is simply too embedded in a lower-middle-class neighborhood for developers or redevelopers to take much interest in it. They have simply ceded the building to the poor.

Inside, off of the main hall marked by high ceilings, marble floors, and columns, are offices assembled out of prefabricated materials and awkwardly inserted to fill the space. The interior of the building was never redesigned specifically for these offices; instead, everything seems temporary and borrowed. The sickle cell association offices have worn, badly fitted carpet, and the materials used to create the walls are cheap.

But the staff is skilled and committed, and the director is determined for his association to become the entity that all sickle cell patients and families in his area turn to for information, support, and services. In the more than two decades that this association has supported sickle cell patients and their families, it has never been solvent. It runs on hope and passion, from the first director, who had sickle cell disease, to his wife, Ebony, to the current businessman, Mr. Porter, who was hired to save the organization. Mr. Porter described the value of his association: "When a child has sickle cell disease, it affects the family because everyone has to adjust to this. Most of our population is from single-parent families. So when the child has to go in for either a transfusion, or if they have a crisis of this nature, then the parent has to accompany that child. . . . We have made available an advocacy group, a parent's group, so that parents will have the opportunity to share with each other some of the issues and concerns that they may have, and which gives us the opportunity to advocate on their behalf.

"They are able to share some of the issues or concerns that they may have as far as how the child is being treated in the hospital, what kind of care are they receiving, what kind of things that they may need to support them, like blood transfusions and holding blood drives. They let us know what some of their social needs are. Their needs may be that they need assistance with their utility bills, paying rent. I'll give you a case in point. A child may have two or three siblings, but that child is the only one who has sickle cell disease, and so those siblings suffer almost as much as the child does because the parent is not able to provide for the total family. So, we make resources available to that family to make sure that everybody in the family is taken care of, not just a child with sickle cell disease, you see. Even though the services that we provide, the state says, 'The only ones that we're concerned with is the child.' But the agency can't be just concerned about the child, it has to be concerned about the family.

". . .We don't *try* to link, we *do* link. We follow up from beginning to end. We have so many different resources at our disposal for that family that the end result is always successful. It's always successful. We just make sure that there is someone, an agency or organization out there that is responsive or responsible for the care of every child in [our area], or in the five counties. . . . The state provides all kinds of services. They do it through other organizations such as our agency. So, we will go to those other agencies that are being supported by the state and say, 'Listen, we have a population that needs food, or needs assistance with

their utility bills, that needs rental assistance, that needs housing . . .'
Maybe a situation where the child doesn't have any clothes, so we go out
and find where can we get some clothes for this child."

Mr. Porter is simply articulating that the health of the patient is contingent on more than the quality of care he or she receives in the hospital. In pediatric care, health care access is built around presumptions
about the time flexibility of the parent, a parent's access to transportation, and the ability of the parent to sustain a certain standard of living
(food, clothing, heat, shelter). From the association's point of view,
health care does not end with diagnosis and medical treatment. If
poverty interferes with what some consider treatment compliance, then
eliminating a family's poverty could, according to this logic, be considered part of health care. Currently we do not consider poverty a health
care issue, but if it compounds the suffering of sickle cell patients, would
it make sense to do so? Knowing that states have limited resources, I
asked Mr. Porter where he defined the limits of his association's role as
a comprehensive social service agency?

Mr. Porter answered, "Well, of course you know, when you use the
word comprehensive, you're all-inclusive . . . to treat the whole person,
you see. And that person may need a variety of things that are available
in the community. Oftentimes we get a situation where we have to call
on the Department of Human Services. We will go to the Department of
Human Services, and we say, 'Listen, we have a family that is in need of
housing because they were either burnt out or they can't pay their rent.'
And they say, 'Listen, you've got to go to the housing authority and
make your case with them.' Or if it's a situation where they need some
type of assistance as far as utilities [are] concerned, 'Well, then you need
to go to the electric company or the gas company and talk with them.'"

Trying to put his answer in context, I said, "I know other associations that are trying to put limits on how far they'll go because they feel
like they just can't rescue everybody."

In response, Mr. Porter defined his vision: "There's a giant pie, and
that pie is cut up in so many different ways. If my agency can't address
an issue, maybe another agency can. If not an agency, then a philan-
thropist could do it, you know. There's an answer to everyone's problems, you just have to research it, and get to it, and do it. We have a
situation we're dealing with now with a person who is threatening to
commit suicide because she just cannot bear being sick any longer. Well,
that's out of our realm. But, we know that if she says she is critical as far
as committing suicide that there is the suicide prevention network that

we can call on. There is an organization of black psychologists and psychiatrists who we can call on to get them some type of assistance. We go
through the hospitals because the hospitals have a responsibility as well
to do something like that. And if that's not addressed, then we go back
to the state, and we say, 'Listen, this is an issue here . . .' "

Responsibility for maintaining the health of individuals, particularly
poor individuals, is divided between various agencies. The association
links individuals to agencies and therefore acts like a primary care physician, diagnosing the problem and determining appropriate interventions. The sixteen-year-old whom Mr. Porter said threatened suicide
because she could no longer bear the pain asked the association for help
rather than the hospital-based medical professionals. This is revealing
of differences between the hospital-based clinics and the associations.
By building bridges between family, education, housing, employment,
and health care, the association acts as a holistic health care agency.
The hospital clinics attempt similar patient support, but while hospitals
employ social workers, psychologists, and child life specialists, these
professionals do not visit homes, and more importantly, the hospital
psychosocial staff is often far more judgmental.

A large part of the responsibility of the psychosocial staff at hospitals
is to improve patient and family compliance to medical authority. The
intervention is geared toward helping the institution run more efficiently
rather than helping a patient or family solve a self-identified problem.
There are hospital psychologists and psychiatrists from which my
informants regularly seek help, but physicians often encourage a patient
to talk to the psychologist or psychiatrist when a patient complains that
his or her pain is not being managed by the medication. For example,
while hospitalized, Dominique, a twenty-two-year-old college student,
demanded to be treated by a different physician because she felt that her
pain was not being managed properly. During the clinic team meeting
the staff discussed their frustration with Dominique. They even briefly
touched on the need to transition her to an adult care provider whose
approach to pain management, they said, was to provide as much pain
medication as the patient demands short of killing him or her. Then
they decided that the best solution was to call the psychiatrist. The psychiatrist then mediated between the patient and the hospital by giving
Dominique strategies for dealing with her pain that did not interfere
with hospital protocols and staff efficiency. The psychiatrist also framed
Dominique's problems to the sickle cell team in a way they could understand given how they define the limits of their role in patient care.

The choice to call the association rather than discuss suicide with medical professionals was strategic on the part of this sixteen-year-old. In the hospital her pronouncement would be seen as an indication of noncompliance, lack of maturity, insufficient education regarding the disease, or perhaps secondary gain and drug seeking. Culturally, hospitals are places where finding rational solutions to problems is held in high regard. A patient's expression of defeat would be treated as a symptom; a physician would attempt to locate responsibility (blame), usually in the individual or the family, and then propose a rational course of action. The idea that no single entity is responsible for her suffering, that there is nothing that needs to be fixed, that perhaps the only solution is to provide this patient with a wealth of resources in order for her to find her own solution to her suffering is not a set of possibilities that health care professionals are taught to consider. The association, on the other hand, treats suicidal thoughts as a reasonable response to severe chronic pain rather than secondary gain or dysfunction. The association also attempts to locate blame, but it looks beyond the individual to social structures.

Describing his client, Mr. Porter said, "This is a child who is threatening to do away with herself because she can't get assistance . . ."

"And the pain medication isn't doing anything?" I asked.

"See, that only works for a period of time. And, I'm glad that you brought that up, because this is something that is critical with our population. Now, for children, it doesn't affect them as much because they have a law in [our state] that says that every child is to receive medical care, and it's a program that the state will finance. So every child who is sick can get medical care, period. Adults, it's a different issue, okay."

Because the disease permanently damages various organs, chronic pain generally strikes older patients, and sixteen-year-old sickle cell patients are included in that older demographic. Mr. Porter addressed the issue of the undermanagement of chronic pain not as the result of patient dysfunction but as a health care access issue. For many patients, shifting blame for chronic pain from self to structural deficits can be empowering. The typical pathologizing that often occurs in hospitals of black patients and families who do not conform to hospital culture and who challenge the authority of biomedicine can be disempowering. Patients resist by failing to comply with doctor-recommended treatments, missing appointments, hiding information from their physician, and in some cases overtly challenging medical authority. Creating an alternative narrative about why a patient may not be getting better—one that shifts the burden of responsibility from patient to health care structure, and to the limits of biomedicine in the case of alternative medicine—gives patients a sense that they are responsible for creating a future that they, in part, design. They recognize that they play a part in shaping their own well-being and suffering.

Aminah, the woman at the association responsible for adolescent transitioning, articulated in an interview how the association shifts power to the patient and family. Aminah was an articulate, energetic woman with a sparkle in her eye and an eager smile. She both performed home visits to parents of newly diagnosed infants and was in charge of the adolescent transitioning program. A Muslim convert who wears *hijab* (covering), Aminah enthusiastically embraced Mr. Porter's mandate to increase the educational credentials of his staff. She attended as many national meetings as she could and became certified in a number of counseling subspecialties, including genetic trait counseling.

The discourse on adolescent transitioning in the medical community focuses on medical compliance. Although the association's transitioning program shares many features with hospital-based transitioning programs, Aminah taught her clients to understand the good and bad of these new discourses and accompanying practices. Aminah taught her clients that by obeying transitioning practices they facilitated their access to health care. But she acknowledged that the discourses are also repressive unless one looks at them as a means toward African American empowerment generally. "I think everyone needs some assistance. You can look back on your high school, and you say, 'If it wasn't for that teacher, I wouldn't have done that. If it wasn't for that counselor, I wouldn't have done that.' Although you have a strong family foundation, although your family wants best for you, outside of that you still have to live. I think with the transition program, it helps you explore. It's a safety net because once you get out there, there's no turning back. You can't go back and be a ten-year-old. You *have* to be a sixteen-year-old, or you *have* to be a twenty-one-year-old. If in fact they stumble, they have something to fall back on. So, if you look at that and say the opposite, if we didn't have it, how many would stumble and fall and never get up?"

Critiquing other transitioning programs, Aminah continued: "We have this whole group of people who say, 'Okay, we're going to do this a, b, and c, and once you're done, you're done, you're out of here.' I think it's a little more complex than that. It's more like going with them from now until death. And you say, 'Well, is that possible?' I think so, as long as you have a good resource network. No matter what comes up, you should be able to assist that person in a systematic way; at the beginning and then, as you go along, the need for you is not so much."

Aminah viewed transitioning as a process not of creating autonomous individuals but of shifting a patient's resource base from family to community and self. The association, she noted, does not have an institutionally defined time frame deeming at what age dependence becomes inappropriate or a sign of dysfunction. From the association's point of view, resource dependence is much more complex given the complicating factors of disease and disability. Aminah described the long-term goals of her intervention: "As we conduct this transition program, we want to make sure that we're not pushing these young people because we know that they have struggles ahead of them. Sometimes we push hard because we know that if we don't do this, it's going to really be devastating. So, that's where that personality comes in, where you have to say, 'Am I doing this because it's part of the program, or am I doing this because I can see later on down the road that this young man is going to have problems, and we have to hold on a little tighter to him?' Especially the young males that come through here. They are African American males, and of course [in] the health care industry or even the medical facilities they confront the biggest struggles, or the biggest problems."

I asked for examples, and Aminah offered one. "Like, um . . . Racism, and um . . . fears. Sometimes you can be afraid and not a racist, and I can't make that call. I don't know who that person is on the other end. We live in an ugly society sometimes, and some of our young adults have not confronted that *yet*. But we're afraid that they are going to confront that because of history telling us that. When you go into an emergency room, somebody may say or do something to you because of the color of your skin and the sex you are. And, if they do, this is what you need to prepare yourself for. But, what if they never [confront racism]? So, we've prepared them for something that didn't happen, that's not going to happen. Should we just go on and prepare them like everybody else should be prepared [and not suggest racism]? So, that's when that personality comes in and you say, 'Did I do that because I feel that this one particular child is not going to be able to be strong enough like some of the other ones?'

"They come up against struggles within the employment industry where they may have to go into a place of employment, and the first thing that they have against them is that they're African American, and they're male. So, you're pretty stern, 'Listen, you've got to wear a suit when you go in there!' 'Listen, you have to talk nicely!' It's like, 'Why should I be saying that to this person? I should be able to instruct him the exact same way that you instruct everybody else across the board.' But, again, you have that gut feeling that someone's going to say something to him, and he's going to get a little bit upset, and they're not going to understand him."

Aminah described a transitioning program that is sensitive to the complexities and uncertainties of race and gender discrimination. She recognized that each of her clients will probably respond differently to miscommunication or racism at work and in the hospital, and therefore she tailored her transitioning to fit each client. She privately wondered, however, if she herself was perpetuating racism and sexism by singling out particular individuals for a more blunt education: "Again, personally, I'm not tough, but I'm more apt to cross my t's and dot my i's with the males than I am with the females. Because, personally, I feel they have a better chance because history has shown me that females with sickle cell disease are more successful than males with sickle cell disease. But, is it because there was no transition program prior? They have no hard evidence to say that that was the case."

To be educated about one's disease and health care services was, for Aminah, not enough. For transitioning to work, Aminah believed she must instruct her clients both about the possibility that racism exists and about the possibility that what they might experience as racism was in fact a misperception. Transitioning for Aminah was about educating her clients about possible future scenarios given the uncertainties of suffering, race (racism), health, and health care.

But what is the proof that transitioning works? If one took an evidence-based approach to community-based health, it would have a very low evidence rating. Many would argue that only social programs that prove that the benefits (usually financial) exceed the costs should receive support. The sickle cell community must not only produce rhetoric about the legitimacy of patient suffering—patients are not malingers or drug seekers but are hardworking and productive—but also must prove that transitioning actually produces more productive citizens.

Describing her first experiences working for the association, Aminah said, "When I first came, the number one thing that I saw people in all of the hospitals, the number one problem that they had with people with sickle cell disease was that they were a burden on the system. . . . In the health care industry, let's take HMOs . . . the cost for them to be in the hospital is like double the amount that they are allotted. Remember, when the standards came in, it's only three days that you should be able to be recovered in a hospital. Well, of course, with sickle cell disease they're in there a lot longer, so you're taking up space. Plus, you're [on] government [disability]. So the people that are paying us money, they're not able to come in the hospital when they need to because you're taking up this space. So, now that's the hospital. Pharmacy . . . if this person cannot take that . . . that . . . that generic, again a burden. And let's not talk about society! You're not contributing because you don't work. Even if you didn't get an education, you're not doing anything. You're uneducated—again, these were in the past— you're drug seeking, you're on welfare. You see what I'm saying?"

I agreed. "Yeah, all of the negative."

After affirming my response, Aminah continued: "But when you turn it around with the transition program, you have people now that are educated. Not just educated, but they can also articulate their disease. They now are becoming productive citizens in this society. They are now being able to understand their bodies more because they are educated, and they may not be in the hospital as much because of their education."

Aminah enlisted the community rhetoric about transitioning to explain why the community embraced it. But, again, all the evidence suggesting that transitioning is effective discounts other social factors. In fact, Aminah asserted that a large part of the reason sickle cell patients are now able to work is not because they have become better citizens but because the Americans with Disabilities Act has granted patients rights that earlier they did not have. Schools also did a poor job accommodating students who were absent due to illness and would hold students back if they missed a set number of days. Now there are laws to make sure that sick children receive an education. Aminah believed that half of the sickle cell patients on Supplemental Security Income (SSI) were held back so much that they eventually dropped out of school. Now schools are much more accommodating of children with disabilities.

But Aminah tried to encourage her clients not to think of themselves as victims: "What we try to talk about is, how much is it your sickle cell and how much of it is you? I'll give you an example. I had a client call here one day, and she got fired. My question was, 'Well, what did you get fired for? Let's go step by step. Does it have anything to do with sickle cell, because if it did, then I can assist you. But if it didn't, then you need to reexamine what happened and figure out what we need to do.' And it just so happened that it was the sickle cell. Some things we have to look at, and I let them know, again, the way you dress, the way you act, you know. I call it work etiquette. How to keep a job, not *how to get a job,* but how to keep a job. There are several things you need to do. One, you need to know your place. You don't walk in the door giving orders. You walk in a door *taking* orders. . . . Work as hard as you can at what you do. Let people know that you love what you're doing, or you're good at what you're doing. Even if you worked at McDonald's, if you're there on time . . . time management is the number one thing that we work on. A lot of young people are not accustomed to getting up early in the morning, especially with sickle cell. It's like, 'I'm on medication, and I had to take some late, and I woke up late.' So those are some of the things that we go over as it relates to the work ethic. But, again, you can do all those things and something can happen. That's just life."

Continuing the story, Aminah said, "That person did end up getting their job back because, actually, one of the things that I do here at the agency is I review the disability laws, the family act of 1983 [and] those types of things. What I did was, I called to find out if . . . because it was a parent of a child. What I found out was that they did terminate her illegally. And also, she didn't know what rights she had as it relates to the union. So, I gave her both of those resources. So, she went to two different people. And as a matter of fact, I didn't even have to advocate on her behalf. It never even made the hearing phase because the person who terminated her, her boss, knew for sure that they had a fight on their hands, so he said, 'Forget it, hire her back.' So, again, we have to look at exactly what happened. What's in the letter that you were given? What are the exact words? You kind of become an investigator. But, as it relates to the transition of young adults, we try and prevent those things from happening by equipping them with the information prior to."

Conversations about transitioning with medical professionals rarely included discussions of legal rights and uncertainty. But community-based health advocates were very sensitive to both of these matters. Aminah, in particular, noted these issues: "Sickle cell affects every last one of the people individually, which means, no matter what you do, you're still going to end up disabled. You can be as healthy as possible. You can eat the right foods, you can rest appropriately, you can dress appropriately for the weather, and still end up with a stroke, because that's just the structure of sickle cell disease. So, you can't overlook that.

You can't say, 'Well, we've got something here for sure that is going to make sure that every person with sickle cell disease ends up healthy, strong, and productive.' It's just not going to happen because you still have to look at the fact that with sickle cell, the way that it affects the human body . . . you're shooting dice. So, again, you have to look at that sickle cell also played a part in causing a person to be disabled at home on SSI and not being able to work. Sickle cell is the chronic illness. How do they go out and work because their crisis is a little more than the average person? Which means, I don't care how educated they are. They could have finished college and the whole nine yards and still the route that the disease took caused them to have to take a back seat."

Aminah best summed up how the hospital and the association function differently in the lives of sickle cell patients. She noted that patients may, according to a hospital's criteria, be classified as functional and mature as long as they are compliant. The result is that patients slip through the cracks. Aminah described how this happens: "With the hospitals you may think that there is no need because this person seemed to be fine. But no one ever talked to this person to find out. One thing that's not in comprehensive care is a psychologist for youth and young adults. They don't exist. We have one, which is over at one of the hospitals, but that person is not dealing with the issues that directly affect them as a result of having sickle cell. I know cancer and thalassemia . . . those chronic illnesses they have that in place for children that are suffering. But, in sickle cell, I could truly say across the board, nationwide, there isn't anything in place. So, no one can say that because this youth or young adult who appears to be functioning very well is functioning very well, because no one took the time to ask them."

Aminah believed that psychosocial support was generally dispensed only when a patient missed appointments or had difficulties in school. Aminah offered a recommendation: "I think somebody needs to sit down and talk to each of them and say, 'How are things going? Whatcha doing? How do you feel about going to this new hospital?' Because you've been at one hospital your whole entire childhood, you've seen one physician, one social worker, and one nurse. Now, all of a sudden, someone told you that you need to go. Where are you going? I will be curious to know if anyone ever took those well-adjusted young people and said, 'When you were changing, what did it make you feel like?'

"I cannot separate this sickle cell transition from any other thing that happens in life because some young people that walk in the door, you can just tell that they're too dependent on their parents or on the hospital.

So they're the ones you really have to hand-hold and tippy-toe with. And, some people say, 'Well, that's just too time-consuming.' As a worker, you just cannot have the time. That's why I'm glad that we're able to do it outside of the hospitals because if it was inside the hospitals, forget it. You're only allotted a certain amount of time and a certain number of days. Here I can at five o'clock say, 'I didn't hear from Joanne today. . . . Hey, Joanne, what's going on? How are you doing? What's happening? I didn't see you last week. We made an appointment, you didn't make it.' It may take me a whole year to get Joanne into the office just to talk about what her future looks like, but it's okay because that's part of getting her to where she wanted to be. I sometimes tell them that they have to get up, they have to be in a controlling mode. It's like this is your life, control it. I work for you, tell me what you want. Tell me how you want me to assist you in getting to *your* goals. I can't set goals for you."

Community-based advocates like Aminah emphasize that the role of the association is not to judge clients or to impose a set of predetermined, socially accepted, age-defined goals. Clients must articulate their own goals, and the association acts as a facilitator. The differences between community-based health and hospital-based health care are not diametric. The clinic at Children's Hospital East would like to hire a psychologist and has built a support network for patients by hiring social workers, nurses, and physicians who feel it is their duty to encourage patients to pursue educational and employment goals. The differences between Aminah, who runs the transitioning program through the association, and Tammy, who runs the clinic-based transitioning program, are not related to their level of concern for patients. Tammy is simply limited by the institutional culture of CHE and by the hegemonic discourses surrounding biomedicine and health care distribution.

When I sat in on team meetings, it became clear that attention is bestowed on patients who disrupt the efficiency and cost-effectiveness of health care delivery. Compliant patients who make few demands on the health care industry but who suffer in silence are invisible in a hospital setting. Mr. Jefferson, the CHE clinic social worker, has a saying: "The hospital doesn't manage care, they manage dollars." At the same time that Mr. Jefferson recognizes the overwhelming mandate of his institution, he has a difficult time separating the way he frames suffering, cultural competence, and patient well-being from the institutional frames. His job performance is, after all, graded on how effectively he shapes patient and family performance to match the needs of the institution.

From the hospital's perspective, health care is expensive enough without adding layers of psychosocial staff. Time is money, so quick survey instruments to test patient psychological well-being and appointment time limits are important business strategies to improve the hospital's bottom line. Hospital culture dictates that responsibility for problematic patients is passed on either to the family or to the patient. Biomedical discourses trump all other discourses, and patients who do not comply are simply deemed irrational. Within this conceptual box, there is very little room to reconsider suffering and the role health care can play in empowering sickle cell patients specifically and black patients generally.

The community-based health association allows clients to define for themselves what they need. While it might seem impractical to incorporate the services provided by the association into a hospital setting, one wonders if the idea of facilitating rather than focusing on results is an approach the hospital could take in dealing with chronically ill children and adults. After I described the enthusiasm around developing quality-of-life measures as a way to improve health care, Aminah bristled: "So, why are we trying to develop a measuring stick for the quality of life for individuals with sickle cell disease when we should be looking at the measuring stick that society has made for African Americans? I can see us having an impact on a person's quality of life, and that's what this transition program is trying to do, have an impact on *that* individual's quality of life. Which means, hopefully, it can have a positive influence. Everything that happens in life has *some* bearings on your quality of life, but how does it affect it? I don't know. So, what confuses me is when you start to get into a measuring thing and say, 'Okay, if you're here, then you have poor quality of life. If you're here, at the top, you have good quality of life.' I'm Muslim, and my husband has the ability to have another wife. I sit home, and my husband takes care of me. Does that mean that my quality of life is less than an ambitious corporate American woman? No. So, how do we measure those two women on this scale? I can see you measuring their productivity in life, but I can't see you measuring their quality of life. Because I might not be as chronic as the next person, but I can feel like I don't want to work. 'I think I'm the happiest person in the world. I think that sickle cell was the best thing that ever happened to me. Because I don't have to work, I can get SSI!' Does that mean that my quality of life is any less?"

Aminah's insistence that quality-of-life measures should not determine the value of intervention is at odds with particular hegemonic discourses within the National Heart, Lung, and Blood Institute and within the sickle cell community. Quality-of-life measures are used to validate treatment protocols and psychosocial intervention strategies, and they have been useful in opening up patient access to health care. But they tend to rate quality of life based on a prior understanding of good and bad, for example, employment is good, and SSI dependence is bad.

Aminah found the community seduced by statistical significance: "Some people said, 'What measuring stick do you have to say that [her program] is affecting the quality of life of this person?' And I think that my response was, 'I'm not looking to change the quality of life of this person. I'm looking to make sure that this person feels or knows that they're a productive citizen in this society.' Not that I have the magic wand and their life is going to change, because if I had a magic wand, sickle cell wouldn't exist, and we wouldn't be having this conversation. But, because I don't have a magic wand, then these individuals that are transitioning need to know that they are part of a society that could care less if they have sickle cell or not, but as long as you're producing, What do you have to contribute? That's what we need to do, not deal with quality of life. That's why I said that I was the wrong person to talk to."

Aminah felt that her opinions ran so counter to the status quo that she needed to apologize: "And it bothers me when I hear these people get up and talk and say, 'Because you have sickle cell doesn't mean that you can't be a doctor and a lawyer.' Well, I don't have sickle cell and *I* can't be a doctor or a lawyer either, 'So tell me *why* you said what you said? Is it because you have some magic wand?'"

The discourses about patient suffering and moral character used to subvert negative stereotypes about sickle cell patients have themselves become repressive discourses. At the national meetings in particular, patients who represent the community's ideal are asked to speak to and for the community. Aminah offered an explanation: "I think what happens is that some people get caught up that every time they're around a certain group of people they hear the negative about sickle cell, and they just want to once hear something positive. So, they took on the challenge and said, 'We're going to make everybody with sickle cell a college graduate.' But, that's false. You cannot take this small group of people and make them something that they're not going to be, only because you're tired of it being the negative disease. We have to make sure that we do these individuals justice by saying, 'You are a part of society whether you're a doctor or a janitor.' Whether you're volunteering, because you can't move but one finger, you are productive. I just have issues with putting up on the stage all of our more successful people and not the mother who has children. The mother who has a husband, who takes care of her family, who doesn't get sick that often. She's productive. She's raising children. She has a very organized family. So, what makes her different than the doctor or the lawyer? And, again, I understand why they feel that way. I just don't think it's fair to the sickle cell community."

The discourses used to suggest that sickle cell patients are not drug seekers or malingers are, Aminah felt, inspired by a similar pressure blacks have felt generally to prove their moral worth. Many blacks, for historical reasons, believe that individual behavior stands in for the whole of their race. Prejudice is built around anecdotal experiences. One or two negative encounters can shape a medical professional's belief that all blacks are a certain way. This is why the community would like all sickle cell patients to know hospital etiquette, be able to intelligently discuss their disease with medical professionals, finish their schooling, and seek employment. Aminah told a story: "I was with a friend one day, and [this friend's a nurse] and she's like, 'I was so embarrassed, this [black] woman comes into the emergency room, her and her friend, they smelled bad. One had one shoe on, the other one had the other one on. They had this baby that was so ragged and dirty and the baby was sick.' And these white doctors were around them, and she said, 'I was so embarrassed for them. This person made me so embarrassed.' And, I'm like, 'How?' First and foremost, what I would have done was like, 'Wait, you need help. C'mon, we need to get you some resources.' But, we still do the same thing. That's how the sickle cell community feels. We make them feel like that each time we say that they're not doing enough: 'It's not enough, you've got to do more.' Now, what about the person sitting in the audience knowing good and well that he never finished high school, or even if they're in their last year of high school but struggling, 'I'll never be a lawyer, so I'll never be any good.' What do you do with those people? You can't toss them aside. We have to make them contributing factors of this society. How do you do that? By dealing with their strengths. I'm so curious to know about this quality-of-life thing."

## ALTERNATIVE MEDICINE

In a city border space, where poor African Americans were being displaced by gentrification or, depending on one's perspective, where wealthy European Americans were finding opportunities to refurbish old brownstones, Dr. Paul Bodhise performed deep pressure massage and chiropractic and holistic therapies on about eighty patients per week. Oasis, Bodhise's treatment center, was just one block from a fairly new Whole Foods, a gourmet natural food store that did brisk business in this neighborhood of young professionals and middle-aged yuppies. In one sense, by encouraging less wealthy African Americans to practice some of the same healing rituals performed by wealthy whites, Dr. Bodhise was essentially building a bridge between the blacks just south of his center and the whites just north of his center. Dr. Bodhise treated and worked with people of all races and ethnicities, but his commitment to facilitate holistic health care access to the African American community was what brought him to this border space.

The building exterior, with metal bars on the windows and peeling paint, masked an interior that Dr. Bodhise worked hard to make sacred. The office, which was no larger than twelve by twelve feet, was divided into three areas. Occupying the first area was his secretary-receptionist, who sat behind a desk just a few feet from the front door. Five feet from the front desk was Dr. Bodhise's office. His office was slightly raised and fully demarcated by a soundproof sliding door. The third space—which I can only describe as the initiation room—was just behind the reception area. Marking its corners were three brass stand-alone shelves decorated with white Christmas lights. The shelves held various products, and each shelf had a different green and white sign. One read, "Aromatherapy," and on that shelf were a number of aromatherapy products that were for sale. Another sign read, "Homeopathy," labeling a shelf that held homeopathic products available for purchase. Other signs and shelves were labeled "Reiki" and "Shiatsu." One brass shelf dedicated to the products sold by Dr. Bodhise's brother were labeled "Workers Compensation" and "Accident Insurance." At first I was taken aback because it seemed to be such a departure from the other signs, but the products were healing treatments for everything from tonsillitis to sore muscles.

It was in this initiation space that new clients were encouraged to watch videos of patient testimonials. I watched the one on deep tissue/ deep pressure massage and its effect on sickle cell pain. In the tape a physician with sickle cell disease described to a small audience how deep pressure massage had helped her with her painful crises. The tape, a third- or fourth-generation copy, was difficult to follow because at times the image and sound dropped out, but the message was clear; even credible medical doctors recognize the benefits of Dr. Bodhise's neuromuscular massage therapy.

To get into the other half of Oasis, one had to walk outside. The space next door was a long, narrow room with wall-to-wall industrial gray carpet. The room had seven Japanese wood and paper dividers, marking off spaces with chairs or tables where patients sat or lay while receiving their one- to two-hour treatment. The space also had a small kitchen hidden by a raised counter. Besides functioning as a place for the healers to wash their hands, clean equipment, and store solutions, the extra space contained objects that helped imbue the room with a sacred ambience, part of the healing ritual. A small rock waterfall, a stereo playing gentle acoustic music, a red light, and an incense burner occupied three of a patient's seven senses while the therapist attempted to encourage the body to heal itself through various forms of noninvasive touch therapy.

I visited the center a couple of times before I interviewed Dr. Bodhise. The first time I went to a support party for a holistic healer who was running for an elected office. The candidate did eventually win the election. Of the twenty people in attendance, about five were Muslim, and almost all practiced or subscribed to some form of alternative medicine. During my third visit to the center, when I went to formally interview Dr. Bodhise, one of the first things he did was apologize. He said that his center used to be in a large space with two floors, but the "inmates" tried to take control of the space, and so he decided that it was time to leave. Tall, dark-skinned, with shoulder-length dreadlocks and wearing a mudcloth vest and loose cotton pants, Dr. Bodhise did not strike me as a confrontational man who would want to waste his time fighting the "inmates."

Although the healing space was, according to Dr. Bodhise, not ideal for his practice, the center's location and condition were symbolic of the economic and social issues confronting this African American healer. Just as his center existed at the margins of a gentrified neighborhood or at the margins of social and economic power, so too did his practice. Dr. Bodhise was a highly respected healer and had received numerous recognitions, including one from the mayor in 2002, but the mainstream medical community had yet to embrace his work. Medical insurance companies often refused to reimburse him for his services, and hospitals have not incorporated him or his approach into any standard of care. Given his recent publication in a peer-reviewed medical journal, one would assume that his holistic approach to sickle cell disease would be more accepted. Bodhise and his colleagues discovered that twenty-four to forty-eight hours after neuromuscular message therapy, pain scores on a scale of 0 to 10 (with 10 being the most severe) diminished from 9.6 to 2.8. His patients spent on average two fewer days per month in an emergency room or hospitalized. All but one of the patients stopped taking opioids; the other was able to reduce her opioid use by 50 percent.[3] Despite his struggle for legitimacy, Dr. Bodhise remained committed.

Describing his journey into holistic medicine, Bodhise said, "The first [sickle cell] patient I was around was my niece. Before I was a doctor. Before I even thought about health care. I was twenty-four, and I saw her writhing in pain on my mother's sofa. For me to see this person that I love in so much pain . . . And there's nothing that anyone can do but kind of like love her and hug her. That was my first experience. It always stayed in the back of my mind that there is nothing that the doctors could do about it."

Bodhise began practicing alternative medicine in the 1970s, when most physicians rejected all treatment modalities outside allopathic medicine. He was working as an insurance claims adjuster in Los Angeles when a chiropractor submitted a bill. The response from his superior was disgust that a chiropractor would even submit a claim. Ironically, Bodhise eventually became a doctor of osteopathy. He described how when he first entered the profession, he was unable to prove through double-blind studies that his treatments were effective. Patient testimonials became his P value: "We saw people coming in with canes and leaving them, and crutches and leaving them, and people who have been in pain for six years. The closest recognition that we had gotten about our effectiveness was a lady who came in who had an auto accident six years ago, fractured her pubic bone. She had been in excruciating pain ever since and was just getting the highest doses of pain reliever, and so she found herself at our door. With our particular technique that we use, I was able to get her out of pain, and she wrote it up and gave it to a community college. Out of that writing, they gave me the alumni of the year award of 1989. So her writing about her experience is probably, prior to this abstract, the only record of what Dr. Bodhise does with this particular healing technique." Describing his technique, he clarified, "It's not a massage, it's a unique muscular, deep pressure, trigger point, healing technique that I have developed over the years. Even the chiropractic profession was against it, in principle [because of] the amount of time and effort that I would use to try and heal someone. You're supposed to be with a patient about ten or fifteen minutes, and that should be all that is necessary to give them chiropractic adjustment and send this person out."

Unlike Aminah at the association, who would have liked to avoid attempts to quantify the benefits of her psychosocial interventions, Dr. Bodhise sought legitimacy from the medical establishment for his treatment methods: "I recognized that there was something about massage that really helped a person, and then utilizing my experience in chiropractic . . . And the science background gave me the understanding that I have to go find the place of the lesion and start working with it. By finding the location of the lesion and working with it, I was able to bring about a faster, more thorough complete healing. This led me to believe that if I could be under some type of microscope that they could see that what I'm doing helped the person. [Then] along came William, Ebony's husband. [Ebony] said, 'Well, maybe you can help him. He's in extreme pain and discomfort. They just keep giving him drug after drug.' So, she literally dragged [her husband] to my center, almost physically dragged him with him in protest. After the first treatment, he knew that it did something wonderful for him. He began to reduce his drug dependency and told his fellow sickle cell patients that you really need to look at this. This is something that he wished he could have done fifty years prior. Then, a small trickle of patients started coming from the sickle cell disease association."

Describing what followed, Dr. Bodhise continued. "Dr. Samir Ballas, who was the chief hematologist for many of these patients, began talking to them. Prior to that, he informed me, all the massage reports that he had gotten were all negative. It wasn't until the patients were coming from me that they were saying, 'No, Dr. Bodhise actually helped me to such an extent that I don't need the morphine, and I don't need a new prescription, and I was not in the hospital as long as I usually have been.' As a result of going to some of the sickle cell meetings and him meeting me, he indicated that perhaps we should do an abstract. Before he would do that, he physically came here when I was working on a patient and actually watched what I was doing and heard my explanation of how I was applying the treatment. He backed our project and told me to give him a figure of the patients who I was seeing. And that's how we came up with the abstract. So, what I see is a combination of . . . of . . . of . . . ignorance from the medical community and just not knowing what it is that many people who do hands-on therapy [do]."

From his perspective, a scientist should be open to all possibilities and should be willing to test alternative therapies. He believed that to reject a potential healing modality based upon prejudice is negligence: "I do not call it a disease, I call it a condition."

I asked why.

"It was a genetic variation to combat malaria. Therefore, it wasn't like a disease organism. Many of the patients that I see, if they maintain a more stringent diet and get their massage therapy, the symptoms of sickle cell are just not there. And that is really what the issue is. The issue is the pain and suffering of a sickle cell patient. Not the fact that they have this genetic variation."

Descriptors such as *anemia, disease,* or *condition* used to classify sickle cell have become powerful tools for conceptualizing the disease and intervention strategies. *Anemia* implies a lack of oxygen-carrying hemoglobin, suggesting blood transfusion therapy or increased iron intake. *Disease* implies a foreign invader like a virus, bacteria, or cancer that must be destroyed or removed from the body. Dr. Bodhise elaborated: "And so the medical approach is try to get rid of the sickle cells by doing all kinds of risky procedures, whether it's bone marrow replacements or other kinds of invasive procedures. What we're interested in is keeping the blood vessels open enough so that you can continue to have circulation and to do whatever you can to increase the oxygenation of the blood so that the person can lead a normal life. If you can do that through noninvasive types of techniques, such as massage therapy and dietary changes, then you've solved the major issue of the sickle cell patient. It's a condition that has not had appropriate attention by our health care authorities due to the politics of medicine."

Bodhise's use of the term *condition* implies that sickle cell is a permanent physiological state requiring noninvasive daily management. Additionally, *condition* implies that with proper daily care, powerful pain relievers that have damaging long-term consequences will be less necessary, and the secondary complications of frequent untreated vascular occlusion will be reduced.

Bodhise wanted to use scans to prove that his message therapy actually generates blood flow in veins that were once occluded. Recognizing that patient subjectivity is not necessarily a criterion for validating treatment, he also wanted to develop a long-term study following patients who regularly receive his muscular therapy. He explained: "I'm firmly convinced that given the proper tools you will have not only the patient saying, 'I feel better,' but you will also have the positive results of electron microscopy saying those vessels are packed [with blood cells] now, whereas before the treatment, they were not. Because, after all, something physiologically has to change in order for the patient to say, 'I feel better.' Even if it's a placebo effect, there's got to be a physiological change going on somewhere even if it's at the mental level. So, not only do you get to feel better, but you get an increased range of motion of those joints, you get decreased inflammation, you get change in temperature of joints and limbs that once were cold and now are warm."

The benefit of alternative healing modalities is not simply feeling better, according to Dr. Bodhise. Patient subjectivity is evidence of treatment efficacy. He also believed that this efficacy would be measurable if a granting agency were only willing to fund a study. In the meantime, he and his patients continued to subscribe to non-evidence-based therapies. The difference between the hospital's approach to suffering and the alternative health community's is that in the hospital, patient subjectivity is treated with suspicion. Evidence-based protocols dictate how patients are treated, and if a patient is dissatisfied with that intervention, it might require another study to prove the patient right. Alternative medicine treats anecdotal experience as authoritative. But can hospitals allow patients to request interventions that have not been statistically proven? Given these real institutional concerns, I said, "Let me play devil's advocate. I'm a hospital administrator, 'You want to spend how long with a patient? I mean, I don't think that we have the staff, and we can't afford it.' Or, 'I'm an insurance company, You want me to pay for . . .' So how do you answer that?"

Enjoying the role-playing, Bodhise retorted, "How much did it cost you, hospital administrator, to handle a sickle cell patient that comes in five or six times a month or stays two to three weeks per stay. So, therefore, they stay two and three months [per year], and you can't be reimbursed after a certain amount of time from these insurance companies for that stay. So now you know that, number one, you have a moral, an ethical, and a federal obligation to keep this patient in this hospital whether you have funds for them or not. And, so, how much have these insurance companies reimbursed you for this sickle cell patient who you call a frequent flyer? Those are people who keep coming in, getting high doses of morphine, using your bed space. Now, how long will that same patient [stay]? My study suggests [he] will not have to frequently fly. So, now, if you are accountable, financially and ethically, then the answer has to be that this noninvasive technique requires attention."

I asked him to explain the spiritual aspects of his practice.

"If you have a doctor, you must know that they have to read tons and tons and tons of books. That being said, I can state as a fact that reviewing those books, I never heard the word *God* unless it had to do with some subjective conversation. There are a few words that relate [to] the spiritual aspect of things. Those words could be *homeostatis* and *innate*. When we look at alternative healing, we use the mind, body, spirit, which has been ignored by the medical profession until you get to those two words: *homeostatis* and *innate intelligence.*"

Needing clarification, I said, "Can you tell me the interaction between innate intelligence and healing?"

Bodhise provided a narrative: "Something I said to a patient who had multiple herniated discs. He's been to a number of neurologists, orthopedists, and getting second, third, and fourth opinions, all of them say, 'The only thing we can do is give you pain medication. We can try a surgical procedure, or you can just live with the pain.' These are their three choices. So, [the patient] said, 'Dr. Bodhise, you know, I may feel a little better, and I'm trying your technique, but can you explain to me, what is it that you expect, and what's going to happen inside of me as a result of this treatment?' And I said to him, 'What I'm doing inside of you is putting my force, my pressure from outside, to affect the mechanisms inside, your structures inside, causing a change in the physiology of that location. And at that point, I'm depending on innate intelligence to take over, to do what it believes is right in that area.' Whether it could be creating scar tissue to [heal the wound]. It could increase muscle mass, to strengthen the area, it could increase bone mass, it could increase circulation in the area to help the healing, it could strengthen supportive muscles and ligaments to take over the work that that particular injured segment was doing. But we want innate intelligence to come in, to have its ability to determine what comes next, not the physician determining that what comes next is a wire, or a screw, or other kinds of mechanical and even biomechanical invasions that oftentimes [are] known to leave very devastating and serious side effects, sometimes worse than what they're using the procedure for. The cliché is the operation went well, but the patient died. That means that what you did worked well from the biomechanical level, but it didn't work well when it comes to the outcome that was intended by the person."

Trying to summarize, I offered, "You believe that the body wants to be well, and it works to strike a balance of some sort."

"Yeah, well, we know that the immune system is operated by this innate intelligence. We know that immunizations stimulate the body's immune system [to create] antibodies. We can use that same innate intelligence to activate a healing potential at the place of the injury."

Trying to make connections, I said, "So, that's very homeopathic. You're adding spirit to it."

Dr. Bodhise clarified, "I don't think that alternative healing works with a different science than medical healing. Impossible. The science remains the same. We're using that same bodily potential to heal itself, just using different modalities with [different] levels of compassion. So, I bring compassion into the picture because I believe that that is part of the spirituality of innate intelligence. To have a sickle cell patient sit in a waiting room for five hours in writhing pain because your staff just does not know what to do with them, and some of them just don't believe them, when many patients die in the waiting rooms just waiting to be acknowledged that this morphine that they need is not because they need a drug hit, but they are really in that much pain."

Bodhise also criticized patients who have been socialized to accept the biomedical rituals of long waits in the emergency room and the use of drugs in place of compassionate care. While many patients are willing to wait six or seven hours in the emergency room and another six or seven hours before they see a doctor on the wards, they often get impatient with Bodhise's one- to two-hour treatments. He even said that many of his patients who spend two or three weeks on morphine in the hospital report that during that time they still had to deal with pain. The morphine changed the quality of their pain but did not eliminate it.

So he wondered why people buy into the rituals and promises of biomedicine: "They don't want to stay. They get edgy after an hour and a half because of this socialization and not understanding that here is where they should be spending those two or three days so that I can give them fresh-squeezed vegetable juice, give them brown rice. That same fast that they had on IV at the hospital, they need to continue it here with that vegetarian diet regimen and constant massage therapy. And we should be paid adequately for housing and maintaining a chronically ill patient like that, instead of . . . you know. Even on an outpatient level, instead of the inhumane approach that the medical profession is using for the pain patients."

Like Aminah, Dr. Bodhise has no proof that compassion for his patients translates into better patient outcomes, but he believes so. Again, differences with respect to traditional biomedicine and holistic care come down to questions of evidence. Within the sickle cell community there are people at both ends of the spectrum: those who believe that sickle cell care should be sensitive to patient subjectivity, and those who want treatment protocols to be standardized based on the best available statistically significant evidence.

In our conversation Bodhise pointed out that there is tremendous proof that standardized treatment protocols that do not require compassion on the part of the medical professional are actually more dangerous than untested alternative treatments. ["My coauthor and I] wrote an article that utilized the AMA records to show that there were 120,000 accidental deaths in hospitals across the United States of America. That was a fact that was buried in their journal, but we brought the fact out and discussed it in a very thorough way in a local newspaper article." The local newspaper picked up their article and a month later published an exposé that eventually was reproduced in several major newspapers across the country. Bodhise found it incredible that alternative therapies that have killed so few people in comparison are considered suspect given that the equivalent of a jumbo jet plane full of people die each day from hospital infections, neglect, or malpractice. He pointed to ephedra, which developed a bad reputation because of two deaths thirty years apart, and to several instances of chiropractic malpractice. But even if one factors in all the other deaths and injuries caused by alternative remedies, he still believes that traditional allopathic medicine is the most dangerous treatment modality. Of course, allopathic physicians deal with very serious conditions where the risks are already much higher. The problem, however, is biomedicine has such hegemony that it is perceived as the only rational risk when in fact it is not.

Bodhise also commented that blacks and the poor are disproportionately affected by hospital neglect, which is why he wrote the article: "But, this matters to us. As a matter of fact, what I was specifically saying to the African American community, in our own code, was that most of the people that die as a result of that are African Americans. Because they are the ones who are being neglected the most in these hospitals. We go to the funerals of our uncles and aunts and brothers and sisters who have died in the hospital as a result of some kind of disease. They have really been dying from malpractice-type issues. But, of course, this was across the board, in many other races, sometimes income-dependent type things."

He also believes that pharmaceutical companies are permitted to sell drugs that have properties similar to those of illegal street drugs. He used the example of Ritalin, which acts like methamphetamine and is often sold, crushed, and snorted by teens. From his perspective, pharmaceutical companies are simply the legal branch of the otherwise illegal international drug trade. Again, he wrote an article that he believes broke the story about teenage abuse of Ritalin. He throws the critique of "subjectivity" back onto the pharmaceutical companies, arguing that attention deficit hyperactivity disorder is a subjective diagnosis. This is particularly troubling to him because while the pharmaceutical companies get rich selling what he calls "kiddie crack," his patient-empowering, holistic approach remains financially unviable. He grudgingly revealed, "We are not in the green, if that's what you mean. We're asking God to keep us afloat, basically, and to do the work that we do. The heart-wrenching work of getting the people who have been spit out of the medical regime and still in extreme pain and saying, 'Well, Dr. Bodhise, I've heard about you and I understand that you can help me.' No more insurance left, the automobile insurance is gone, they're out of work, they don't have any group insurance, under the Medicaid, Medicare system some of them. Many of them you have to prove beyond a reasonable doubt that they needed therapy, and most of them do not pay for maintenance, which is what most of the people need. So as far as the medical community is concerned, they have to live with that pain. The only time that you can treat them, doctor or chiropractor, is when that pain intensity rises above what that constant pain intensity normally is. Group insurance, or any other insurance, they don't pay for maintenance therapy. They only pay for therapy that is aggravated. Most of the people who come here are in that maintenance therapy place because they still experience extreme pain and discomfort to a very serious level. That makes them seek out help, and they come to us and they seek out our help. So, we die back there with the patients, until their rebirth. They're happy, they're sending more patients, they leave their canes and crutches. But we have not been acknowledged appropriately until this letter came from *Hematology* [the medical journal that accepted his article]."

Our conversation ended very much as it began, with Bodhise stressing the importance of getting published in a major medical journal. For him, holistic medicine is scientifically valid and should not be considered distinct from biomedicine. He does not dispute that traditional biomedicine can be effective; however, he believes that physicians and patients are so socialized to accept the rituals and drug regimens of biomedicine that they blind themselves to some obvious disconfirming evidence: more than 100,000 hospital-caused deaths per year, senseless emergency room waits, pain relievers that do not relieve pain, and finally the disproportionate neglect of black patients. For Bodhise, biomedicine should incorporate any treatment modality that works. But the system generally funds a narrow range of studies and thus is self-legitimating and self-reproducing. If the system paid less homage to drug regimens and more to patient care, he believes, health care not only would be affordable but also would help eliminate some of the racial health care disparities.

With respect to race and medicine, there are two major problems with health care, according to Bodhise: the science, which includes the rituals of health care, and the financing. While the alternative health community is on the right track with respect to scientific experimentation and openness to new ideas, it has not been sensitive to how treatment pricing has virtually shut out communities that need it the most. Bodhise described how this is changing for the African American community: "Let me tell you something. I was invited to go to a meeting down in Maryland [at] the acupunctural school that accredits acupuncturists for the state of Maryland. They brought together a big meeting last fall for all of these alternative [healers] all around the country, and I sent my credentials in. All white . . . I was probably the only black guy in a room with about sixty or seventy academics from various hospital administrations, in that mainstream. And, I went down there with this negative feeling, like, another gathering that just ignores the plight of African Americans, but I'm just going to be in there anyway, but the topic was . . . the guy who opened it up, an administrator at the acupuncture school, and he opened it up with a statement similar to this, 'The reason why we are here is that we are stating that alternative healing for the new millennium is actually ineffective and obsolete and is irrelevant to health care if it cannot reach the people who need it the most. And, those are the people who cannot afford it, and those that have not been given access to it. And those are mostly minority people.' You could have picked me off the floor. I was completely blown away. Completely."

## RELIGION AND HEALTH: DOMINIQUE

At our first encounter in 2001, Dominique was twenty and in between colleges. The first college she went to for one semester was not fully wheelchair accessible and, from her perspective, caused a decline in her health. By spring she had already been accepted to another four-year college and so was taking a semester off to take care of a number of health issues. In many ways she had defied the odds. She was born two months premature; she had severe sickle cell disease, meaning she had three or more crises per year; and she had cerebral palsy, which required her to use a wheelchair. The cause of her cerebral palsy remained a mystery, but Dominique speculated that her pain was so severe that when she was an infant she simply refused to walk: "But my sickle cell crises are always hitting me in my feet. I guess I got it, like, subconsciously in my mind that I'm not going to do this because it's going to make my legs hurt, 'I'm not going to get up and walk.' So, by me not using those muscles. . . . And like they tried everything, therapy, testing my brain to see if it was something up there. And everything came out normal. It was just something, I guess, I had just got. I said I'm not going to do it, 'cause I was a child, I didn't really understand. All I knew was pain, and if I bear this weight on my feet, I'm going to get this pain that I don't like to have. By me not using the muscles in my legs I developed spastic cerebral palsy, which put me in the wheelchair."

Dominique had a dark chocolate complexion and huge, expressive eyes that seemed to reach out to whomever she was speaking to. She was phenomenally positive and ambitious despite what some might consider a difficult life. About her high school career Dominique said, "I'm in the national honor society, and I was senior class president of my class, newspaper editor, I was cheerleading captain for, like, three years." She also received a full four-year scholarship to the Catholic college she was about to attend. That does not mean she does not have dark moments when she lamented her predicament. She described how she makes sense of it: "I've realized that, you know, with going to church and things like that, that God, he does things the way he wants them to go." For Dominique, God worked through medicine to heal her from sickness and relieve her suffering. Displacing responsibility for her health and well-being from science onto God meant that the time she spent singing and praying was time spent healing and finding strength to pursue her goals. Recognizing the importance Dominique placed on religion, I thought it would be helpful to understand how the experience of church brought her a sense of well-being.

On a crisp summer morning, when the sky was a beautiful powder blue with sculpted clouds that, in the words of my seven-year-old son, looked "like plastic," I drove down to the city to attend church. The pastor of the church was Dominique's grandmother, Essie. Dominique had told me while she was in the hospital, "I like to go to church. I like to sing." Later she told me it was her *favorite* thing to do. Singing and praying for Dominique lasted anywhere from four to eight hours every Sunday.

Hobbies, a neglected area of research, have always intrigued me. Karl Marx argued that men must recognize the artificial division between the political sphere and civil society. Human consciousness, for Marx, was the recognition that people are social beings and therefore dependent on one another. Accordingly, all work should be the fulfillment of one's species-being, where the spiritual and the political are indistinguishable from the material relations of society. For Marx, the exploitation of workers is wrong because it denies both the oppressed and the oppressor his species-consciousness. As he writes in the essay "On the Jewish Question": "Human emancipation will only be complete when the real, individual man has absorbed into himself the abstract citizen; when as an individual man, in his everyday life, in his work, and in his relationships, he has become a *species-being;* and when he has recognized and organized his own powers (*forces propres*) as *social* powers so that he no longer separates this *social* power from himself as *political* power."[4]

A hobby or chosen labor replicates, albeit in a limited sense, Marx's understanding of emancipation. At an experiential level, how might emancipated labor contribute to healing? In Dominique's case, religion was her hobby, but at a physical level, was it liberating? Did church help relieve her anxieties? If so, which ones? Did church encourage her to keep trying in the face of tremendous odds? Was church a place of social, personal, and political healing? Did her pain subside during church?

The Baptist church that Dominique attended was in a northern part of the city pockmarked by two decades of deindustrialization. Beautiful old brick factories, long abandoned, were being gentrified for risk-taking entrepreneurs and artists inspired by gritty poverty. This shift seemed to be proceeding slowly, but if the predictions of a local holistic healer and traffic court judge were correct, as a result of gentrification this predominantly black neighborhood would develop an entirely new racial makeup within a few years. In the meantime, this area represented an interesting mix of the poor and lower middle class. Within the two-block radius around this Baptist church there were more than six storefront churches, with a mosque a stone's throw away. Three of the churches were run by women pastors. Most of the churches offered more than one service every Sunday, and Dominique's grandmother, Essie, gave two three- to four-hour services, beginning at noon and ending at seven or eight at night.

Essie's church was aesthetically one of the most welcoming churches in the area. The outside doors were glass. Entering the church, one was

greeted immediately by women dressed in traditional white nurses' uni-
forms, white gloves, and lacy head coverings that look like yarmulkes.
When I entered, a man was testifying, and so I was asked to wait and fill
out a card with my name, address, and whether I wanted a private meeting with the pastor, to which I responded no. The congregation space
was long and narrow, about fifteen by thirty-five feet, with walls painted
a virginal white. The burgundy and gray industrial carpet looked fairly
new, and the red vinyl chairs were organized in ten rows of six chairs
each, divided to make room for an aisle.

There was a wooden lectern framed by two microphones. Behind the
lectern sat the choir, composed of eleven adolescents and young adults,
including Dominique and two of her three sisters. To the right of the
pastor's dais and lectern sat the drummer, an adolescent boy who
responded musically to the emotional climate of the room; to the left of
the pastor was the keyboardist, a middle-aged woman equally responsive to the emotional climaxes and lulls that marked the service.

I arrived an hour late to what in the end amounted to a four-hour
service. When I arrived, the congregation was just coming down from
personal testimonies, and a couple continued to exclaim, "Thank you,
Jesus" and "Hallelujah," punctuating the relative quiet. Then a very
light-skinned older lady in a straw hat with flowers got up to announce
the upcoming events. As she approached the microphone, half the congregants pulled out their calendars and marked the dates for numerous
events, from vacation Bible school to a trip to a local amusement park.
Then she welcomed me, and I was given a small brown envelope for a
quarter blessing and a large envelope for the church offering. For the
next twenty minutes the choir sang as the fifty congregants were mar-
shaled back and forth to the altar for each donation.

Then an older lady in a large beige hat with gold trimming gave a
prayer suffused with "Thank you, Jesus," "Hallelujah," and "Amen."
Following this prayer, Essie emerged from the back. The room was quiet.
Essie wore a white cotton sport coat over a white-and-gray-striped cotton
shirt. Similar to all the women, she wore nylons under a skirt that fell well
below her knees. For shoes she wore white satin ballet slippers, and she
carried a large, white lace handkerchief, which she used to dab the sweat
from her forehead and neck. Her sermon began with several short sentences followed by about twenty seconds of silence. She would say something like, "I just want to say Hallelujah and thank Jesus," and the
congregation was electrified. After each sentence a man in front would
throw his hands out before him, stamp his feet, and say "Hallelujah," and

a woman repeated, "Oh, thaaank ya thaaank ya thank ya." Essie looked
hard at the congregation, as if she were looking right into the souls of
each member. She appeared thoughtful and intelligent, but perhaps more
important for the congregation, she seemed to be touched by the Holy
Spirit. As proof, after about five minutes of preaching, she broke into
song, using a rich and powerful voice that was more beautiful than that
of any of the choir members. It was clear from the response of the congregation that Essie was a charismatic authority who with the smallest
signifying gesture could produce a cascade of emotions.

Essie's relationship to this storefront congregation was both unique
and fairly typical. Many such congregations consist of extended families
and close friends, and in this respect Essie's congregation was similar.
Essie's children and grandchildren made up about 20 percent of the congregation. Then there were extended family members and finally
friends. Ironically, the only people who sat together as a family were
mothers with young children. Husbands did not sit with wives, and
grown children did not sit with their parents. From one vantage, Essie
seemed to be ministering to individuals as opposed to families; from
another, she seemed to be ministering to one big family. Although not
all female Baptist preachers have female-dominated congregations,
Essie's congregation was about 80 percent female. The informal gender
segregation, the men sitting in the chairs behind the drummer, reminded
me of a mosque. Unlike in most mosques, however, the women occupied positions of leadership, from deacons to attendants.

Following Essie's singing, she had a middle-aged man who regularly
threw his hands in the air and shouted "Jesus!" read from Mark, verse
46. The man read in a manner that made me question his education
and/or his intelligence but not his sincerity. Clearly Essie picked him for
a reason. After only a couple sentences, Essie stopped him, and she
began to speak about Bartimaeus, the blind beggar who spoke to Jesus
on the road leaving Jericho. In the story Jesus asks the blind man what
he wants, and he responds, "Rabbi, I want to see you." With that, his
vision was restored. Essie spoke about the need for deliverance and how
one needs to know what one needs deliverance from in order to receive
it. In more than thirty minutes, Essie was able to get through only six
sentences from the book of Mark, but her exegesis of the short passage
touched the congregation deeply.

Then came her public ministering of individuals. I was surprised by
her candor and a bit fearful that she would call me up. She told Bernice
to watch out for the devil, who will rot her soul. She told Janice that she

was a very sweet person and not to let others hurt her. She told Alice
that she did not deserve her pain, but "What comes around goes
around." Alice erupted into tears. Essie comforted her by rubbing Alice's
back and then taking her own hand away and shaking it as though symbolically extracting this woman's hurt and flinging it away. To another
woman, Paige, she said, "You have been pushing and you need to keep
on pushing." Essie touched Paige and told her to continue her fight. The
woman began to weep. Then Paige threw her hands out to her sides and
began shaking and crying. Paige's chair rocked precariously backward
and forward, and her rectangular glasses flew to the floor. She repeated,
"It's the hurt, Jesus. It's the hurt, Jesus." A thin older woman in a black
wig and magenta suit had a stack of paper towels, and she handed a
towel to each of the crying women.

Finally, a very short older woman was invited forward. Essie said to
her, "The problem is not with what's in your bed, it's with you. You
know what I mean by your bed, your daughter and your husband. The
problem is with you." The woman started crying, and then she started
dancing and shouting the name of Jesus. The band went with the energy
being generated by this woman and played louder. Suddenly the woman
in the magenta suit began dancing, as did the woman in the gold hat.
Then the women who were ministered to began crying; one began
chanting, "Jesus, Jesus, Jesus. . . ," which she repeated for thirty minutes, sometimes so quickly that "Jesus" slipped into "seje, seje."

As her congregation caught the Holy Spirit, Essie stood in front, head
bowed, with her elbows on the lectern and her hands opened up to God.
She seemed to be praying but did not herself go into trance. The meeting officially ended when the very short older woman ran from the altar
to the front door, symbolically pushing the devil out the door. She did
this twice, signifying that the congregation was purified and that they
had asked for and received forgiveness for their sins. Now they could
confront their drug addictions, infidelities, employment failures, problems with ex-spouses and children, and sickle cell disease. In the course
of four hours, hope had been renewed. This was Dominique's weekly,
sometimes twice-weekly, healing.

BEYOND HEALTH CARE

In order to conclude that racial health disparities can be transformed
through medicine, one must first presume that health care is *the* domain
in which bodies are restored to health. The preceding three examples

demonstrate that healing and a sense of wellness for most sickle cell patients rely on more than access to allopathic medicine. Access to bio-medicine remains an essential ingredient for ameliorating racial health inequities, but health care access should be made simple and unfettered. Moral complexity should be removed as much as possible from health care access, and the public should cease using medicine as a tool of social control or a stage on which to adjudicate issues of moral charac-ter and citizenship. Dr. Benjamin recognizes that what biomedicine does well is treat disease at the pathophysiological level. She does not believe that social workers, psychologists, or psychiatrists should be excluded from health care, but she delineates clear borders between medical care access and psychosocial support.

Anthropologist Joe Dumit argues that the current approach by phar-maceutical companies of expanding diagnostic criteria creates "surplus health," a term that borrows from Karl Marx's distinction between use-value and surplus-value. For Marx, use-value is the value of a commod-ity based purely on the labor put into the production of the good. Surplus-value equals the exchange-value, the cost determined by the seller of the commodity, minus the cost of labor or use-value. Surplus-value allows capitalists to become rich off the exploitation of labor. Playing with Marx's notion of surplus-value, Dumit argues that when a pharmaceutical company finds a way to convince 10 million people that they need a drug when in fact only 1 million truly benefit from the drug, it has created surplus-health.

The public and the health care system continue to invest more and more in surplus-health, drawing more and more money away from community-based health care. One could argue, using another Marxist concept, that biomedicine has become fetishized, or it is being worshiped well beyond its use-value. If some of the 15 percent of the gross domestic product spent on health care went toward, for example, reimbursing Dr. Bodhise, creating affordable housing and good jobs in Dominique's neighborhood, and investing in more community-based organizations such as the sickle cell disease association, one can only imagine how this would improve health in poorer black communities.

# Conclusion

During my fieldwork, I observed many incidents that threw a complicated light on a very distressing problem, but the problem with relying on stories to understand health care inequities is that they are anecdotal and therefore easily dismissed. While I could instead build my story about health care disparities using statistics, as done successfully in *Unequal Treatment,* the same statistics can be narrated to tell very different stories.[1] For example, the first draft of the "National Healthcare Disparities Report," issued in December 2003 by the Department of Health and Human Services, opened: "The overall health of Americans has improved dramatically over the last century. Just in the last decade, the United States has seen significant reductions in infant mortality, record-high rates of childhood vaccinations, declines in substance abuse, lower death rates from coronary heart disease, and promising new treatments for cancer."[2] After this version was publicly ridiculed for ignoring disparities, the revised report not only highlighted inequalities, it stated: "Inequalities in health care that affect some racial, ethic, socioeonomic, and geographical subpopulations in the United States ultimately affect every American. From a societal perspective, we aspire to equality of opportunities for all our citizens. Persistent disparities in health care are inconsistent with our American values."[3] Using the same statistical data, either statement can be interpreted as correct, demonstrating that statistics can be used to tell different stories.[4]

Under the watchful eye of Tommy Thompson, the Agency for Healthcare Research and Quality (AHRQ) chose to emphasize that some Native American groups have some of the lowest detected rates of cancer. Left out of the report is the fact that these same groups also have some of the shortest life expectancies in the United States. The choice of variable can make minor social problems seem widespread and can be used to hide contradictory data.[5] In terms of the AHRQ report, distinguishing blacks from Latinos from whites was for Thompson unimportant with respect to policy. For him, the object of concern was the health of the entire nation. By redefining the objects that matter, in this case any improvements in the health and well-being of the entire nation, racial health care disparities actually became a story of hope. For those who objected to the report, who called it "politically sanitized," the object of moral concern was the relative differentials in health outcomes of racial and ethnic groupings.[6]

To address health care disparities for this book, I considered it essential not to rely too much on statistics. From my perspective, *Unequal Treatment* and the final version of the AHRQ report prove that racial and ethnic health and health care disparities matter. Throughout my research, my goal has never been to reproduce the statistical literature but to understand how racial disparities are made through the deployment of scientific discourses and hegemonic notions of citizenship.

The sickle cell community relies heavily on discourses about individualism and responsibility when it comes to teaching patients how to be taken seriously by health care professionals. It also relies heavily on scientific objectivity when it comes to pushing the medical community to take sickle cell suffering seriously. The community attempts to develop consensus regarding what forms of suffering require medical intervention and what forms of suffering are the responsibility of the patient, knowing that science and citizenship are powerful discourses that inform what Hannah Arendt calls the politics of pity.

Although I try throughout this book to remain agnostic with respect to ethics and policy, I do believe that eliminating racial and ethnic health disparities is a noble goal. Unfortunately, my most significant contribution to discussions about health care inequities is that in America we must change our unwritten social contract. Health care is fetishized in the United States. Long life stands in for a life well lived. In the meantime, people are suffering as a result of multiple forms of social neglect. At the risk of sounding clichéd, I believe that health care needs to be rightfully positioned next to education as something that we all need in order to improve our lives. By overinflating the value of health care and treating it as a scarce resource, Americans allow insurance companies and pharmaceutical companies to exploit the system and to exploit them. Within the sickle cell community, the most vocal social justice advocates encourage patients to look beyond health care to occupation, diet, spirituality, and alternative health regimens for better health. They also encourage the state to invest in individuals and families—education, housing, jobs, neighborhoods—so that all people can determine, to a certain extent, their quality of life and their future health.

This book is not an indictment of the sickle cell community. Because of its hard work, many good things are happening. The community is creating an effective counterdiscourse that works both internally and externally to author new meanings about sickle cell disease and race. What is striking in this bid to create a community with a shared mission and clear rules is how difficult it is to develop consensus given the levels of uncertainty. While the Enlightenment thinkers believed that locating causation for suffering was possible given the right methodological tools, the levels of uncertainty that the sickle cell community deals with illustrate how difficult locating blame can be. Ultimately, this book challenges the current approaches to managing health disparities almost solely through the health care system. Suffering even for sickle cell patients involves much more than DNA and pathophysiology, and to eliminate racial health care disparities, social factors must be considered.

## NOTIONS OF MEDICAL CITIZENSHIP

The implicit social contract undergirding the American health care system emerges from discourses about the rights and duties of individuals to society and society to individuals. There are financial rights and duties (if you pay for insurance you are entitled to certain types of health care), and there are ethical rights and duties that are culturally informed, implicit, and open to negotiation. Americans do not require the health care system to mitigate all forms of suffering. In fact, we institutionalize sacrifice by identifying some suffering as being the result of a private rather than a public harm.[7] The discourses of patient suffering developed by the sickle cell community are intended to shift what is considered private suffering into the public realm. In terms of pain, for example, the discourse turns what was once treated as self-inflicted suffering, "drug addiction," or "malingering" into something natural, "disease," "pseudoaddiction," or "drug dependence." The latter descriptors narrate a different story about the patient's agency, shifting the reason for patient demands for strong opioids from a personal moral weakness onto something society could and therefore should mitigate. This discursive strategy on the part of the sickle cell community demonstrates how language has the power to mediate how we classify and conceptualize the world around us.[8]

By creating discourses of suffering, the sickle cell community attempts to control language about the disease to shape a public consciousness about how patients should be treated. The question then becomes, Why must the community prove that sickle cell patients suffer? In other countries, debates about increasing or decreasing health care access are usually separated from issues of patient worthiness. For example, limiting care to infants born more than twelve weeks prematurely or limiting extraordinary care to adults over the age of sixty-five are practices based on a moral calculus that considers overall benefits to society, and social equality, paramount. This calculus is of course an idealization; many countries with national health care also allow people to purchase private health insurance. Nevertheless, the ideals upon which any system is based matter. Idealizations and implicit social contracts are hegemonic and normative. Reformers must borrow from these powerful discourses in order to make calls for change seem rational. This scaffolding explains why reform discourses rarely stray far from *doxa*. Resignification, as Judith Butler argues, is never revolutionary. In the United States, suffering has an interesting historical relationship to rights of citizenship, which is why the sickle cell community continues to rely on discourses of suffering to improve health care access.

## MAKING CHANGE DESPITE UNCERTAINTY

When Mamie Till Mobley put her fourteen-year-old son's lynched, mutilated body on display for the nation in 1955, the effect was the equivalent of the bursting of a dam. Before the photographs of Emmett Till circulated throughout the country, many in the black community willingly sat on the sidelines of a growing civil rights movement. Some rejected the need for integration; others believed that blacks needed to take responsibility for the community's economic, social, and political status. Parity, they believed, would result from hard work, both moral and physical. Possibilities for dignity and economic success existed during segregation, making it difficult to determine what the civil rights struggle should be about. In hindsight, the relationship between segregation and suffering seems clearer, but before 1955 there was tremendous uncertainty about black suffering, its origins, and how to ameliorate it.[9]

Negro uplift movements in the nineteenth and twentieth centuries focused more on improving the moral character of blacks and encouraging self-sufficiency than on condemning the judicial, economic, and social forces arrayed against the community. Historian Evelyn Higginbotham describes the Black Baptist Convention's excoriation of shiftless blacks.[10] Similarly, Marcus Garvey, Elijah Muhammad, and social scientist E. Franklin Frazer all disparaged black people for being complicit in their own oppression. These perspectives can easily be compared to the recent comments made by comedian Bill Cosby, who condemned African American youth culture at the NAACP's celebration of the fiftieth anniversary of *Brown v. Board of Education*.

At the turn of the twenty-first century, a number of social critics have written books either absolving or incriminating blacks for the current crises in black America. Popular books that implicate blacks include Juan Williams's *Enough! The Phony Leaders, Dead-End Movements, and Culture of Failure That Are Undermining Black America—and What We Can Do about It;* Shelby Steele's *White Guilt: How Blacks and Whites Together Destroyed the Promise of the Civil Rights Era;* and John McWhorter's *Winning the Race: Beyond the Crisis in Black America.* There are far fewer books in the popular press that relieve blacks of responsibility. Aside from Michael Eric Dyson's *Is Bill Cosby Right? Or Has the Black Middle Class Lost Its Mind?,* most texts that blame structures for continued inequality are scholarly and seldom read outside of the academy. Despite inequalities in health, educational outcomes, and rates of imprisonment, the black community is far more sympathetic to the argument that fault lies within itself than to the argument that the disparities are the result of structural inequalities alone. Sociologist Orlando Patterson, editorializing on inequities in the justice system, wrote, "But there is another equally important cause: the simple fact that young black men commit a disproportionate number of crimes, especially violent crimes, which cannot be attributed to judicial bias, racism or economic hardships. The rate at which blacks commit homicides is seven times that of whites."[11] Uncertainties about the causes of black suffering, for example, whether high crime rates caused by social forces or individual pathology, thwart collective action.

But in 1955, Emmett Till's adolescent body was understood to be innocent, and therefore undeserving of torture and execution, and for the next ten years the discourse of black people's complicity in their own economic, political, and social degradation was muted, at least in the black community. Black subjectivity and suffering shifted from an "I" framing to a "we" framing, which effectively galvanized the civil rights movement. In the struggle that followed, the black body continued to be a signifier of collective disfranchisement, and after civil rights legislation was passed in 1965, the focus of many black activist groups centered around the social neglect of the black body.

The successful coding of the black body as a metaphor for the suffering of the black community produced an explosion of debates that forced the government to place a symbolically rich but hardly plentiful array of health issues on the national agenda. For example, the National Sickle Cell Anemia Control Act was passed in 1972 to help alleviate the "deadly and tragic burden" of having sickle cell disease.[12] The body as a metaphor of black victimhood did not, however, last. With forced integration, the black body stopped being viewed as a mere object of oppression (akin to Till's adolescent body) and was again viewed as agentive. Questions about whether blacks were deserving reemerged as their work ethic, intelligence, and morality were once again brought into question in the late 1960s and 1970s. By 1980, presidential candidate Ronald Reagan denied that blacks were entitled to any social reparations in the form of affirmative action, essentially arguing that blacks were responsible for their diminished social status.

Reading African American history, I have been struck by the instability of discourses of suffering and racial injustice. There seem to be moments such as Emmett Till's lynching when individuals agree on the origins of suffering and collective expressions of blame and responsibility are ratified. These moments are generally brief and followed by longer periods of uncertainty about who has the right to claim victim status and who should be assigned blame.

Uncertainties about the causes of racial health disparities have generated a similar policy paralysis. One paper argues that there are biases in patient treatment,[13] another that black patients make different medical choices.[14] Some papers argue that blacks are resourceful when it comes to illness and discerning when it comes to the medical system.[15] Others argue that blacks practice cultural behaviors that increase rates of illness,[16] that they are less compliant,[17] and that high rates of illiteracy among blacks impact morbidity and mortality.[18] None of these identified causes, however, is an independent variable. The fact that black people are lumped together as a "people," for example, is connected to a rich social history. The fact that black patients may not always trust their physicians or follow their recommendations is tied to that same history.[19] Similarly, rates of literacy in the United States are tied to class, which is tied to race. In other words, observations of racial differences, themselves often based on questionable presumptions, have no detectable point of origin, and therefore the statistically significant data on health disparities can be read in multiple ways.

The community is profoundly uncertain not only about the sources of inequality but also about what should be done about the fact that they even exist. There is no symbolic equivalent of Emmett Till's body to make Americans and the medical community say, "Stop! There may be multiple reasons for health disparities, but if we eliminate health care access barriers tied to class differences, we can at least disentangle discourses of worthiness and entitlement from health care." Looking back on revolutionary moments in American history, including the American Revolution, the Civil War, and the civil rights movement, none of these movements relied on statistically significant studies to identify the problems and propose a solution. So why is the medical community waiting for the definitive study to decide what needs to be done to alleviate health disparities?

The reason has to do with the fact that we have a health care system that rations care by cost, which means that poor people without access to insurance get less care. Black people are proportionately less well off than whites, meaning blacks are more likely to have reduced health care access. Beyond issues of rationing, having health care access related to ability to pay and often connected to employment means that cultural notions about hard work, social value, and deservedness get entangled with patient care. For poor or disabled patients, two currencies are available in the health care system: the currency of insurance (tied to wealth and employment) and the currency of suffering. By creating discourses about how sickle cell patients suffer, hematologists provide them with a useful form of currency for negotiating health care.

Unfortunately, discourses of suffering are contingent, meaning they must be backed up with performances. The sickle cell community recognizes that patients must be taught how to act in the clinic in order to maintain the respect of the medical professionals. This is why transitioning programs for adolescents are considered necessary. These programs are meant to cultivate in patients particular dispositions toward illness and to impart knowledge. At their most empowering, they teach patients about medical uncertainty and the culture of medicine. At their worst, they teach patients to submit to medical authority without question, and conversations about race and disfranchisement are replaced with repressive narratives about cultural competence, compliance, and rationality. Given that for the poor, health care exists in the domain of charity rather than social justice, transitioning programs teach patients necessary performance strategies for negotiating the medical system.

In the United States, the term *scientific hegemony* is essentially redundant. Scientific methods are considered objective, and because Americans privilege objectivity, science has the power to shape common sense. Even creationists use science to disprove evolution.[20] When health care consumers read that a scientific study determined that eating five servings of vegetables daily reduces the chance of getting certain cancers, or that the aggressive use of statins by people with high cholesterol reduces the risk of heart attack, they accept that information as fact—until another study refutes them. Rarely do health care consumers ask to see the results of competing studies, question the credentials of the scientists, or, as Joel Best shows in *Damned Lies and Statistics,* question the statistical data.[21] In addition to science, there are other authorized or legitimated discourses, including particular religious discourses and historical narratives, that we accept without question. Entangled in American origin myths, either religious or historical, are ideas about the values of independence, freedom, and democracy. This list represents only some of the discourses that exist in the realm of the unquestioned, common sense, or what Pierre Bourdieu calls *doxa.*[22] Then there are discourses that have recently moved from the realm of heterodoxy and opinion into the realm of *doxa;* these include feminism, multiculturalism, and civil rights.

It takes tremendous conceptual scaffolding to move ideas from one realm to another. Marilyn Strathern, in *Reproducing the Future: Anthropology, Kinship, and the New Reproductive Technologies,* describes how conceptual scaffolding has been used in England to naturalize technologically assisted reproduction: "The anthropological analysis of culture points to the general human facility for making ideas out of other ideas. We make fresh concepts by borrowing from one domain of life the imagery by which to structure other areas—as Darwin apparently did by finding in nineteenth-century ideas about degrees of kinship and affinity the vocabulary for his nascent theory of natural selection. But images pressed into new service acquire new meanings."[23]

Within medicine, the conceptual scaffolding used to move scientific ideas from the realm of heterodoxy into *doxa* is revealed in interesting ways at the national sickle cell meetings. The meetings are designed to transform uncertainty into certainty so physicians feel secure about their treatment decisions, psychologists adopt newer diagnostic instruments, and social workers develop effective patient programs.

In my seven years of research, my focus shifted away from trying to locate racism in health care to examining how the sickle cell community discusses, organizes, censors, embraces, or attempts to eradicate uncertainty.[24] Its power as a community depends on developing consensus about the disease and developing appropriate treatments. Certainty leads to legitimacy, which translates into institutional support. After completing a book describing the various ways a community of Muslim women discuss, organize, censor, embrace, and attempt to eradicate ambivalence with respect to faith, I found myself fascinated by the same discursive processes taking place within medicine.

## CONCLUDING THOUGHTS

I am not a health care policy analyst, and anthropologists rarely tell people what to do, so I include these recommendations with a bit of trepidation. I do so because I believe the cultural and ideological underpinnings of unequal treatment, my area of expertise, seem to blind Americans from being able to imagine a number of hopeful solutions. For example, few people consider how significant it is that health care for the poor is situated more in the domain of charity than social justice. Because charity is given to people deemed worthy for whatever reason, perceptions about a patient's work ethic, citizenship, entitlement, and social value become embedded in ideas about health care resource distribution, fairness, and efficiency. These conceptual entanglements have a huge impact on how we imagine the future and our biotechnical embrace.

A belief that someone is moral and good is typically reinforced materially. For instance, we often think that people who are wealthy do not take drugs, do not abuse their children, are smart, and work hard. Why else would they be wealthy? The flip side, of course, is that we presume that lower-income people are poor because they are lazy, dumb, bad parents, or engaged in illicit activities. The quality of someone's insurance or lack thereof becomes part of this conceptual matrix. Therefore, the best way to ameliorate racial health disparities is to equalize the distribution of health care resources such that patients are never placed into these categories.

That said, my first recommendation is to create a single-payer, tax-based, universal health care system. The current system is broken, and our market-based approach produces enormous inequities in health care access and is morally bankrupt. This does not mean that a universal health care system will be perfect, just better. Ideas about patient worthiness are the unintended consequences of a system that rations health care by cost and allocates resources based in part on discourses of suffering. Because African Americans are disproportionately poor and because the suffering of black people is often questioned, this form of health care rationing only exacerbates racial inequality.

My second recommendation is to decenter mainstream health care by giving patients the option to create a health care program that works for them. For example, often out of necessity, sickle cell patients find healing outside of formal health care settings such as churches, holistic health centers, or disease advocacy organizations. These organizations provide valuable long-term disease education in a less hurried manner and in more accessible settings in which the power dynamics that exist in the clinic, and the demands placed on patients to comply with protocols that sometimes increase patient suffering, are absent. Simply put, these organizations provide the tools for patients to participate more actively in their care.

Expanding access to traditional health care resources represents only a partial solution. Less fettered access to mainstream medicine must be coupled with more funding to local patient organizations. When sickle cell patients receive continuing education about everything from disease etiology to employment counseling, they are less likely to use hospital services. The mounting demands being placed on urban hospitals to treat the growing number of chronically ill patients should encourage states to provide greater support to legitimate disease advocacy and alternative health care centers. These centers, financed on hope, are often holes-in-the wall dressed up with new carpeting and paint. But, located in run-down neighborhoods, these centers are accessible and are responsible for transforming the practices and dispositions of not only poor inner-city folk but also chronically ill physicians, entrepreneurs, and legislators who also utilize them.

Policy makers must not dismiss the nontraditional places that poor, sick people go for information and treatment. Instead, they need to find ways to make these places more viable. As resource poor as we pretend health care is, its deficits pale in comparison to the state of education in poor neighborhoods, to the lack of social investment in people rather than prisons, and to the retrograde approach to creating urban communities that are environmentally and socially unhealthy. Decentering the medical establishment by supporting local health centers and initiatives is simply another way of looking at health and well-being as a social rather than a purely medical issue.

My third and final recommendation is to the sickle cell disease community. A number of wonderful and dedicated social scientists and psychologists in the community have been working for years to improve adolescent transitioning. They need more resources to create effective transitioning services. Educating patients such that they are able to appropriately challenge medical authority is the best form of empowerment for teens and young adults. Educate the patients by pulling back the curtain to reveal the wizard's tricks. Organize teen leaders to attend NIH and association meetings so that they can become aware of medical uncertainty. Instead of having forums where patients present their personal narratives, have physician and nurse forums where medical professionals speak about how difficult and frustrating it is to treat sickle cell disease and sickle cell patients. Teach adolescents that professionals are as vulnerable as they are when it comes to demands made by the medical system coupled with the limits of available treatments and resources. Finally, respect that adolescent sickle cell patients have endured enough suffering to participate in informed decisions about their care.

# Notes

INTRODUCTION

1. Transcribed interview with Eva, April 2001, Children's Hospital East.

2. U.S. Department of Health and Human Services 2000.

3. Alexander and Sehgal 1998; Ayanian et al. 1999; Brancati et al. 1992; Ellison et al. 1993; Epstein et al. 2000.

4. Kasiske et al. 2002.

5. The initiative was announced in 1998 and is entitled *Healthy People 2010*.

6. Smedley, Stith, and Nelson 2003: 290–383.

7. Agamben 1998; Foucault 1977b; Petryna 2002.

8. Smedley, Stith, and Nelson 2003.

9. Betancourt 2004.

10. Children's Hospital West (CHW) is a pseudonym for a hospital located in California.

11. Gottfredson 2004.

12. Klick and Satel 2006.

13. Sickle cell disease is often used as proof of genetic dissimilarity even though the incidence of sickle cell trait and disease various tremendously on the continent of Africa and around the Mediterranean.

14. Kelley 1997.

15. In *Deciding Who Lives: Fateful Choices in the Intensive-Care Nursery*, Renee R. Anspach describes one doctor who presumed that because the family was Hispanic they were Catholic, and because they were Catholic they did not understand euthanasia. The surgeon says, "Well, it's difficult to talk to the parents because of their background. They don't have a concept of euthanasia." Anspach 1993: 107.

16. Good 1994; Mattingly 1994; Ricoeur 1985; Schulz and Mullings 2005.

17. "National Survey of Drug Use and Health: National Findings," http://www.oas.samhsa.gov/nsduh/2k5nsduh/2k5Results.pdf, published by the United States Department of Health and Human Services, Substance Abuse and Mental Health Services Administration, Office of Applied Sciences, September 2006, p. 71.

18. "Punishment and Prejudice: Racial Disparities in the War on Drugs," http://www.hrw.org/reports/2000/usa/Rcedrg00.htm#II.%20THE%20EXTENT%20OF%20U.S., by Human Rights Watch, May 2000, vol. 12, no. 2 (G), "Summary and Recommendations." It is important to note that 77.5 percent of drug offenses are nonviolent. See "Who Goes to Prison for Drug Offenses? A Rebuttal to the New York State District Attorneys Association," http://www.hrw.org/campaigns/drugs/ny-drugs.htm, Human Rights Watch, 1999.

19. Klick and Satel 2006; Smedley, Stith, and Nelson 2003.

20. Klick and Satel 2006: 27.

21. Betancourt 2004; Kleinman and Benson 2006.

22. Klick and Satel 2006.

23. Cohen 1999; Schulz and Mullings 2005.

24. Cosby and Poussaint 2007; McWhorter 2005; Steele 2007; Williams 2006. Black and white reviewers on Amazon.com rate the works of these scholars highly. They appreciate the fact that the writers openly criticize the black community. Khalil Muhammad, a professor of history at Indiana University, wrote a thoughtful critical review of Cosby and Poussaint's thesis that collapses race and culture. Khalil received harsh responses from both blacks and whites (Muhammad 2007). Having spent two decades interviewing and working with poor and low-income blacks, I find the presumptions that they are bad parents, that they do not care about education, and that they lack a work ethic profoundly disturbing. From my perspective this is a new form of racism sold as truth-telling. A parent's wealth and social connections remain the two most important keys to economic success in the United States.

25. Tapper 1999.

26. Hine 1989.

27. Tapper 1999; Wailoo 1997.

28. Mason 1922; Taliaferro and Huck 1923.

29. Tapper 1999: 17.

30. Wailoo 1997: 135.

31. Tapper 1999: 27–54.

32. Hodges 1950: 804–10.

33. Wailoo 2001: 187.

34. Best et al. 2002.

35. Armstrong 2003; Duster 2003; Leavitt and Numbers 1997; Rosenberg and Golden 1992; Wailoo and Pemberton 2006.

36. It is important to note that resident physicians receive very poor training in dealing with cultural differences (Weissman et al. 2005).

37. Teen support group, Children's Hospital West, 1998.

38. What anthropologists do with contrasting perceptions is accept each perspective as representational of something. We shy away from calling that something "truth" or "reality," but anthropologists accept that individual subjectivity

is tied to cultural and material objects (shared beliefs and practices, insurance, disease, technology, etc.). For anthropologists, the messiness of "truth" provides the fertile ground for cultural change. It is because of the uncertainties that people are able to change cultural beliefs and practices through persuasion or resignification.

39. Card, Dobkin, and Maestas 2004.
40. Committee on the Consequences of Uninsurance 2004.
41. Chen et al. 2001; Carlisle, Leake, and Shapiro 1997.
42. Scheper-Hughes 1992: 22–23.
43. Scheper-Hughes 1992: 529–30.
44. Scheper-Hughes 1992: 530.
45. Farmer 2003: 236.
46. Farmer 2003: 19.
47. Behar 1997; Rapp 2000; Rapp and Ginsburg 2001.
48. Powers and Faden 2006; Rouse 2007.
49. Cultures have different moral discourses, and in order to challenge oppression people employ the discourses that resonate with those around them, the "vein of enthusiasm and commitment" (Farmer 2003: 19). Members of the sickle cell community employ moral discourses to resignify what and who matters in the clinic and, given those priorities, what should be done. Resignification is a process not of radical subversion, as Judith Butler notes in *Bodies That Matter: On the Discursive Limits of "Sex"* (2003: 237), but of rearticulating practices by inhabiting particular norms. Within the clinic various norms and moral discourses dominate, operate, compete, or come together to form something new.
50. See the literature review in Smedley, Stith, and Nelson 2003: 285–383.
51. Good 2001.
52. Klick and Satel 2006.

## CHAPTER 1. RACE AND UNCERTAINTY

1. *The Management of Sickle Cell Disease* 2002: 60–61.
2. *The Management of Sickle Cell Disease* 2002: 61.
3. Betancourt 2004.
4. Interview with Max and Vanessa (both pseudonyms), May 1999, Children's Hospital West.
5. "Personality disorder," in American Psychiatric Association 2000: 685–730.
6. Geertz 1983: 85.
7. Rhodes 2004.
8. Farmer 1999, 2003.
9. Coombs et al. 1993; Leiderman and Grisso 1985; Dans 2002. "Ger" was a term described to me by one of my students who spent a summer working at Bellevue Hospital in New York.
10. Dans 2002: 26.
11. Smedley, Stith, and Nelson 2003; Strakowski et al. 1996.
12. Life expectancy for sickle cell patients has tripled in the last twenty years, from fifteen to forty-five years, and many cities have yet to develop comprehensive adult sickle cell clinics. This city was no exception.

13. Alderman 2000: 673.
14. Alderman 2000: 679.
15. Wacquant 2005: 128.
16. Foucault 1995: 308.
17. Kristeva 1982: 135.
18. Cheng 2005: 569.
19. Agamben 1998.
20. Douglas 1966: 3–4.
21. The *Primal Source,* a conservative Tufts University newspaper, published a racist screed to be sung to the tune of the Christmas carol "O Come All Ye Faithful." Meant to break the silence about the intellectual and scholastic inferiority of black students, the song, published in December 2006, described the fifty-two black Tufts freshmen as "boisterous" and "born in to oppression." The lyrics were as follows:

O COME ALL YE BLACK FOLK (sung to the tune of O Come All Ye Faithful)
O Come All Ye Black Folk
Boisterous, yet desirable
O come ye, O come ye to our university
Come and we will admit you,
Born in to oppression;
O come, let us accept them,
O come, let us accept them,
O come, let us accept them,
Fifty-two black freshmen.
O sing, gospel choirs,
We will accept your children,
No matter what your grades are F's D's or G's
Give them privileged status; We will welcome all
[refrain]
Fifty-two black freshmen.
All come! Blacks, we need you, born into the ghetto.
O Jesus! We need you now to fill our racial quotas.
Descendents of Africa, with brown skin arriving:
[refrain]
Fifty-two black freshmen

What is particularly troubling in the case of this aggressive hate speech is the assumption on the part of the *Primal Source* staff that their black cohort had lower high school grades and lower test scores than they did. When Don Imus was fired from CBS for his comment that the Rutgers women's basketball team were "nappy-headed hos," the public learned that one of the women on the team was a high school valedictorian and one was a straight-A student at Rutgers. The other students were also described as extremely competitive both in the classroom and on the court. On a whole, the LSAT and SAT test scores of blacks are lower than those of whites and Asians, but individual tests scores are different than aggregates. The inability on the part of the *Primal Source* staff, and many others, to differentiate blacks speaks to a lack of race consciousness.

22. Adorno was a member of a group of Marxian scholars who began asking why socialism had failed so miserably in Europe in the twentieth century. He belonged to the Institute for Social Research, known commonly as the Frankfurt school, which began at the University of Frankfurt in 1923. Other scholars have contributed to a study of late modern capitalism and what is known as the crisis in historical materialism. Antonio Gramsci, modern French historiographers and philosophers, including Michel Foucault and Walter Benjamin, and members of the Birmingham school, including Stuart Hall, have all explored how inequality is reproduced at the cultural, psychological, and structural level.

23. Crenshaw 1995: 103.

24. Murray 1984: 18.

25. Wacquant 2002.

26. Ford 2008.

## CHAPTER 2. SICKLE CELL DISEASE IN THE CLINIC

1. LaTasha was not sure why they were doing a pelvic exam.

2. Green et al. 2007.

3. *The Management of Sickle Cell Disease* 2002.

## CHAPTER 3. HEALTH CARE ACCESS AND MEDICAL UNCERTAINTY

1. Pernick 1983: 26.

2. Bloche 2001: 96–97, 121.

3. Bloche 2001: 120–21.

4. One can find information regarding the NIH Consensus Development Program on the Internet at http://consensus.nih.gov/about/about.htm.

5. Interview with Dr. Allen at his office at Children's Hospital West, January 1999.

6. Green et al. 2003; Maxwell, Streetly, and Bevan 1999; Pletcher et al. 2008; Todd 2001; Todd et al. 2006.

7. Sutton et al. 1999.

8. Bourdieu 1977: 164.

9. Harding 1986, 1993; Kuhn 1970; Latour and Woolgar 1979; Wailoo 1997; Wailoo and Pemberton 2006.

10. Mol and Elsman 1996.

11. The racial composition of the clinic staff is unusual for any hospital including CHE, but the relationship between their treatment approach and the racial correspondence between the staff and patients are complicated.

12. Maxwell, Streetly, and Bevan 1999.

13. Weber 1930: 80. In *The Protestant Ethic and the Spirit of Capitalism*, Weber describes Martin Luther's notion of duty: "It is true that certain suggestions of the positive valuation of routine activity in the world, which is contained in this conception of the calling, had already existed in the Middle Ages, and even in late Hellenistic antiquity. We shall speak of that later. But at least one thing was unquestionably new: the valuation of the fulfillment of duty in

worldly affairs as the highest form which the moral activity of the individual could assume. This it was which inevitably gave every-day worldly activity a religious significance, and which first created the conception of a calling in this sense. . . . The only way of living acceptably to God was not to surpass worldly morality in monastic asceticism, but solely through the fulfillment of the obligations imposed upon the individual by his position in the world. That was his calling."

14. Chris Feutner describes how diabetes treatment has been profoundly shaped over the last century by these same physician determinations; see Feutner 2003.

15. Latour and Woolgar 1979.

16. Hacking 1992.

17. Harris 2005.

18. Foucault 1980, 170.

19. Greenhouse 1996. These diverse, often suppressed, iterations about time disrupt any attempts on the part of the state to create a monotheistic biomedical regime connected to the state's linear model of (productive) time.

20. Foucault 1977a.

21. Harris 2005.

22. Rosen 2007: 844–46.

23. Nissen and Wolski 2007: 2457–71.

24. Rosen 2007: 844.

25. Notably, even my presentation of the treatment variables is in no way value-neutral. The order in which I present the information; the language I use, including "suppression" and "destruction"; and the information I leave out, which in this case might be stories told by patients describing their experiences with any of these therapies, will produce a different understanding of the relative risks and benefits of any treatment.

26. It is important to note that Dr. Vichinsky, also an expert in the treatment of thalassemia, built his career in the 1980s developing safer blood transfusion protocols. See Vichinsky 1980, 1982, 1991.

27. Chronic blood transfusion is the oldest effective treatment, but while transfusions have been used to treat symptoms of sickle cell disease since the 1970s, hydroxyurea is credited by the NIH as being "the first effective therapy for severely affected adults with sickle cell disease; painful episodes were reduced by 50 percent" ("Sickle Cell Research for Treatment and Cure," NIH, September 2002: 10). Distinguishing hydroxyurea as a therapy, or a cure, is, I will argue, making a statement about the relative qualities of either treatment because hydroxyurea does not in fact cure sickle cell disease any more than blood transfusions do. I will discuss the relevance of these delineations in the section on time.

28. *The Management of Sickle Cell Disease* 2002.

29. Goodman 1999.

30. Goodman 1999: 996.

31. Goodman 1999: 1001.

32. Conversation with Joe Dumit, Princeton University, 2005.

33. Goodman 1999: 1002.

34. Bunkle 1988, 1993.

35. Hackney-Stephens and Vichinsky 2002.

36. Baudrillard 1988: 166.

37. "Use of Hydroxyurea in Patients with Sickle Cell Disease: The Multicenter Study of Hydroxyurea in Sickle Cell Anemia (MSH)," revised April 22, 1998, http://sickle.bwh.harvard.edu/hyguid.html.

38. Charache et al. 1995: 1317.

39. Greenhouse 1996: 4.

40. Goodman 1999: 996.

## CHAPTER 4. THE AFFECTIVE DIMENSIONS OF PAIN

1. Obeyesekere 2002: 135.

2. There are, of course, wealthy patients with sickle cell disease. Their experiences deserve more attention given that racial health care disparities cross class lines. These patients are uniquely situated, and their experiences can offer us insights into when class does and does not matter in the clinic. Unfortunately, I did not focus on this subsection of the population.

3. Good et al. 1994.

4. *The Management of Sickle Cell Disease* 2002; Benjamin et al. 1999; Benjamin, Swinson, and Nagel 2000.

5. Millman 1993.

6. Rapp 2000.

## CHAPTER 5. UNCERTAIN EFFICACY

1. Good 1995: 199.

2. Wailoo 2001: 199.

3. Wailoo 2001: 165.

4. Wailoo 2001: 170–74.

5. Levine et al. 2001: 480–81.

6. Smedley, Stith, and Nelson 2003: 38–71.

7. Wailoo 2001: 166–67.

8. Then Job answered: "Listen carefully to my words, and let this be your consolation. 3 Bear with me, and I will speak, and after I have spoken, mock on. 4 As for me, is my complaint against man? Why should I not be impatient? 5 Look at me, and be appalled, and lay your hand upon your mouth. 6 When I think of it I am dismayed, and shuddering seizes my flesh. 7 Why do the wicked live, reach old age, and grow mighty in power? 8 Their children are established in their presence, and their offspring before their eyes. 9 Their houses are safe from fear, and no rod of God is upon them. 10 Their bull breeds without fail; their cow calves, and does not cast her calf. 11 They send forth their little ones like a flock, and their children dance. 12 They sing to the tambourine and the lyre, and rejoice to the sound of the pipe. 13 They spend their days in prosperity, and in peace they go down to Sheol. 14 They say to God, 'Depart from us! We do not desire the knowledge of thy ways. 15 What is the Almighty, that we should serve him? And what profit do we get if we pray to him?' 16 Behold, is not their prosperity in their hand? The counsel of the wicked is far from me."

9. Johnson 1998b: 2.

10. Napier 1999: 4.

11. Long 2005.

12. Johnson 1998a: 1–2.

13. Armstrong, Carpenter, and Hojnacki 2006: 759.

14. Committee on the NIH Research Priority-Setting Process, Institute of Medicine 1998: 43–52.

15. Committee on the NIH Research Priority-Setting Process, Institute of Medicine 1998.

16. Gross, Anderson, and Powe 1999: 1881–87.

17. Kleinman and Kleinman 1997: 14.

18. Dresser 2000: 411.

19. Edelman 1985: 193.

20. Although the largest, the NIH is only one of several federal agencies that funds health care research. Others include the Centers for Disease Control and Prevention, the Agency for Health Care Policy Research, the Indian Health Services, the Health Care Financing Administration, the Heath Resources Services Administration, the Substance Abuse and Mental Health Administration, and the Food and Drug Administration. The NIH budget for 2004 can be found at http://www.aaas.org/spp/rd. Also, the National Science Foundation funds research that often has health care applications.

21. Noted medical sociologist Betsy Armstrong has observed grassroots attempts to alter the capital flows in health care, but given the virtual public handout to pharmaceutical and insurance companies in the form of the Medicare Reform Act, it is difficult to predict what reform, if any, is possible.

22. Weber 1930: 53. "It might thus seem that the development of the spirit of capitalism is best understood as part of the development of rationalism as a whole, and could be deduced from the fundamental position of rationalism on the basic problems of life" (76).

23. Moss 1996.

24. Numbers 1997: 269–83.

25. Numbers 1997: 276.

26. Numbers 1997: 277.

27. "These are quotes from members of the Consortium for Eliminating Health Care Disparities Through Community and Hospital Partnerships, and the National Advisory Panel. Members' quotes are from a meeting held on November 5, 2003, to articulate the rationale for developing a uniform framework for data collection and the importance of collecting data." Health Research and Educational Trust, http://www.hretdisparities.org/hretdisparities/html/makingthecase.html.

28. Rouse 2004.

29. Rosenberg 2003: 502.

30. Larrimore 2001; Weber 1946: 275.

31. Obeyesekere 2002: 135.

32. Larrimore 2001: xix.

33. Larrimore 2001, 149.

34. Discussion of Hobbes in Halpern 2002: 113.

35. Thomas 1979: 120–21, 143.

## CHAPTER 6. UNCERTAIN SUFFERING

1. Smedley, Stith, and Nelson 2003.
2. Chen et al. 2001: 1443–49; Carlisle, Leake, and Shapiro 1997: 263–67.
3. Ballas 1998: 52.
4. Parsons 1991.
5. Ballas 1998.
6. Young 2000.
7. Ballas 1998: 51; see also Smith et al. 2008.
8. Malinowski 1973; Murdock 1949; Parsons 1955; Radcliffe-Brown 1940.
9. Nietzsche 1968: 13.
10. Scarry 1985: 13.
11. Green 1997: 6.
12. Asch 1999: 2000.
13. Peter A. Ubel, George Loewenstein, Norbert Schwarz, and Dylan Smith, "Misimagining the Unimaginable: The Disability Paradox and Healthcare Decision Making" (working paper presented at Princeton University, 2004).
14. Albrecht and Devlieger 1999.
15. Lee 1984; Shostak 1983; Turnbull 1962.
16. Asch 1999, 2000.
17. Livingston 2005; Rapp 1988.
18. Das 1990; Kleinman and Kleinman 1991; Lock 1996.
19. Temkin 1963.
20. Chuengsatiansup 2001: 34–35.
21. Kleinman, Das, and Lock 1997.
22. Arendt 1990: 85, 86.
23. Rouse 2004b.
24. Sharp 2006: 307–8.
25. As of 2004, two such programs are Healthy Kids in California, which extends health care to children aged five and under whose parents do not earn enough to pay for insurance, and Kidcare in Florida.
26. Renowned pain researcher J. Bonica notes that the percentage of patients who report pain is greater in sickle cell patients (more than 95 percent) than in bone cancer (85 percent), oral cancer (80 percent), genitourinary cancer (75 percent), lymphomas (20 percent), and leukemias (5 percent). Bonica, Ventafridda, and Twycross 1990: 400–460. In an article on treatment of pain in children, Charles B. Berde and Navil Sethna describe similar pain treatments for sickle cell pain and cancer pain: "We routinely prescribe basal infusions for children with cancer or sickle cell disease" (2002: 1099). Even though they draw the comparison in terms of treatment, they recommend "Children with sickle cell disease who have vaso-occlusive episodes should receive opioids as needed to relieve pain. Studies emphasize oral dosing of potent opioids and NSAIDs, home treatment, and reduced reliance on emergency departments or inpatient admission" (1101).
27. OxyContin, an extremely powerful pain reliever, received federal drug approval in 1995. The pill is designed to release the drug slowly into the system, but when it is crushed, it produces a powerful high. By the late 1990s, OxyContin had became a popular drug of choice, particularly in rural America. As a result,

it is associated with drug addiction, and users are treated with suspicion. For more information on how OxyContin is now marketed, see Government Accounting Office 2003.

28. Gamble 1997.

29. *The Burden of Chronic Diseases and Their Risk Factors: National and State Perspectives 2004*, Section II, "The Burden of Heart Disease, Stroke, Cancer, and Diabetes," National Center for Chronic Disease Prevention and Health Promotion, part of the Centers for Disease Control, www.cdc.gov/nccdphp/burdenbook2004/Section02/heart.htm.

30. Rouse 2007.

31. Sickle cell anemia and sickle cell disease are the same thing. The name change was motivated by a desire to convey the seriousness of the condition.

32. Dr. Allen, e-mail correspondence, January 2002.

33. Interview with Dr. Taylor, Children's Hospital North, October 2002.

34. Habermas 1989.

## CHAPTER 7. FINDING A WAY OUT OF *DOXA:* ANTHROPOLOGY OF THE IMAGINATION

1. Kleinman 1977; Good and Good 1980.

2. Kleinman 1980: 107; see Horton 1967. The amount of time a physician spends with a patient is important depending on the disease. Sickle cell patients, for example, require a tremendous amount of time because physicians are trying to determine which symptoms are traceable to the disease and which might be traceable to other ailments. The problem in this case is not one of empathy but of which services are "billable" and which are not. Insurance companies will, for example, pay when a physician prescribes insulin or antihypertensive medication during an office visit for an obese patient. They will not pay the physician for a visit designed to help the patient lose weight in order to eliminate the need for the medications.

3. Biehl 2005; Das et al. 2000; Das et al. 2001; Farmer 1999.

4. Good 1994.

5. Baer, Singer, and Susser 2003: 21.

6. I would like to thank in particular Mary-Jo Good, Peter Guarnaccia, and the Russell Sage Foundation for the opportunity to think outside *doxa*, or the box. The workshops examining racial health care disparities were very helpful in developing the thesis for *Uncertain Suffering*.

7. Smedley, Stith, and Nelson 2003: 15–16.

8. Minino and Smith 2001.

9. Jesse D. McKinnon and Claudette E. Bennett, *We the People: Blacks in the United States*, in Census 2000, Special Report, 2005, Census Bureau, www.census.gov/prod/2005pubs/censr-25.pdf.

10. *Unemployed Persons by Marital Status, Race, Hispanic or Latino Ethnicity, Age, and Sex*, Department of Labor, Bureau of Labor Statistics, 2008, http://www.bls.gov.web/cpseea29.pdf.

11. Poverty 2005, U.S. Census, http://www.census.gov/hhes/www/poverty/poverty05/table5.html.

12. *United States: Punishment and Prejudice: Racial Disparities in the War on Drugs,* May 2000, vol. 12, no. 2(G), http://www.hrw.org/legacy/reports/2000/usa/; *Race and Incarceration in the United States,* Human Rights Watch, February 27, 2002, http://www.hrw.org/legacy/backgrounder/usa/race/.

13. Interview with Dr. Taylor, Children's Hospital North, October 2002.

14. National Heart, Lung, and Blood Institute 2002.

15. Wailoo 2001.

16. This is taken from the National Sickle Cell Anemia Control Act of 1972, Sections 2(a)(1) and 2(a)(2).

17. Wailoo 2001: 170.

18. Baer, Singer, and Susser 2003.

19. Rousseau 1997.

20. Arendt 1990: 88.

21. Boltanski 1999.

22. Interview with Dr. Achebe, Children's Hospital East, October 2001.

## CHAPTER 8. ADOLESCENT TRANSITIONING: ACCULTURATING PATIENTS TO THE CULTURE OF MEDICINE

1. Interview with Dr. Sorral and Ms. Barns, Camp Freedom, August 2003. Emma's reasons for sticking herself with a needle were never discussed, and as an observer I chose not to interrupt. I assumed her sticking herself was akin to cutting oneself to relieve anxiety and/or take control of one's pain.

2. Interview with Dr. Achebe, Camp Freedom, August 2003.

3. Blum et al. 1993: 570.

4. Guinier and Torres 2002.

5. Interview with Mr. Jefferson, Children's Hospital East, July 2001.

6. Gremillion 2003.

7. Interview with Mr. Jefferson, Children's Hospital East, July 2001.

8. Alegria et al. 2004; Green et al. 2003; Killion 2007; Lopez and Guarnaccia 2000.

9. Gardner 1984.

10. Hall 1904.

11. Kimmel and Weiner 1985: 3.

12. Elder 1980; Katz 1975.

13. Kimmel and Weiner 1985: 10–11.

14. Chodorow 1991; Inhelder and Piaget 1958; Piaget 1932; Vygotsky 1994.

15. Bloche 2007: 1173.

16. According to the *Federal Register,* the Bush administration, on October 2, 2002, extended health insurance coverage to fetuses under the State of Children's Health Insurance Program (SCHIP). This regulation does not extend to pregnant women. In 2007, President Bush vetoed two bills to extend SCHIP.

17. In the well-publicized case of the first sickle cell patient to be treated with unrelated donor bone marrow, the twelve-year-old miracle patient Keone Penn developed graft-versus-host-disease nine months after treatment. Penn's setback could have been due to lack of compliance to posttreatment drug regimens, or perhaps GVHD was inevitable. At an NIH meeting on bone marrow

transplant protocols, the team that transplanted him said they are pushing to transplant patients before they become teenagers so that their parents are responsible for medical compliance. This move would make a bone marrow transplant not a decision based upon autonomy or free will but one made entirely by physicians and parents.

18. Telfair et al. 2004: 446.

19. Telfair et al. 2004: 449.

20. Telfair et al. 2004: 458.

21. Telephone interview with Joseph Telfair, July 2003.

22. For an in-depth discussion of the role of adolescent "maturity" in judicial bypass hearings and in adolescent decision making, see Levesque 2000: 111–37. Columbia Law School professor Carol Sanger, in a working paper entitled "Compelling Narrative: Judicial By-pass Hearings and the Misuse of Law," discusses the arbitrariness of judicial decisions to deny adolescents the right to abort without parental consent. A judge's decision always involves some standard performance of maturity that the minor failed to live up to. Paper presented by Carol Sanger at Princeton University's Department of Anthropology, November 2003.

23. Barbara Ehrenreich, in *The Hearts of Men* (1983), describes how some psychologists from the 1950s to the 1980s pathologized a young man's refusal to assume traditional adult roles, such as marriage, career, and family. In the literature, these men were diagnosed as immature, and their masculinity was questioned.

24. The Centre for Contemporary Cultural Studies (CCCS) was initiated at the University of Birmingham, England, in 1963. The scholars explore the role of culture in the reproduction of the relations of production. One very important work to emerge from what some call cultural Marxism was Paul Willis's *Learning to Labor: How Working Class Kids Get Working Class Jobs* (1977). Similar to other studies of youth, *Learning to Labor* positions youth as creative agents who, in an attempt to resist their own oppression, end up reproducing it.

## CHAPTER 9. THOUGHT EXPERIMENT: WHAT DOES IT MEAN TO SAVE A LIFE?

1. I use these data for a chapter in an edited volume entitled *A Death Retold: Jesica Santillan, the Bungled Transplant, and Paradoxes of Medical Citizenship;* see Rouse 2006: 329–48.

2. Sharp 2006: 301.

3. Good 2001: 395–410.

4. Each participant signed a consent form, interviews were taped and transcribed, and each participant was offered a gift of See's candies following the interview. The association let me use one of its booths in the hotel typically reserved for pharmaceutical companies. Instead of paying $2,500 for the booth, I was asked to donate $50.

5. I posed the same questions during my interview with Eva and Flora three months later.

6. Sickle cell disease and other hemoglobinopathies exist in countries around the Mediterranean and in the Middle East and Asia. The large international presence of

medical professionals and patients from Israel, India, Ghana, Nigeria, Liberia, Britain, and Jamaica is therefore not surprising. The racial and ethnic diversity at a medical conference in the United States is, however, a bit unusual.

7. Walters et al. 2000.

8. Vermylen 2003.

9. It should be noted that as medical procedures shift from being considered experimental to being considered standard, the pressure on the patient and family to accept a procedure becomes greater. Kidney transplants, for example, once considered "life-enhancing," are now considered "lifesaving" because the long-term outcomes for patients on dialysis are worse than for those who receive a transplant. Bone marrow transplants for sickle cell patients might follow this trajectory.

10. Unrelated donor transplants are much riskier than related donor matches. Dr. Kassim's paper addressed the question, If sickle cell disease can be treated through chronic transfusion therapy and hydroxyurea (and other less significant therapies), is transplantation a legitimate option?

11. Parsons 1991.

12. Hanisco 2000: 906.

13. Hanisco 2000: 922.

14. Hanisco 2000: 908–9.

15. Hanisco 2000: 921.

16. Hanisco 2000: 928–29.

17. Hanisco 2000: 905.


CHAPTER 10. RETHINKING SUFFERING: COMMUNITY-BASED HEALTH CARE, ALTERNATIVE MEDICINE, AND FAITH

1. Elijah Muhammad, the founder of the Nation of Islam, advocated alternative eating practices as part and parcel of liberation. The use of alternative medicine by African American Sunni Muslims therefore seems very much like an outgrowth of this earlier history. See Curtis 2002; Rouse and Hoskins 2004.

2. Curtis 2002; Rouse and Hoskins 2004.

3. Bodhise et al. 2004: 236. (Note: I could not hide the identity of Dr. Bodhise with a pseudonym because of the need to cite his publication.)

4. Marx 1978: 46.


CONCLUSION

1. Best 2001.

2. Agency for Healthcare Research and Quality 2003.

3. Agency for Healthcare Research and Quality 2004.

4. National Medical Association press release, "NMA Appalled over Distorted HHS Disparities Report," January 22, 2004.

5. Harding 1993.

6. National Medical Association, "NMA appalled over distorted HHS disparities report," press release, January 22, 2004.

7. Rosenberg 2003; Temkin 1963.

8. Bakhtin 1981; Sontag 1989.

9. The relationship between segregation and oppression is again in question given that forty years after the Civil Rights Act of 1964 the gains made by blacks, particularly in education, remain elusive.

10. Higginbotham 1993.

11. Patterson 2007.

12. National Sickle Cell Anemia Control Act (P.L. 92–294) of 1972. This quotation comes from section 2 of the Sickle Cell Control Act. The first part of section 2 reads, "The Congress finds and declares (1) that sickle cell anemia is a debilitating, inheritable disease . . . that afflicts approximately two million American citizens and has been largely neglected; (2) that the disease is a deadly and tragic burden which is likely to strike one-fourth of the children born to parents who both bear the sickle cell trait; (3) the efforts to prevent sickle cell anemia must be directed toward increased research in the cause and treatment of the disease, and the education, screening, and counseling of carriers of the sickle cell trait."

13. Melfi et al. 2000.

14. Margolis et al. 2003; McCann et al. 2005.

15. Phillips et al. 1997; Lillie-Blanton et al. 2000.

16. Williams and Jackson 2005.

17. Eberhardt et al. 1994; Auslander et al. 1997.

18. Klick and Satel 2006: 42–47.

19. Griggs and Engel 2005.

20. In 2007 our department's UPS driver struggled in the summer heat to deliver hundreds of copies of *Atlas of Creation* by Harun Yahya. The gratis copies of this book, each weighing more than thirty pounds, were delivered to academics across the country. Yahya's atlas attempts to dispel the idea of evolution by representing in scientific detail how species preserved in fossils, described by scientists as being millions of years old, are in fact identical to species found today. This, for Yahya, is proof that species have not evolved. Creation museums in the United States similarly use science to disprove evolution.

21. Best 2001.

22. Bourdieu 1977: 159–71.

23. Strathern 1992: 15.

24. The sickle cell community includes patients, medical professionals, families, local associations, and advocates.

# References

Abraham, Laurie Kaye. 1993. *Mama Might Be Better Off Dead: The Failure of Health Care in Urban America*. Chicago: University of Chicago Press.

Agamben, Giorgio. 1998. *Homo Sacer: Sovereign Power and Bare Life*. Stanford, Calif.: Stanford University Press.

Agency for Healthcare Research and Quality. 2003. *National Healthcare Disparities Report*. Pub. no. 04–0034.

———. 2004. *National Healthcare Disparities Report*. Pub. no. 05–0014. Rockville, Md. AHRQ, 2004.

Albrecht, G. L., and P. J. Devlieger. 1999. The Disability Paradox: High Quality of Life against all Odds. *Social Science and Medicine* 48:977–88.

Alderman, Derek H. 2000. A Street Fit for a King: Naming Places and Commemoration in the American South. *Professional Geographer* 52: 672–84.

Alexander, G. Caleb, and Ashwini R. Sehgal. 1998. Barriers to Cadaveric Renal Transplantation among Blacks, Women, and the Poor. *Journal of the American Medical Association* 280:1148–52.

Algeria, Margarita, David Takeuchi, Glorisa Canino, Naihua Duan, Patrick Shrout, Xiao-Li Meng, William Vega, et al. 2004. Considering Context, Place, and Culture: The National Latino and Asian American Study. *International Journal of Psychiatric Research* 13:208–20.

American Psychiatric Association. 2000. *Diagnostic and Statistical Manual of Mental Disorders*. 4th ed., text revision. Washington, D.C.: American Psychiatric Association.

Anspach, Renee. 1993. *Deciding Who Lives: Fateful Choices in the Intensive-Care Nursery*. Berkeley: University of California Press.

Arendt, Hannah. 1990. *On Revolution*. London: Penguin Books.

Armstrong, Elizabeth. 2003. *Conceiving Risk, Bearing Responsibility: Fetal Alcohol Syndrome and the Diagnosis of Moral Disorder*. Baltimore: Johns Hopkins University Press.

Armstrong, Elizabeth M., Daniel P. Carpenter, and Marie Hojnacki. 2006. Whose Death Matters? Mortality, Advocacy, and Attention to Disease in the Mass Media. *Journal of Health Politics, Policy and Law* 31:729–72.

Asch, Adrienne. 1999. Prenatal Diagnosis and Selective Abortion: A Challenge to Practice and Policy. *American Journal of Public Health* 89:1649–57.

———. 2000. Why I Haven't Changed My Mind about Prenatal Diagnosis: Reflections and Refinements. In *Prenatal Testing and Disability Rights*, edited by Erik Parens and Adrienne Asch, 234–58. Washington, D.C.: Georgetown University Press.

Auslander, Wendy F., Sanna J. Thompson, Daniele Dreitzer, Neil H. White, and Julio V. Santiago. 1997. Disparities in Glycemic Control and Adherence between African-American and Caucasian Youths with Diabetes: Family and Community Contexts. *Diabetes Care* 20:1569–75.

Ayanian, John Z., Paul D. Cleary, Joel S. Weissman, and Arnold M. Epstein. 1999. The Effect of Patients' Preferences on Racial Differences in Access to Renal Transplantation. *New England Journal of Medicine* 341:1661–69.

Ayanian, John Z., I. Steve Udvarhelyi, C. A. Gatsonis, C. L. Pasho, and A. M. Epstein. 1993. Racial Differences in the Use of Revascularization Procedures after Coronary Angiography. *Journal of the American Medical Association* 269:2642–46.

Bach, Peter B., Laura D. Cramer, Joan L. Warren, and Colin B. Begg. 1999. Racial Differences in the Treatment of Early-Stage Lung Cancer. *New England Journal of Medicine* 341:1198–1205.

Baer, Hans A., Merrill Singer, and Ida Susser. 2003. *Medical Anthropology and the World System*. Westport, Conn.: Praeger.

Bakhtin, Mikhail. 1981. *Discourse in the Novel*. Austin: University of Texas Press.

Ballas, Samir. 1998. *Sickle Cell Pain: Progress in Pain Research and Management*. Vol. 11. Seattle, Wash.: International Association for the Study of Pain.

———. 2001a. Iron Overload Is a Determinant of Morbidity and Mortality in Adult Patients with Sickle Cell Disease. *Seminars in Hematology* 1 (suppl.): 30–36.

———. 2001b. Sickle Cell Disease: Current Clinical Management. *Seminars in Hematology* 38:307–14.

Barnes, Barry. 1974. *Scientific Knowledge and Sociological Theory*. London: Routledge and Kegan Paul.

Baszanger, Isabelle. 1995. *Inventing Pain Medicine: From the Laboratory to the Clinic*. New Brunswick, N.J.: Rutgers University Press.

Baudrillard, Jean. 1988. Simulacra and Simulations. In *Jean Baudrillard: Selected Writings*, edited by Mark Poster, 166–84. Stanford, Calif.: Stanford University Press.

Behar, Ruth. 1997. *The Vulnerable Observer: Anthropology That Breaks Your Heart*. Boston: Beacon Press.

Benjamin, Lennette J., Carlton D. Dampier, and Ada Jacox, Victoria Odesina, David Phoenix, Barbara Shapiro, Maureen Strafford, and Marsha Treadwell. 1999. *Guideline for the Management of Acute and Chronic Pain in Sickle-Cell Disease.* Glenview, Ill.: American Pain Society.

Benjamin, Lennette, Gwendolyn I. Swinson, and Ronald L. Nagel. 2000. Sickle Cell Anemia Day Hospital: An Approach for the Management of Uncomplicated Painful Crises. *Blood* 95:1130–37.

Bennett, Michael, and Vanessa D. Dickerson. 2001. Introduction. In *Recovering the Black Female Body: Self-Representations by African American Women,* edited by Michael Bennett and Vanessa D. Dickerson, 1–15. New Brunswick, N.J.: Rutgers University Press.

Berde, Charles B., and Navil Sethna. 2002. Analgesics for the Treatment of Pain in Children. *New England Journal of Medicine* 347:1094–1103.

Berg, Marc, and Annemarie Mol. 1998. *Differences in Medicine: Unraveling Practices, Techniques and Bodies.* Durham, N.C.: Duke University Press.

Best, Joel. 2001. *Damned Lies and Statistics: Untangling Numbers from the Media, Politicians, and Activists.* Berkeley: University of California Press.

Best, M., C. Marker, C. Cruz, J. Kwiatkowski, K. Ohene-Frempong, and J. Radcliffe. 2002. Neuropsychological Functioning in Infants and Young Children with Sickle Cell Disease. Paper presented at the thirtieth anniversary of the National Sickle Cell Disease Program, National Heart, Lung, and Blood Institute, National Institutes of Health and the Sickle Cell Disease Association of America, Inc., September 2002, Washington, D.C. Abstract No. 4.

Betancourt, Joseph R. 2004. Cultural Competence: Marginal or Mainstream Movement? *New England Journal of Medicine* 351:953–55.

Biehl, Joao. 2005. *Vita: Life in a Zone of Social Abandonment.* Berkeley: University of California Press.

Bloche, M. Gregg. 2001. Race and Discretion in American Medicine. *Yale Journal of Health Policy, Law and Ethics* 1:95–131.

———. 2007. Health Care for All? *New England Journal of Medicine* 357:1173–75.

Blum, Robert W., Dale Garell, Christopher H. Hodgman, Timothy W. Jorissen, Nancy A. Okinow, Donald P. Orr, and Gail B. Slap. 1993. Transition from Child-Centered to Adult Health-Care Systems for Adolescents with Chronic Conditions: A Position Paper of the Society for Adolescent Medicine. *Journal of Adolescent Health* 14:570–76.

Bodhise, Paul Brown, Marjorie Dejoie, Zemoria Brandon, Stanley Simpkins, and Samir K. Ballas. 2004. Non-pharmacological Management of Sickle Cell Pain. *Hematology* 9:235–37.

Boltanski, Luc. 1999. *Distant Suffering: Morality, Media and Politics.* Cambridge: Cambridge University Press.

Bonham, Vence L. 2001. Race, Ethnicity, and Pain Treatment: Striving to Understand the Causes and Solutions to Disparities in Pain Treatment. *Journal of Law, Medicine and Ethics* 29:52–68.

Bonica, John J., V. Ventafidda, and R. G. Twycross. 1990. Cancer Pain. In *The Management of Pain,* edited by John Bonica, 400–460. Philadelphia: Lea and Febiger.

Bourdieu, Pierre. 1977. *Outline of a Theory of Practice*. Richard Nice. Cambridge: Cambridge University Press.

Brancati, Frederick L., Jeffery C. Whittle, Paul K. Whelton, A. J. Seidler, and Michael J. Klag. 1992. The Excess Incidence of Diabetic End-Stage Renal Disease among Blacks: A Population-Based Study of Potential Explanatory Factors. *Journal of the American Medical Association* 268:3079–84.

Broome, Marion E., and Deborah J. Richards. 2003. The Influence of Relationships on Children's and Adolescents' Participation in Research. *Nursing Research* 52:191–97.

Buchanan, Allen, Dan Brock, Norman Daniels, and Daniel Wikler. 2000. *From Chance to Choice: Genetics and Justice*. Cambridge: Cambridge University Press.

Bunkle, Phillida. 1988. *The Politics of Women's Health in New Zealand*. Oxford: Oxford University Press.

———. 1993. Calling the Shots? International Politics of Depo-Provera. In *The "Racial" Economy of Science: Toward a Democratic Future*, edited by Sandra Harding, 287–302. Bloomington: Indiana University Press.

Butler, Judith. 1993. *Bodies That Matter: On the Discursive Limits of "Sex."* New York: Routledge.

Byrd, W. Michael, and Linda Clayton. 2003. Racial and Ethnic Disparities in Healthcare: A Background History. In *Unequal Treatment: Confronting Racial and Ethnic Disparities in Health Care*, edited by Brian D. Smedley, Adrienne Y. Stith, and Alan R. Nelson, 455–527. Washington, D.C.: National Academies Press.

Card, David, Carlos Dobkin, and Nicole Maestas. The Impact of Nearly Universal Insurance Coverage on Health Care Utilization and Health: Evidence from Medicare. March 2004. http://ssrn.com/abstract=516706.

Carlisle, David M., Barbara D. Leake, and Martin F. Shapiro. 1997. Racial and Ethnic Disparities in the Use of Cardiovascular Procedures: Associations with Type of Health Insurance. *American Journal of Public Health* 87:263–67.

Charache, Samuel, Michael L. Terrin, Richard D. Moore, George J. Dover, Franca B. Barton, Susan V. Eckert, Robert P. McMahon, and Duane R. Bonds. 1995. Effect of Hydroxyurea on the Frequency of Painful Crises in Sickle Cell Anemia. *New England Journal of Medicine* 332:1317–22.

Chen, Jersey, Saif S. Rathore, Martha Radford, Yun Wang, and Harlan M. Krumholz. 2001. Racial Differences in the Use of Cardiac Catheterization after Acute Myocardial Infarction. *New England Journal of Medicine* 344:1443–49.

Cheng, Anne Anlin. 2005. Passing, Natural Selection, and Love's Failure: Ethics of Survival from Chang-Rae Lee to Jacque Lacan. *American Literary History* 17:553–74.

Chin, M. H., J. X. Zhang, and K. Merrel. 1998. Diabetes in the African-American Medicare Population: Morbidity, Quality of Care, and Resource Utilization. *Diabetes Care* 21:1090–95.

Chodorow, Nancy. 1991. *Feminism and Psychoanalytic Theory*. New Haven, Conn.: Yale University Press.

Chuengsatiansup, Komatra. 2001. Marginality, Suffering, and Community. In *Remaking a World: Violence, Social Suffering, and Recovery,* edited by Veena Das, Arthur Kleinman, Margaret Luck, Mamphela Ramphele, and Pamela Reynolds, 31–75. Berkeley: University of California Press.

Cohen, Cathy. 1999. *The Boundaries of Blackness: AIDS and the Breakdown of Black Politics.* Chicago: University of Chicago Press.

Committee on the Consequences of Uninsurance. 2004. *Insuring America's Health: Principles and Recommendations.* Washington, D.C.: National Academies Press.

Committee on the NIH Research Priority-Setting Process, Institute of Medicine. 1998. *Scientific Opportunities and Public Needs: Improving Priority Setting and Public Input at the National Institutes of Health.* Washington, D.C.: National Academies Press.

Coombs, R. H., S. Chopra, D. R. Schenk, and E. Yutan. 1993. Medical Slang and Its Functions. *Social Science and Medicine* 36:987–98.

Cosby, Bill, and Alvin F. Poussaint. 2007. *Come on People: On the Path from Victims to Victors.* Nashville, Tenn.: Thomas Nelson.

Crenshaw, Kimberle. 1995. Race, Reform, and Retrenchment: Transformation and Legitimation in Antidiscrimination Law. In *Critical Race Theory: The Key Writings That Formed the Movement,* edited by Kimberle Crenshaw, Neil Gotanda, Gary Peller, and Kendall Thomas, 103–22. New York: New Press.

Csordas, Thomas. 1990. Embodiment as a Paradigm for Anthropology. *Ethos* 18:5–47.

Cunningham, W. E., D. M. Mosen, and L. S. Morales. 2000. Ethnic and Racial Differences in Long-Term Survival from Hospitalization for HIV Infection. *Journal of Health Care for the Poor and Underserved* 11:163–78.

Curtis, Edward E. 2002. *Islam in Black America: Identity, Liberation and Difference in African American Islamic Thought.* Albany: State University of New York Press.

Daly, Jeanne, ed. 1996. *Ethical Intersections: Health Research, Methods and Researcher Responsibility.* Boulder, Colo.: Westview Press.

Daniels, Norman, Bruce P. Kennedy, and Ichiro Kawachi. 1999. Why Justice Is Good for Our Health: The Social Determinants of Health Inequalities. *Daedalus* 128:215–51.

Dans, Peter. 2002. The Use of Pejorative Terms to Describe Patients: "Dirtball" Revisited. *BUMC Proceedings* 15:26–30.

Das, Veena. 1990. Moral Orientations to Suffering: Legitimation, Power, and Healing. In *Health and Social Change in International Perspective,* edited by Lincoln C. Chen, Arthur Kleinman, and Norma C. Ware, 139–70. Boston: Harvard University Press.

Das, Veena, Arthur Kleinman, Mamphela Ramphele, and Pamela Reynolds, eds. 2000. *Violence and Subjectivity.* Berkeley: University of California Press.

Douglas, Mary. 1966. *Purity and Danger: An Analysis of the Concepts of Pollution and Taboo.* New York: Routledge.

Dresser, Rebecca. 2000. Government Priorities for Biomedical Research: What Does Justice Require? In *Current Legal Issues: Law and Medicine,* edited by

Michael Freeman and Andrew Lewis, 399–419. Oxford: Oxford University Press.

Duster, Troy. 2003. *Backdoor to Eugenics*. 2nd ed. New York: Routledge.

Dyson, Michael Eric. 2005. *Is Bill Cosby Right? Or Has the Black Middle Class Lost Its Mind?* New York: Basic Civitas Books.

Eberhardt, Mark S., D.T. Lakland, F.C. Wheeler, R.R. German, and S.M. Teutsch. 1994. Is Race Related to Glycemic Control? An Assessment of Glycosylated Hemoglobin in Two South Carolina Communities. *Journal of Clinical Epidemiology* 47:1181–89.

Edelman, Murray. 1985. *The Symbolic Uses of Politics*. Urbana: University of Illinois Press.

Ehrenreich, Barbara. 1983. *The Hearts of Men: American Dreams and the Flight from Commitment*. New York: Doubleday.

Eichler, Thomas P. 2005. *Incarceration: A Preliminary Consideration*. Wilmington: Delaware Center for Justice and Metropolitan Urban League.

Elder, G.H., Jr. 1980. Adolescence in Historical Perspective. In *Handbook of Adolescent Psychology*. New York: Wiley.

Ellison, Mary D., T.J. Breen, T.G. Guo, P.R. Cummingham, and O.P. Daily. 1993. Blacks and Whites on the UNOS Renal Waiting List: Waiting Times and Patient Demographics Compared. *Transplantation Proceedings* 25: 2462–66.

Epstein, Arnold M. 2000. Racial Disparities in Access to Renal Transplantation. *New England Journal of Medicine* 343:1537–44.

Epstein, Arnold M., John Z. Ayanian, Joseph H. Keogh, Susan J. Noonan, Nancy Armistead, Paul D. Cleary, Joel S. Weissman, et al. 2000. Racial Disparities in Access to Renal Transplantation: Clinically Appropriate or Due to Underuse or Overuse? *New England Journal of Medicine* 343: 1537–44.

Epstein, Helen. 2003. Enough to Make You Sick? *New York Times Magazine*, October 12.

Epstein, Steven. 1996. *Impure Science: AIDS Activism and the Politics of Knowledge*. Berkeley: University of California Press.

Farmer, Paul. 1999. *Infections and Inequalities: The Modern Plagues*. Berkeley: University of California Press.

———. 2003. *Pathologies of Power: Health, Human Rights, and the New War on the Poor*. Berkeley: University of California Press.

Federici, Michael. 1991. *The Challenge of Populism: The Rise of Right-Wing Democratism in Postwar America*. New York: Praeger.

Feutner, Chris. 2003. *Bittersweet: Diabetes, Insulin, and Transformation of Illness*. Chapel Hill: University of North Carolina Press.

Ford, Richard Thompson. 2008. *The Race Card: How Bluffing about Bias Makes Race Relations Worse*. New York: Farrar, Straus and Giroux.

Foucault, Michel. 1977a. *The Archaeology of Knowledge and the Discourse on Language*. Trans. A.M. Sheridan Smith. New York: Pantheon Books.

———. 1977b. *Discipline and Punish: The Birth of the Prison*. Trans. Alan Sheridan. New York: Vintage Books.

———. 1980. *Power/Knowledge: Selected Interviews and Other Writings, 1972–77*. Ed. Colin Gordon. New York: Pantheon Books.

————. 1990. *The History of Sexuality: An Introduction.* Vol. 1. New York: Vintage Books.

————. 1994. *The Birth of the Clinic: An Archaeology of Medical Perception.* New York: Vintage Books.

————. 1995. *Discipline and Punish: The Birth of the Prison.* 2nd Vantage edition. Trans. Alan Sheridan. New York: Random House.

Frayn, Michael. 1998. *Copenhagen.* New York: Anchor Books.

Gaertner, Samuel L., and John F. Dovidio. 1986. The Aversive Form of Racism. In *Prejudice, Discrimination, and Racism,* edited by John F. Dovidio and Samuel L. Gaertner, 61–89. Orlando, Fla.: Academic Press.

Gamble, Vanessa Northington. 1997. Roots of the Black Hospital Reform Movement. In *Sickness and Health in America: Readings in the History of Medicine and Public Health,* edited by Judith Walzer Leavitt and Ronald L. Numbers, 369–91. Madison: University of Wisconsin Press.

Gardner, Howard. 1984. The Development of Competence in Culturally Defined Domains: A Preliminary Framework. In *Culture Theory: Essays on Mind, Self, and Emotion,* edited by Richard Shweder and Robert A. LeVine. Cambridge: Cambridge University Press.

Geertz, Clifford. 1983. Common Sense as a Cultural System. In *Local Knowledge: Further Essays in Interpretive Anthropology.* New York: Basic Books.

Giddens, Anthony. 1991. *Modernity and Self-Identity: Self and Society in the Late Modern Age.* Cambridge, UK: Polity Press.

Giles, W. H., R. F. Anda, M. L. Casper, L. G. Escobedo, and H. A. Taylor. 1995. Race and Sex Differences in Rates of Invasive Cardiac Procedures in U.S. Hospitals. *Archives of Internal Medicine* 155:318–24.

Good, Byron. 1994. *Medicine, Rationality and Experience.* Cambridge: Cambridge University Press.

Good, Byron, and Mary-Jo DelVecchio Good. 1980. The Meaning of Symptoms: A Cultural Hermeneutic Model for Clinical Practice. In *The Relevance of Social Science for Medicine,* edited by Leon Eisenberg and Arthur Kleinman, 165–96. Boston: Reidel.

————. 1981. The Semantics of Medical Discourse. In *Science and Cultures: Sociology of the Sciences,* vol. 5, edited by E. Mendelsohn and Y. Elkana, 177–212. Dordrecht: Reidel.

————. 1993. Learning Medicine: The Construction of Medical Knowledge at Harvard Medical School. In *Knowledge, Power and Practice: The Anthropology of Medicine and Everyday Life,* edited by Shirley Lindenbaum and Margaret Lock, 81–107. Berkeley: University of California Press.

Good, Mary-Jo DelVecchio, ed. 1992. *Pain as Human Experience: An Anthropological Perspective.* Berkeley: University of California Press.

————. 1995. *American Medicine: The Quest for Competence.* Berkeley: University of California Press.

————. 2001. The Biotechnical Embrace. *Culture, Medicine and Psychiatry* 25:395–410.

Good, Mary-Jo DelVecchio, Paul E. Brodwin, Byron J. Good, and Arthur Kleinman. 1994. *Pain as Human Experience: An Anthropological Perspective.* Berkeley: University of California Press.

Good, Mary-Jo DelVecchio, Cara James, Byron J. Good, and Anne E. Becker. 2002. The Culture of Medicine and Racial, Ethnic and Class Disparities in Health Care. In *Unequal Treatment: Confronting Racial and Ethnic Disparities in Health Care*, edited by Brian D. Smedley, Adrienne Y. Stith, and Alan R. Nelson, 594–625. Washington, D.C.: National Academies Press.

Goodman, Steven N. 1999. Toward Evidence-Based Medical Statistics. 1: The P Value Fallacy. *Annals of Internal Medicine* 130:995–1004.

Gorman, Kathleen. 1999. "Do You Doubt Your Patient's Pain?" *American Journal of Nursing* 99(3):38–43.

Gottfredson, Linda S. 2004. Intelligence: Is It the Epidemiologists' Elusive "Fundamental Cause" of Social Class Inequalities in Health? *Journal of Personality and Social Psychology* 86:174–99.

Green, Alexander R., Dana R. Carney, Daniel J. Pallin, Long H. Ngo, Kristal L. Raymond, Lisa I. Iezzoni, and Mahzarin R. Banaji. 2007. Implicit Bias among Physicians and Its Prediction of Thrombolysis Decisions for Black and White Patients. *Journal of General Internal Medicine* 22:1231–38.

Green, Carmen R., Karen O. Anderson, Tamara A. Baker, Lisa C. Campbell, Shiela Decker, Roger B. Fillingim, Donna A. Kaloukalani, et al. 2003. The Unequal Burden of Pain: Confronting Racial and Ethnic Disparities in Pain. *Pain Medicine* 4:277–94.

Green, Ronald M. 1997. Parental Autonomy and the Obligation Not to Harm One's Child Genetically. *Journal of Law, Medicine and Ethics* 6:5–15.

Greenhouse, Carol J. 1996. *A Moment's Notice: Time Politics across Cultures.* Ithaca, N.Y.: Cornell University Press.

Gregg, Bloche M. 2001. Race and Discretion in American Medicine. *Yale Journal of Health Policy, Law and Ethics* 1:95–121.

Gremillion, Helen. 2003. *Feeding Anorexia: Gender and Power at a Treatment Center.* Durham, N.C.: Duke University Press.

Griggs, Jennifer J., and Jerome Engel. 2005. Epilepsy Surgery and the Racial Divide. *Neurology* 64:8–9.

Gross, Cary P., Gerard F. Anderson, and Neil R. Powe. 1999. The Relation between Funding by the National Institutes of Health and the Burden of Disease. *New England Journal of Medicine* 340:1881–87.

Guinier, Lani, and Gerald Torres. 2002. *The Miner's Canary: Enlisting Race, Resisting Power, Transforming Democracy.* Cambridge, Mass.: Harvard University Press.

Habermas, Jürgen. 1989. Social Action and Rationality. In *Jurgen Habermas on Society and Politics: A Reader,* edited by Steven Seidman, 142–64. Boston: Beacon Press.

Hacking, Ian. 1992. The Self-Vindication of the Laboratory Sciences. In *Science as Practice and Culture,* edited by Andrew Pickering, 29–64. Chicago: University of Chicago Press.

Hackney-Stephens, Ekua, and Elliott Vichinsky. 2002. The Spiritual Needs of Sickle Cell Families. In *Medicine, Science and Community: Working Together for a Cure,* 122. Program and abstracts for the 30th Anniversary of the National Sickle Cell Disease Program and the Sickle Cell Disease Association of American, Inc. September 17–21.

Hall, G. Stanley. 1904. *Adolescence: Its Psychology and Its Relations to Physiology, Anthropology, Sociology, Sex, Crime, Religion, and Education.* New York: Appleton.

Hall, Stuart. 1996. Gramsci's Relevance for the Study of Race and Ethnicity. In *Critical Dialogues in Cultural Studies,* edited by David Morley and Kuan-Hsing Chen, 411–40. New York: Routledge.

Hall, Tom, and Heather Montgomery. 2000. Home and Away: "Childhood," "Youth" and Young People. *Anthropology Today* 16(3):13–15.

Halpern, Cynthia. 2002. *Suffering, Politics, Power: A Genealogy in Modern Political Theory.* Albany: State University of New York Press.

Hanisco, Christine M. 2000. Acknowledging the Hypocrisy: Granting Minors the Right to Choose Their Medical Treatment. *New York Law School Journal of Human Rights* 16:899–932.

Harding, Sandra. 1986. *The Science Question in Feminism.* Ithaca, N.Y.: Cornell University Press.

———, ed. 1993. *The "Racial" Economy of Science: Toward a Democratic Future.* Bloomington: Indiana University Press.

Harris, Gardiner. 2005. F.D.A. Moves toward More Openness with the Public. *New York Times,* February 20, 28.

Harry, Collins, and Trevor Pinch. 1982. *The Social Construction of Extraordinary Science.* London: Routledge and Kegan Paul.

Herrnstein, Richard, and Charles Murray. 1994. *The Bell Curve: Intelligence and Class Structure in American Life.* New York: Free Press.

Herskovits, Melville. 1930a. *The American Negro.* New York: Knopf.

———. 1930b. *The Anthropometry of the American Negro.* New York: Columbia University Press.

———. 1990. *The Myth of the Negro Past.* New York: Beacon Press.

Higginbotham, Evelyn. 1993. *Righteous Discontent: The Women's Movement in the Black Baptist Church, 1880–1920.* Cambridge, Mass.: Harvard University Press.

Hilbert, Richard A. 1984. The Acultural Dimension of Chronic Pain: Flawed Reality Construction and the Problem of Measuring. *Social Problems* 31:365–78.

Hine, Darlene Clark. 1989. *Black Women in White: Racial Conflict and Cooperation in the Nursing Profession, 1890–1950.* Bloomington: Indiana University Press.

Hodges, John H. 1950. The Effect of Racial Mixtures upon Erythrocytic Sickling. *Blood* 5:804–10.

Hoffmann, Diane E., and Anita Tarzian. 2001. The Girl Who Cried Pain: A Bias against Women in the Treatment of Pain. *Journal of Law, Medicine, and Ethics* 29:13–27.

Honkasalo, Marja-Liisa. 2001. Vicissitudes of Pain and Suffering: Neurasthenia, Depression, and Pain in Modern China. *Medical Anthropology Quarterly* 19:319–53.

hooks, bell. 1993. *Sisters of the Yam: Black Women and Self-Recovery.* Boston: South End Press.

Horton, Robin. 1967. African Traditional Thought and Western Science. *Africa* 37(1–2):50–71.

Inhelder, Bärbel, and Jean Piaget. 1958. *The Growth of Logical Thinking from Childhood to Adolescence: An Essay on the Construction of Formal Operational Structures*. Trans. Anne Parsons and Stanley Milgram. New York: Basic Books.

Institute of Medicine's Committee on the Consequences of Uninsurance. 2004. *Insuring America's Health: Principles and Recommendations*. Washington, D.C.: National Academies Press.

Jackson, Derrick Z. 2004. Deleting the Truth on Health Care. *Boston Globe*, February 25.

Johnson, Judith A. 1998a. *Cancer Research: Selected Federal Spending and Morbidity and Mortality Statistics*. CRS Report to Congress 96–253 SPR.

————. 1998b. *Disease Funding and NIH Priority Setting*. CRS Report to Congress 97–917 STM.

Jones, James. 1993. *Bad Blood: The Tuskegee Syphilis Experiment*. New York: Free Press.

Kahneman, Daniel, and Amos Tversky. 1979. Prospect Theory: An Analysis of Decision under Risk. *Econometrica* 47:263–92.

Kasiske, Bertram L., Jon J. Snyder, Arthur J. Matas, Mary D. Ellison, John S. Gill, and Annamaria T. Kausz. 2002. Preemptive Kidney Transplantation: The Advantage and the Advantaged. *Journal of the American Society of Nephrology* 13:1358–64.

Katz, M. B. 1975. *The People of Hamilton, Canada West: Family and Class in a Mid–Nineteenth Century City*. Cambridge, Mass.: Harvard University Press.

Kawai, Tatsuo, A. Benedict Cosimi, Thomas R. Spitzer, Nina Tolkoff-Rubin, Manikkam Suthanthiran, Susan L. Saidman, Juanita Shaffer, et al. 2008. HLA-Mismatched Renal Transplantation without Maintenance Immunosuppression. *New England Journal of Medicine* 358:353–61.

Kelley, Robin D. G. 1997. *Yo' Mama's Disfunktional! Fighting the Culture Wars in Urban America*. Boston: Beacon Press.

Killion, Cheryl M. 2007. Patient-Centered Culturally Sensitive Health Care. *Counseling Psychologist* 35:726–34.

Kimmel, Douglas C., and Irving B. Weiner. 1985. *Adolescence: A Developmental Transition*. Mahwah, N.J.: Erlbaum.

Kleinman, Arthur. 1977. Lessons from a Clinical Approach to Medical Anthropological Research. *Medical Anthropology Newsletter* 8:5–8.

————. 1980. *Patients and Healers in the Context of Culture: An Exploration of the Borderland between Anthropology, Medicine, and Psychiatry*. Berkeley: University of California Press.

————. 1986. *Social Origins of Distress and Disease: Neurasthenia, Depression and Pain in Modern China*. New Haven, Conn.: Yale University Press.

Kleinman, Arthur, and Peter Benson. 2006. Anthropology in the Clinic: The Problem of Cultural Competency and How to Fix It. PLOS Med 3(10): e294 doi:10.1371/journal.pmed.0030294.

Kleinman, Arthur, Veena Das, and Margaret M. Lock. 1997. *Social Suffering*. Berkeley University of California Press.

Kleinman, Arthur, and Joan Kleinman. 1991. Suffering and Its Professional Transformation: Toward an Ethnography of Interpersonal Experience. *Culture, Medicine and Psychiatry* 15:275–301.

———. 1997. The Appeal of Experience, the Dismay of Images: Cultural Appropriations of Suffering in Our Times. In *Social Suffering,* edited by Arthur Kleinman, Veena Das, and Margaret M. Lock, 1–24. Berkeley: University of California Press.

Klick, Jonathan, and Sally Satel. 2006. *The Health Disparities Myth: Diagnosing the Treatment Gap.* Washington, D.C.: American Enterprise Institute.

Koenig, Barbara. 1988. The Technological Imperative in Medical Practice: The Social Creation of "Routine" Treatment. In *Biomedicine Examined,* edited by Margaret Lock and Deborah Gordon, 465–95. Dordrecht: Kluwer.

Kristeva, Julia. 1982. *The Power of Horror: An Essay on Abjection.* New York: Columbia University Press.

Kuhn, Thomas. 1962. *The Structure of Scientific Revolutions.* Chicago: University of Chicago Press.

———. 1970. *The Structure of Scientific Revolutions.* 2nd ed. Chicago: University of Chicago Press.

Lakoff, George, and M. Johnson. 1980. *Metaphors We Live By.* Chicago: University of Chicago Press.

Larrimore, Mark, ed. 2001. *The Problem of Evil: A Reader.* Oxford: Blackwell.

Latour, Bruno, and Stephen Woolgar. 1979. *Laboratory Life: The Social Construction of Scientific Facts.* London: Sage.

Leavell, S. R., and C. V. Fong. 1983. Psychopathology in Patients with Sickle Cell Disease. *Psychosomatics* 24:23–25.

Leavitt, Judith Walzer, and Ronald L. Numbers, eds. 1997. *Sickness and Health in America.* 3rd ed. Madison: University of Wisconsin Press.

Lebra, Takie. 1995. Skipped and Postponed Adolescence of Aristocratic Women in Japan: Resurrecting the Culture/Nature Issue. *Ethos* 23:79–102.

Lee, Richard B. 1984. *The Dobe !Kung.* Fort Worth, Tex.: Holt, Rinehart and Winston.

Leiderman, Deborah, and Jean-Anne Grisso. 1985. The Gomer Phenomenon. *Journal of Health and Social Behavior* 26:222–32.

Levesque, Roger J. R. 2000. Sexually Active Adolescents. In *Adolescents, Sex, and the Law: Preparing Adolescents for Responsible Citizenship,* edited by R. J. Levesque, 111–37. Washington, D.C.: American Psychological Association.

Levine, Robert S.; James E. Foster, Robert E. Fullilove, Mindy T. Fullilove, Nathaniel C. Briggs, Pamela C. Hull, Baqar A. Husaini, and Charles H. Hennekens. 2001. Black-White Inequalities in Mortality and Life Expectancy, 1933–1999: Implications for Healthy People 2010. *Public Health Reports* 116:474–83.

Lillie-Blanton, M., M. Brodie, D. Rowland, D. Altman, and M. McIntosh. 2000. Race, Ethnicity, and the Health Care System: Public Perceptions and Experiences. *Medical Care Research and Review* 51 (suppl. 1): 218–35.

Livingston, Julie. 2005. *Debility and Moral Imagination in Botswana: Disability, Chronic Illness, and Aging.* Bloomington: Indiana University Press.

Lock, Margaret. 1996. Displacing Suffering: The Reconstruction of Death in North America and Japan. *Daedalus* 125:207–44.

Lock, Margaret, and Deborah Gordon, eds. 1988. *Biomedicine Examined.* Dordrecht: Kluwer.

Lock, Margaret, and Patricia Kaufert. 1998. *Pragmatic Women and Body Politics.* Cambridge: Cambridge University Press.

Lock, Margaret, Allan Young, and Alberto Cambrosio, eds. 2000. *Living and Working with the New Medical Technologies: Intersections of Inquiry.* Cambridge: Cambridge University Press.

Loesch, D. E. 2002. Waiting to Inhale. *St. Louis Magazine,* August, 92–95.

Long, Thomas L. 2005. *AIDS and American Apocalypticism: The Cultural Semiotics of an Epidemic.* Albany: State University of New York Press.

Lopez, Steve, and Peter Guarnaccia. 2000. Cultural Psychopathology: Uncovering the Social World of Mental Illness. *Annual Review of Psychology* 51:571–89.

———. 2005. Cultural Dimensions of Psychopathology: The Social World's Impact on Mental Illness. In *Psychopathology: Foundations for a Contemporary Understanding,* edited by James E. Maddox and Barbara A. Winstead, 19–38. New York: Routledge.

Lynch, Michael. 1993. *Scientific Practice and Ordinary Action: Ethnomethodology and Social Studies of Science.* Cambridge: Cambridge University Press.

Malinowski, Bronislaw. 1973. The Group and the Individual in Functional Analysis: Personality, Organization, and Culture. In *High Points in Anthropology,* edited by Paul Bohannan and Mark Glazer, 275–93. New York: Knopf.

*The Management of Sickle Cell Disease.* 2002. Bethesda, Md.: National Institute of Medicine.

Margolis, Mitchell L., Jason D. Christie, Gerard A. Silvestri, Larry Kaiser, Silverio Santiago, and John Hansen-Flaschen. 2003. Racial Differences Pertaining to a Belief about Lung Cancer Surgery: Results of a Multi-center Study. *Annals of Internal Medicine* 139:558–63.

Markowitz, F. 2000. *Coming of Age in Post-Soviet Russia.* Urbana: University of Illinois Press.

Martin, Emily. 1987. *The Woman in the Body: A Cultural Analysis of Reproduction.* Boston: Beacon Press.

———. 1994. *Flexible Bodies: The Role of Immunity in American Culture from the Days of Polio to the Age of AIDS.* Boston: Beacon Press.

Marx, Karl. 1978. *The Marx-Engels Reader.* Ed. Robert C. Tucker. New York: Norton.

Mason, Verne. 1922. Sickle Cell Anemia. *Journal of the American Medical Association* 79:1318–19.

Mattingly, Cheryl. 1994. The Concept of Therapeutic "Emplotment." *Social Science and Medicine* 38:811–22.

Mauss, Marcel. 1979. *Sociology and Psychology Essays.* Trans. Ben Brewster. London: Routledge and Kegan Paul.

Maxwell, Krista, Allison Streetly, and David Bevan. 1999. Experience of Hospital Care and Treatment Seeking for Pain from Sickle Cell Disease: Qualitative Study. *British Medical Journal* 318:1585–90.

McCann, Jennifer, Vasken Artinian, Lisa Duhaime, Joseph W. Lewis Jr., Paul A. Kvale, and Bruno DiGiovine. 2005. Evaluation of the Causes for Racial

Disparity in Surgical Treatment of Early Stage Lung Cancer. *Chest* 128: 3440–46.

McNeil, Barbara. 2001. Hidden Barriers to Improvement in the Quality of Care. *New England Journal of Medicine* 345:1612–20.

McWhorter, John. 2005. *Winning the Race: Beyond the Crisis in Black America.* New York: Gotham Books.

Mead, Margaret. 1949. *Coming of Age in Samoa: A Psychological Study of Primitive Youth for Western Civilization.* New York: New American Library.

Mechanic, David. 1989. *Painful Choices: Research and Essays on Health Care.* New Brunswick, N.J.: Transaction.

Melfi, C. A., T. W. Droghan, M. P. Hanna, and R. L. Robinson. 2000. Racial Variation in Antidepressant Treatment in a Medicaid Population. *Journal of Clinical Psychiatry* 61:16–21.

Merleau-Ponty, Maurice. 1962. *Phenomenology of Perception.* Ed. Colin Smith. London: Routledge.

Merskey, H. 1987. Pain, Personality and Psychosomatic Complaints. In *Handbook of Chronic Pain Management,* edited by G. Burrows, D. Elton, and G. Stanley, 137–46. Amsterdam: Elsevier Science.

Millman, Michael, ed. 1993. *Access to Health Care in America.* Washington, D.C.: National Academies Press.

Minino, Arialdi M., and Betty L. Smith. 2001. Deaths: Preliminary Data for 2000. *National Vital Statistics Report* 49(12):1–40.

Minuchin, S., B. Tosman, and L. Baker. 1978. The Relationship of Chronic Pain to Depression, Marital Adjustment, and Family Dynamics. *Pain* 5:285–92.

Mol, AnneMarie, and Bernard Elsman. 1996. Detecting Disease and Designing Treatment: Duplex and the Diagnosis of Diseased Leg Vessels. *Sociology of Health and Illness* 18:609–31.

Moss, David A. 1996. *Socializing Security: Progressive-Era Economists and the Origins of American Social Policy.* Cambridge, Mass.: Harvard University Press.

Muhammad, Khalil G. 2007. White May Be Might, but It's Not Always Right. *Washington Post,* December 9, B03.

Murdock, George. 1949. *Social Structure.* New York: Macmillan.

Murray, Charles. 1984. *Losing Ground: American Social Policy, 1950–1980.* New York: Basic Books.

Napier, Kristine. 1999. The Politics of Pathology. *The World and I* 14. http://www.worldandimisto.cz/_MAIL_/article/ciapr99.html.

Nietzsche, Friedrich. 1968. *The Will to Power.* Ed. Walter Kaufmann. New York: Vintage Books.

———. 2003. *The Genealogy of Morals.* Mineola, N.Y.: Dover.

Nissen, S. E., and K. Wolski. 2007. Effect of Rosiglitazone on the Risk of Myocardial Infarction and Death from Cardiovascular Causes. *New England Journal of Medicine* 356:2457–71.

Numbers, Ronald. 1997. The Third Party: Health Insurance in America. In *Sickness and Health in America: Readings in the History of Medicine and Public Health,* edited by Judith Walzer Leavitt and Ronald L. Numbers, 269–83. Madison: University of Wisconsin Press.

Obeyesekere, Gananath. 2002. *Imagining Karma: Ethical Transformation in Amerindian, Buddhist, and Greek Rebirth*. Berkeley: University of California.

Omi, Michael, and Howard Winant. 1994. *Racial Formation in the United States: From the 1960s to the 1990s*. New York: Routledge.

Paris, Peter. 1985. *The Social Teaching of the Black Churches*. Philadelphia: Fortress Press.

Parsons, Talcott. 1955. The American Family: Its Relationship to Personality and to the Social Structure. In *Family Socialization and Interactional Process*, edited by Talcott Parsons and Robert F. Bales, 3–34. Glencoe, Ill.: Free Press.

———. 1991. *The Social System*. London: Routledge.

Patterson, Orlando. 2007. Jena, O.J., and the Jailing of Black America. *New York Times*, September 30.

Pernick, Martin S. 1983. The Calculus of Suffering in Nineteenth-Century Surgery. *Hasting Center Report* 13(2):26–36.

———. 1985. The Calculus of Suffering in 19th-Century Surgery. In *Sickness and Health in America: Readings in the History of Medicine and Public Health*, edited by Judith Walzer Leavitt and Ronald L. Numbers, 98–112. Madison: University of Wisconsin Press.

Petersen, E.D., L.K. Shaw, E.R. DeLong, D.B. Pryor, R.M. Califf, and D.B. Mark. 1997. Racial Variation in the Use of Coronary-Vascularization Procedures: Are the Differences Real? Do They Matter? *New England Journal of Medicine* 336:480–86.

Petryna, Adriana. 2002. *Life Exposed: Biological Citizens after Chernobyl*. Princeton, N.J.: Princeton University Press.

Phillips, Russell S., Mary Beth Hamel, Joan M. Teno, Paul Bellamy, Steven K. Broste, Robert M. Califf, Humberto Vidaillet, et al. 1997. Race, Resource Use, and Survival in Seriously Ill Hospitalized Adults. *Journal of General Internal Medicine* 11:387–96.

Piaget, Jean. 1932. *The Moral Judgment of the Child*. London: Kegan Paul, Trench, Trubner.

Pickering, Andrew, ed. 1992. *Science as Practice and Culture*. Chicago: University of Chicago Press.

Pletcher, Mark J., Stefan Kertesz, Michael A. Kohn, and Ralph Gonzales. 2008. Trends in Opioid Prescribing by Race/Ethnicity for Patients Seeking Care in US Emergency Departments. *Journal of the American Medical Association* 299:70–78.

Powers, Madison, and Ruth Faden. 2003. Racial and Ethnic Disparities in Healthcare: An Ethical Analysis of When and How They Matter. In *Unequal Treatment: Confronting Racial and Ethnic Disparities in Health Care*, edited by Brian Smedley, Adrienne Stith, and Alan Nelson, 722–38. Washington, D.C.: The National Academies Press.

———. 2006. *Social Justice: The Moral Foundations of Public Health and Health Policy*. Oxford: Oxford University Press.

Radcliffe-Brown, A.R. 1940. On Joking Relationships. *Africa* 13:195.

Rapp, Rayna. 1988. Chromosomes and Communication: The Discourse of Genetic Counseling. *Medical Anthropology Quarterly* 2:143–57.

———. 2000. *Testing Women, Testing the Fetus: The Social Impact of Amniocentesis in America*. New York: Routledge.

Rapp, Rayna, and Faye Ginsburg. 2001. Enabling Disability: Rewriting Kinship, Reimagining Citizenship. *Public Culture* 13:533–56.

Ren, Xinhua S., Benjamin C. Amick, and David R. Williams. 1999. Racial/Ethnic Disparities in Health: The Interplay between Discrimination and Socioeconomic Status. *Ethnicity and Disease* 9:151–65.

Rhodes, Lorna. 2004. *Total Confinement: Madness and Reason in the Maximum Security Prison*. Berkeley: University of California Press.

Ricoeur, Paul. 1985. *Time and Narrative*. Vol. 2. Chicago: University of Chicago Press.

Rosen, Clifford J. 2007. The Rosiglitazone Story: Lessons from an FDA Advisory Committee Meeting. *New England Journal of Medicine* 357: 844–46.

Rosenberg, Charles E. 1992. Framing Disease: Illness, Society, and History. In *Framing Disease: Studies in Cultural History*, edited by Charles Rosenberg and Janet Golden, xiii–xxvi. New Brunswick, N.J.: Rutgers University Press.

———. 2003. What Is Disease? In Memory of Owsei Temkin. *Bulletin of the History of Medicine* 77:491–505.

Rosenberg, Charles, and Janet Golden, eds. 1992. *Framing Disease: Studies in Cultural History*. New Brunswick, N.J.: Rutgers University Press.

Rouse, Carolyn. 2004a. "If She's a Vegetable, We'll Be Her Garden": Embodiment, Transcendence, and Citations of Competing Metaphors in the Case of a Dying Child. *American Ethnologist* 31:514–29.

———. 2004b. Paradigms and Politics: Shaping Health Care Access for Sickle Cell Patients through the Discursive Regimes of Biomedicine. *Culture, Medicine and Psychiatry* 28:369–99.

———. 2006. Jesica Speaks? Adolescent Consent for Transplantation and Ethical Uncertainty. In *A Death Retold: Jesica Santillan, the Bungled Transplant, and Paradoxes of Medical Citizenship*, edited by Keith Wailoo, Julie Livingston, and Peter Guarnaccia, 329–48. Chapel Hill: University of North Carolina Press.

———. 2007. Crossing Borders: Kwaku Ohene-Frempong. *Journal of Health Care for the Poor and Underserved* 18(1):1–5.

Rouse, Carolyn, and Janet Hoskins. 2004. Purity, Soul Food, and Islam: Explorations at the Intersection of Consumption and Resistance. *Cultural Anthropology* 19:226–49.

Rouse, Joseph. 1987. *Knowledge and Power: Toward a Political Philosophy of Science*. Ithaca, N.Y.: Cornell University Press.

Rousseau, Jean-Jacques. 1997. *The Discourses and Other Early Writings*. Cambridge: Cambridge University Press.

Sarich, Vincent, and Frank Miele. 2004. *Race: The Reality of Human Difference*. Boulder, Colo.: Westview Press.

Scarry, Elaine. 1985. *The Body in Pain: The Making and Unmaking of the World*. New York: Oxford University Press.

Scheper-Hughes, Nancy. 1992. *Death without Weeping: The Violence of Everyday Life in Brazil*. Berkeley: University of California Press.

Scheper-Hughes, Nancy, and Margaret Lock. 1987. The Mindful Body: A Prolegomenon to Future Work in Medical Anthropology. *Medical Anthropology Quarterly* 1:6–41.

Schneider, E. C., L. L. Leape, J. S. Weissman, R. N. Piana, C. Gatsonis, and A. M. Epstein. 2001. Racial Differences in Cardiac Revascularization Rates: Does "Overuse" Explain Higher Rates among White Patients? *Annals of Internal Medicine* 135:328–37.

Schulz, Amy J., and Leith Mullings, eds. 2005. *Gender, Race, Class and Health: Intersectional Approaches.* San Francisco: Jossey-Bass.

Shapiro, B., L. Benjamin, R. Payne, and G. Heidrich. 1997. Sickle Cell–Related Pain Perceptions of Medical Practitioners. *Journal of Pain and Symptom Management* 14:168–74.

Shapiro, M. F., S. C. Morton, D. F. McCaffrey, J. W. Senterfitt, J. A. Fleishman, J. F. Perlman, L. A. Athey, J. W. Keesey, D. P. Goldman, S. H. Berry, and S. A. Bozette. 1999. Variations in the Care of HIV-Infected Adults in the United States: Results from the HIV Cost and Services Utilization Study. *Journal of the American Medical Association* 281:2305–75.

Sharp, Lesley. 2006. Babes and Baboons: Jesica Santillan and Experimental Pediatric Transplant Research in America. In *A Death Retold: Jesica Santillan, the Bungled Transplant, and Paradoxes of Medical Citizenship,* edited by Keith Wailoo, Julie Livingston, and Peter Guarnaccia, 299–328. Chapel Hill: University of North Carolina Press.

Shostak, Marjorie. 1983. *Nisa: The Life and Words of a !Kung Woman.* New York: Vintage Books.

Shweder, Richard. 1982. Beyond Self-Constructed Knowledge: The Study of Culture and Morality. *Merrill-Palmer Quarterly* 28:41–69.

———. 1991. *Thinking through Cultures: Expeditions in Cultural Psychology.* Cambridge, Mass.: Harvard University Press.

Smedley, Brian, Adrienne Stith, and Alan Nelson, eds. 2003. *Unequal Treatment: Confronting Racial and Ethnic Disparities in Health Care.* Washington, D.C.: National Academies Press.

Smith, Wally R., Lynne T. Penberthy, Viktor E. Boyberg, Donna K. McClish, John D. Roberts, Bassam Dahman, Imoigele P. Aisiku, James L. Levenson, and Susan D. Roseff. 2008. Daily Assessment of Pain in Adults with Sickle Cell Disease. *Annals of Internal Medicine* 148:94–101.

Sontag, Susan. 1989. *Illness as Metaphor and AIDS and Its Metaphors.* New York: Picador.

Steele, Shelby. 2007. *White Guilt: How Blacks and Whites Together Destroyed the Promise of the Civil Rights Era.* New York: Harper Perennial.

Stein, Howard. 1990. *American Medicine as Culture.* Boulder, Colo.: Westview Press.

Stone, Reese, and Alisa Mosley. 2004. NMA Appalled over Distorted HHS Disparities Report. http://www.nmanet.org/pr_012204.htm, accessed June 9, 2004.

Strakowski, Stephen M., Michael Flaum, Xavier Amador, H. Steven Bracha, Anand K. Pandurangi, Delbert Robinson, and Mauricio Tohen. 1996. Racial

Differences in the Diagnosis of Psychosis. *Schizophrenia Research* 21: 117–24.

Strakowski, Stephen M., Paul E. Keck, Lesley M. Arnold, Jacqueline Collins, Rodgers M. Wilson, Davis E. Fleck, Kimberly B. Corey, Jennifer Amicone, and Victor R. Adebimpe. 2003. Ethnicity and Diagnosis of Inpatients with Affective Disorders. *Journal of Clinical Psychiatry* 64:747–54.

Strathern, Marilyn. 1992. *Reproducing the Future: Anthropology, Kinship, and the New Reproductive Technologies.* New York: Routledge.

Sutton, Millicent, George F. Atweh, Teresa D. Cashman, and William T. Davis. 1999. Resolving Conflicts: Misconceptions and Myths in the Care of the Patient with Sickle Cell Disease. *Mount Sinai Journal of Medicine* 66:274–78.

Taliaferro, William H., and John G. Huck. 1923. The Inheritance of Sickle-Cell Anemia in Man. *Genetics* 8:594–98.

Tapper, Melbourne. 1999. *In the Blood: Sickle Cell Anemia and the Politics of Race.* Philadelphia: University of Pennsylvania Press.

Tate, Claudia. 1998. *Psychoanalysis and Black Novels: Desire and the Protocols of Race.* Oxford: Oxford University Press.

Telfair, Joseph, Leah R. Alexander, Penny S. Loosier, Patty L. Allerman-Velez, and Julie Simmons. 2004. Providers' Perspectives and Beliefs Regarding Transition to Adult Care for Adolescents with Sickle Cell Disease. *Journal of Health Care for the Poor and Underserved* 15:443–61.

Temkin, Owsei. 1963. Scientific Approach. In *Scientific Change: Historical Studies in the Intellectual, Social, and Technical Conditions for Scientific Discovery and Technical Invention from Antiquity to the Present,* edited by Alistair C. Crombie, 629–47. New York: Basic Books.

Thomas, William. 1979. *The Philosophical Radicals: Nine Studies in Theory and Practice, 1817–1841.* Oxford: Clarendon Press.

Todd, K. H. 2001. Influence of Ethnicity on Emergency Department Pain Management. *Emergency Medicine* 13:274–78.

Todd, K. H., C. Green, V. L. Bonham, and C. Haywood. 2006. Sickle Cell Disease Related Pain: Crisis and Conflict. *Journal of Pain* 7:453–58.

Turnbull, Colin M. 1962. *The Forest People.* New York: Simon and Schuster.

Tversky, Amos, and Daniel Kahneman. 1974. Judgment under Uncertainty: Heuristics and Biases. *Science,* September 27, 1124–31.

U.S. Department of Health and Human Services. 2000. Chronic Kidney Disease. In *Healthy People 2010: Understanding and Improving Health.* Washington, D.C.: U.S. Government Printing Office.

Van Gennep, Arnold. 1960. *The Rites of Passage.* Chicago: University of Chicago Press.

Van Ryn, M., and J. Burke. 2000. The Effect of Patient Race and Socio-economic Status on Physicians' Perceptions of Patients. *Social Science and Medicine* 50:813–28.

Vermylen, Christiane. 2003. Hematopoietic Stem Cell Transplantation in Sickle Cell Disease. *Blood Reviews* 17:163–66.

Vichinsky, Elliott. 1980. Current Treatment of Sickle Cell Disease. *Current Problems in Pediatrics,* October 10, 1–64.

————. 1982. Multidisciplinary Approach to Pain Management in Sickle Cell Disease. *American Journal of Pediatric Hematology/Oncology* 4: 328–33.

————. 1991. Comprehensive Care in Sickle Cell Disease: Its Impact on Morbidity and Mortality. *Seminars in Hematology,* July 28, 220–26.

Vygotsky, Lev. 1994. *Vygotsky Reader.* Ed. Rene Van der Veer and Jaan Valsiner. Oxford: Blackwell.

Wacquant, Loic. 2002. From Slavery to Mass Incarceration. *New Left Review* 13(January–February):41–60.

————. 2005. Race as Civic Felony. *International Social Science Journal* 57:127–42.

Wailoo, Keith. 1997. Detecting "Negro Blood": Black and White Identities and the Reconstruction of Sickle Cell Anemia. In *Drawing Blood: Technology and Disease Identity in Twentieth-Century America,* 134–61. Baltimore: Johns Hopkins University Press.

————. 2001. *Dying in the City of the Blues: Sickle Cell Anemia and the Politics of Race and Health.* Chapel Hill: University of North Carolina Press.

Wailoo, Keith, and Stephen Pemberton. 2006. *The Troubled Dream of Genetic Medicine: Ethnicity and Innovation in Tay-Sachs, Cystic Fibrosis, and Sickle Cell Disease.* Baltimore: Johns Hopkins University Press.

Walters, Mark C., Rainer Storb, Melinda Patience, Wendy Leisenring, Terri Taylor, Jean E. Sanders, George E. Buchanan, et al. 2000. Impact of Bone Marrow Transplantation for Symptomatic Sickle Cell Disease: An Interim Report. *Blood* 95:1918–24.

Weber, Max. 1930. *The Protestant Ethic and the Spirit of Capitalism.* Trans. Talcott Parsons. London: Routledge.

————. 1946. The Social Psychology of the World Religions. In *From Max Weber: Essays in Sociology,* edited by H.H. Gerth and C. Wright Mills, 267–301. New York: Oxford University Press.

Weisse, Carol S., Paul C. Sorum, Kafi N. Sanders, and Beth L. Syat. 2001. Do Gender and Race Affect Decisions about Pain Management? *Journal of General Internal Medicine* 16:211–17.

Weissman, Joel S., Joseph Betancourt, Eric G. Campbell, Elyse R. Park, Minah Kim, Brian Clarridge, David Blumenthal, Karen C. Lee, and Angela W. Maina. 2005. Resident Physicians' Preparedness to Provide Cross-Cultural Care. *Journal of the American Medical Association* 294:1058–67.

Western, Bruce. 2006. *Punishment and Inequality in America.* New York: Russell Sage Foundation.

Wexler, Alice. 1995. *Mapping Fate: A Memoir of Family, Risk, and Genetic Research.* Berkeley: University of California Press.

Williams, David R., and Pamela Braboy Jackson. 2005. Social Sources of Racial Disparities in Health. *Health Affairs* 24:325–34.

Williams, David R., and Toni D. Rucker. 2000. Understanding and Addressing Racial Disparities in Health Care. *Heath Care Financing Review* 21(4):75–90.

Williams, Juan. 2006. *Enough: The Phony Leaders, Dead-End Movements, and Culture of Failure That Are Undermining Black America—and What We Can Do about It.* New York: Crown.

Williams, Raymond. 1977. *Marxism and Literature*. New York: Oxford University Press.

Willis, Paul. 1977. *Learning to Labor: How Working Class Kids Get Working Class Jobs*. New York: Columbia University Press.

Witt, Doris. 1999. *Black Hunger: Food and the Politics of U.S. Identity*. Oxford: Oxford University Press.

Wright, Douglas. 2002. *State Estimates of Substance Use from the 2000 National Household Survey on Drug Abuse*. Vol. 1, *Findings*. DHHS Publication no. SMA 03–03775, NHSDA Series H-19. Rockville, Md.: Substance Abuse and Mental Health Services Administration Office of Applied Sciences.

Wright, P., and A. Treacher, eds. 1982. *The Problem of Medical Knowledge: Examining the Social Construction of Medicine*. Edinburgh: Edinburgh University Press.

Young, Allan. 2000. History, Hystery and Psychiatric Reasoning. In *Living and Working with the New Medical Technologies: Intersections of Inquiry*, edited by Margaret Lock, Allan Young, and Alberto Cambrosio, 135–62. Cambridge: Cambridge University Press.

Zola, I. K. 1972. Medicine as an Institution of Social Control. *Sociological Review* 20:487–504.

# Index

*Unequal Treatment* (Institute of
    Medicine), 7–8, 123, 155, 258
Union Pacific Railway Company v.
    Botsford, 212
U.S. Supreme Court, 212–13
universal health care, xii, 5, 14, 121,
    167, 266
utilitarianism, 119, 121, 130–31

Vichinsky, Elliott, 81–83, 96, 99
victimhood, 116, 117, 232–33. *See also*
    discourses of suffering; politics of pity

Wacquant, Loic, 41
Wailoo, Keith, 10, 12, 108

Wall, Patrick, 69
Washington, Harriet, 42
wealth: health care as, 114–15; racial
    disparities in, 155–56, 275n2
Weber, Max, 114, 273n13, 276n22
Weiner, Irving, 174–75
Willis, Paul, 280n24
Wittgenstein, Ludwig, 91–92, 165
Wong-Baker Faces Pain Rating Scale.,
    24–25
Woolgar, Stephen, 75
work ethic, 114–17

Yahya, Harun, 282n20

Text: 10/13 Sabon
Display: Sabon
Compositor: International Typesetting and Composition
Indexer: Marcia Carlson
Printer and binder: Maple-Vail Book Manufacturing Group